W9-DFE-190

CARDIOVASCULAR EVALUATION OF ATHLETES

TOWARD RECOGNIZING

ATHLETES AT RISK

OF SUDDEN DEATH

EDITED BY BRUCE F. WALLER, M.D.
AND W. PROCTOR HARVEY, M.D.

*"Dedicated to
the memories of my
beloved sons,
W. Proctor Harvey, Jr.
and
Blair Burns Harvey."*

— W. Proctor Harvey

*"To Lynn, Greta, Sasha,
Allegra and Brock
who sacrificed
many special occasions
and events because
I was always working."*

— Bruce F. Waller

CONTRIBUTORS

Michael H. Crawford, MD
Department of Medicine (Cardiology)
University of New Mexico, Albuquerque

Pamela S. Douglas, MD
Harvard Medical School
Beth Israel Hospital
Cardiovascular Section
Boston, Massachusetts

Gerald F. Fletcher, MD
Professor and Chairman
Department of Rehabilitation Medicine
Emory University School of Medicine
Atlanta, Georgia

Brian Hainline, MD
Director, Clinical Neurology Service
and Sports Neurology
Hospital for Joint Diseases
New York, New York

Assistant Professor of Neurology
New York University School of Medicine

W. Proctor Harvey, MD
Professor of Medicine
Division of Cardiology
Georgetown University Medical Center

Donald M. Knowlan, MD
Team Physician
Washington Redskins
National Football League

Professor of Medicine
Georgetown University Medical Center

Robert M. Jeresaty, MD
Professor of Medicine
University of Connecticut School of Medicine

Chief, Section of Cardiology
Saint Francis Hospital and Medical Center
Hartford, Connecticut

Jacqueline O'Donnell, MD
Associate Professor of Medicine
Department of Medicine/Division of Cardiology
Krannert Institute of Cardiology
Indiana University School of Medicine
Indianapolis, Indiana

Mary L. O'Toole, PhD
University of Tennessee
Campbell Clinic
Department of Orthopaedic Surgery
Memphis, Tennessee

Charles Presti, MD
Fort Wayne Cardiology
Fort Wayne, Indiana

Lawrence D. Rink, MD
Clinical Professor of Medicine
Indiana University School of Medicine
Bloomington, Indiana

Team Physician
Indiana University Basketball
Team Physician
United States Olympic Team

David S. Starr, MD, JD
Georgetown, Texas

Bruce F. Waller, MD
Clinical Professor of Pathology and Medicine
Indiana University School of Medicine

Director, Cardiovascular Pathology Registry
St. Vincent Hospital
Indianapolis, Indiana
Cardiologist, Nasser, Smith, Pinkerton Cardiology
Indianapolis, Indiana

John C. Weistart, JD, LLD
Professor of Medicine
Duke University School of Medicine
Durham, North Carolina

CONTENTS

PREFACE

The Problem

Exercise-related sudden death or cardiovascular complications associated with exercise are apparently becoming more widespread. Increased *popularity* of regular exercise, increased *intensity* of exercise, and increased *numbers* of people of all ages who are exercising competitively, all contribute to this problem.

Considering the very large number of athletes in our country and throughout the world, sudden death of athletes is not common. However, when it does occur, it usually represents a shock to the local community, and often to the entire nation; to think that a presumably ultra-healthy young athlete can die suddenly is difficult to comprehend. This is especially true for the millions of sports fans who recently witnessed the sudden death of a basketball player. He died in plain view as millions watched the game on national TV. All were shocked, stunned, and saddened.

Sudden death in young, highly competitive, apparently healthy individuals is a major tragedy for the family, community, schoolmates, and the coaching and training staff. Frequently, coaches blame themselves for "overpushing" an athlete, for "not paying attention to minor physical complaints," and members of organizational athletic committees ask themselves: "What could we have done to have prevented this death and what can we do to prevent such tragedies in the future?"

The rarity of sudden death in athletes has been used as an argument against the usefulness of large scale, appropriate screening programs. Of course, similar arguments have been used in the past during the early development of Pap smears for cervical cancer and use of mammography for breast cancer. Both of these screening programs have proved extremely successful in the detection of early disease and precursors of serious disease. Some authorities believe that to spot these athletes prone to sudden death would require echocardiography, exercise testing, Holter monitoring, and even nuclear studies. Obviously, the cost of such laboratory tests on a screening basis would be so high (possibly several thousand dollars for each athlete), that it would be too expensive and impractical.

On the other hand, what *is* practical, inexpensive, and efficient is a very careful clinical evaluation. Of most importance is the cardiovascular physical examination, which can be performed in any physician's office or in special examination areas.

Suggestions Toward a Solution to the Problem

The editors believe that with the right kind of cardiovascular training, emphasizing the clinical skills of the examining physician and key medical personnel, that many of the athletes prone to serious medical complications, including sudden death, can be detected or at least suspected on simple, inexpensive screening examination. Appropriate preventive measures and advice can then be given to the athlete, family, and school or team administrative staff.

It is apparent that a careful history and physical examination are of the greatest importance in the initial medical evaluation. And expert auscultation of the heart is a must.

The examining physician can continue to sharpen his or her expertise in this respect by attending and participating in postgraduate courses stressing the patient and physical diagnosis. Already under way are plans by the American College of Cardiology to sponsor such courses, some of which are already available. It cannot be stressed too strongly that one of the most important aspects of prevention of sudden death in athletes is the expertise of the examining physician.

The Purpose of this Book

Can sudden death in athletes be prevented? We believe that in many, and probably most cases, the answer is yes.

Can those athletes who are candidates for sudden death be spotted or screened on routine, preparticipation physical examination? Again, we believe that, in many, the answer is yes. The editors and contributors to this book suggest their approaches to the problem, based on their own clinical experience.

In addition to the suggestions for routine cardiovascular evaluation and screening of athletes, the more specialized examinations that might be needed in individual cases are outlined in separate chapters; these include: exercise treadmill testing, echocardiography, and Holter monitoring. We have also included chapters on such specialized athletic activities as scuba diving and ultraendurance athletics, as these have become increasingly popular sporting activities. The legal aspects for physicians involved in screening athletes are also discussed.

The reader will note that the editors (Bruce F. Waller, MD and W. Proctor Harvey, MD) have inserted "Editor's Notes" liberally throughout the book. From past experience with previous publications, the editors have employed this format to help unify a book that is purposely diversified. These comments, which sometimes agree and sometimes disagree with the author of the particular chapter, add a personal touch and provide extra food for thought.

The editors believe that, with special care in performing a proper and complete precordial auscultation, physicians and others involved in screening athletes can detect the cardiac signs of athletes who may be at risk of serious cardiac dysfunction.

As a rule, if done carefully, by the time the history and physical evaluation are completed, the examining physician will either have diagnosed a cardiac condition or have spotted clues to the possible presence of a cardiac problem that could result in serious problems or even sudden death. In such cases, additional tests, a consultation, or a second opinion can be obtained.

Bruce F. Waller, MD
W. Proctor Harvey, MD

CHAPTER 1

EXERCISE-RELATED SUDDEN DEATH IN ATHLETES: THE MOST COMMON CAUSES

Bruce F. Waller, MD

Clinical Professor of Pathology and Medicine
Indiana University School of Medicine
Director, Cardiovascular Pathology Registry
St. Vincent Hospital, Indianapolis
Cardiologist, Nasser, Smith, Pinkerton,
Cardiology, Inc., Indianapolis

The popularity of regularly performed exercise continues to increase annually. In the United States, running or jogging is the most popular form of exercise, and is estimated to involve about 20 million Americans. The number of runners has more than tripled in the last 15 years. Although participation in sports and exercise is higher in younger age groups, nearly 40% of all middle-aged Americans are said to exercise regularly. The intensity of exercise and the number of persons exercising competitively also have risen. Although most American runners cover less than 10 miles per week, champion marathoners run 100 miles or more.[1, 2] More than 50,000 Americans have successfully completed one standard marathon race, and an estimated 8 to 10% have covered the 26.2 miles in less than three hours.[3]

Running or jogging is not the only form of exercise that has increased in popularity. Tennis now involves about 10 million regular players, and racquetball has grown from 50,000 players in 1972 to more than 5 million today.

Several motivations have been cited for this interest in regular, vigorous exercise:[4-7]
• Improved fitness
• Positive effects on mental health
• Weight reduction
• Increased leisure time
• Intense efforts by public and private agencies to promote exercise and sports.

Sudden Death Related to Exercise

With increasing numbers of individuals participating in all forms of exercise and sport have come numerous reports of cardiovascular complications, including sudden death during or shortly after exercise.[8-44] While sudden death in the conditioned person may not be a major public health issue, such events in well known individuals such as Jim Fixx, "Pistol Pete" Maravich, and, most recently, Hank Gathers, focuses tremendous public attention on this problem. Fortunately, the incidence of premature sudden death in athletes is low: one death per 50,000 player-hours of rugby,[17] one death per 13,000 to 26,000 person-hours of cross-country skiing,[37] and one jogging death per 7620 joggers (0.01%, or one death per 396,000 person-hours of jogging).[32]

Even in a community with intense interest and activity focused on athletes and sports, the incidence of sudden death is very low. In Marion County (Indianapolis), Indiana, of 6492 deaths in a recent year, 1225 (19%) were subject to coroner's investigations (that is, they were sudden, unusual, unexplained, or violent). Of these, four deaths occurred during or immediately after athletic training, an incidence of only 0.3% of coroner's investigations or 0.06% of all deaths in the county (Figure 1-1).

Burke et al[45] found that 34 of 690 cases of sudden death (5%) in young adults (14 to 40 years of age) were sports related.

The Nature of the Connection

It has been argued that no proof exists that exercise is dangerous for anyone, since there is, in everyone, a per-hour risk of sudden death from occult coronary atherosclerotic disease (CAD), and that sudden death during exercise is a chance event, not a causal occurrence. One estimate[19] is that about 100 deaths per year should occur during jogging, simply by chance alone.

While this argument has statistical validity, Thompson[32] found that the rate of death from CAD during jogging in Rhode Island was seven

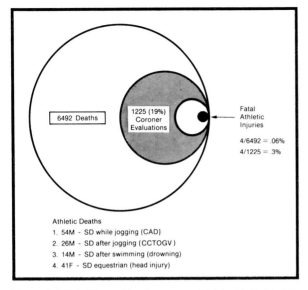

Figure 1-1: Fatalities – The frequency of fatal athletic injuries during training in Marion County, Indianapolis, Indiana, during 1985. The coroner's office records show that, of 6492 total deaths in the county, two were sudden death in athletes who showed cardiac disease. (CAD = coronary artery disease; CCTOGV = congenitally corrected transposition of great vessels.)

times the estimated death rate from CAD during more sedentary activities. Similarly, the sudden death rate in community cross-country skiing events in Finland is about four times the rate for such individuals at rest.[37] These data suggest that exercise contributes to sudden death in susceptible persons.

In an early study of 100 fatalities from CAD in young soldiers,[19] more than 50% died during vigorous effort or while performing chores, while only 10% of the deaths occurred during sleep. In another study of sudden coronary deaths in 115 soldiers,[18] death occurred during or immediately after strenuous physical exertion in nearly 30%, almost twice the frequency expected by chance. In a British study of 100 sudden deaths,[xx] only 10% of the subjects were exercising strenuously before death, but the victims were more active just before death than a control group of patients with nonfatal myocardial infarctions.

The Indiana University National Registry of Exercise-Related Sudden Death

Ten years ago, a national registry of exercise-related sudden death was established at Indiana

University School of Medicine to determine what cardiac abnormalities, if any, might be responsible for these deaths. Specific criteria were established for entry into this registry:

• Each subject died suddenly and unexpectedly during or shortly after vigorous exercise.
• Each subject had been active and conditioned (regularly exercising several times per week) for at least one year before death.
• Each subject had a complete autopsy examination, including toxicology.
• The entire heart was available for restudy, not simply a few selected slides.

Specimens are retrieved nationally and re-examined by a single cardiovascular pathologist. Since 1982, 57 hearts of conditioned subjects have been examined in the registry: 26 subjects older than 30 years of age, and 31 subjects younger than 30. Definite or probable cardiac disease was established in 55 (96%) of these cases.

Five other conditioned subjects who died suddenly also have been examined, to serve as a control group. In three, the sudden death resulted from cocaine overdose; two were hit by automobiles while running.

Causes of Death During Exercise

All of the subjects reviewed in this chapter had no previous clinical symptoms of cardiovascular disease when they started to exercise, and all died during or shortly after vigorous physical activity. These criteria *exclude* patients in cardiac rehabilitation exercise programs.

The data of the Indiana University registry demonstrate the usefulness of separating the subjects into two age categories, based upon distinct anatomic and pathologic conditions occurring almost exclusively in these age subgroups: 1. Conditioned subjects who die suddenly at age 30 years or less, and 2. those who die suddenly at an age older than 30 years.

• **Sudden Death in Athletes Aged 30 Years or Less: The Indiana University Registry Findings** – Of the 57 sudden-death victims studied by the Indiana Unviersity registry, 31 (54%) were aged 13 to 29 years; of these, 26 (84%) were males. Of the 31, 22 had been members of an organized athletic team (high school, college, or professional) for at least one year. (The single professional athlete was a member of a National Football League Team). The types of exercise performed included running or jogging (18), football (9), basketball (8), soccer (3), baseball (4), tennis (4), swimming (3), wrestling (1), and boxing (1). Most of the athletes participated in more than one form of exercise. Three of the runners had completed a standard marathon race.

In retrospect, symptoms suggesting heart disease (chest pain and syncope) were present in seven of these subjects, but sudden death appears to have been the first manifestation of cardiac disease in the remaining 24.

• **Necropsy Findings** – Heart weights ranged from 340 to 650 grams (mean 468). One heart had transmural myocardial necrosis (acute myocarditis), and one heart had transmural fibrosis (hyper-

trophic cardiomyopathy). All of the subjects had clean epicardial coronary arteries. Unequivocal structural cardiac disease was identified in 23 (74%) subjects, and probable heart disease in another 6 (19%). No identifiable cardiac abnormalities were seen in the remaining two subjects; the death of one was attributed to acute bronchial asthma, and the cause of death in the other remains uncertain.

Of the 23 subjects with definite heart disease, the structural abnormalities found included:
• Hypertrophic cardiomyopathy (13) (Figures 1-2, 1-3)
• Congenital coronary artery anomalies (5) (Figure 1-4)
• Floppy mitral valve (3) (Figure 1-5)
• Ebstein's anomaly of tricuspid valve (1) (Figure 1-6)
• Acute myocarditis (1).

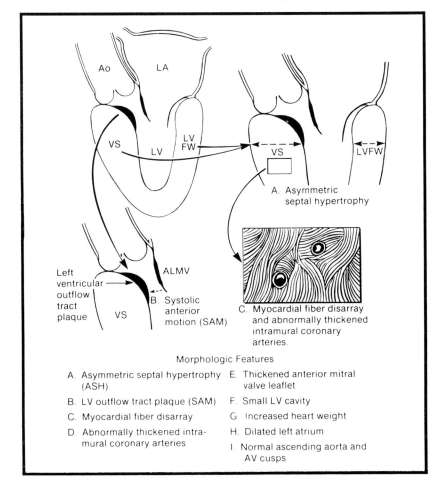

Morphologic Features

A. Asymmetric septal hypertrophy (ASH)
B. LV outflow tract plaque (SAM)
C. Myocardial fiber disarray
D. Abnormally thickened intramural coronary arteries

E. Thickened anterior mitral valve leaflet
F. Small LV cavity
G. Increased heart weight
H. Dilated left atrium
I. Normal ascending aorta and AV cusps

Figure 1-2: Hypertrophic Cardiomyopathy – The morphologic features of hypertrophic cardiomyopathy. ALMV = anterior leaflet mitral valve, Ao = aorta, LA = left atrium, LV = left ventricle, LVFW = left ventricular free wall, VS = ventricular septum.

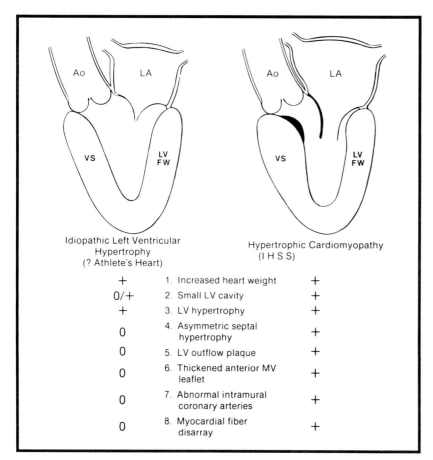

	Idiopathic Left Ventricular Hypertrophy (? Athlete's Heart)			Hypertrophic Cardiomyopathy (I H S S)
	+	1. Increased heart weight	+	
	0/+	2. Small LV cavity	+	
	+	3. LV hypertrophy	+	
	0	4. Asymmetric septal hypertrophy	+	
	0	5. LV outflow plaque	+	
	0	6. Thickened anterior MV leaflet	+	
	0	7. Abnormal intramural coronary arteries	+	
	0	8. Myocardial fiber disarray	+	

Figure 1-3: A comparison of morphologic features of idiopathic left ventricular hypertrophy (left) and hypertrophic cardiomyopathy (IHSS) (right). Ao = aorta, LA = left atrium, LVFW = left ventricular free wall, VS = ventricular septum.

The six subjects with probable heart disease had gross and histologic evidence of left ventricular hypertrophy without other anatomic features of hypertrophic cardiomyopathy. These are tentatively classified as "idiopathic left ventricular hypertrophy." (Figure 1-3).

One major purpose of necropsy examinations is to provide morphologic information that might be useful clinically in the prospective premortem diagnosis, detection, treatment, and management of disease processes prone to cause sudden death. Multiple case reports and several large series of exercise-related sudden death are now available for analysis. Using the results of a *single* cardiovascular pathology registry to provide us with this morphologic information may be biased. The *manner of case accession* (local or national derived material, one form of exercise versus many types of exercise), the *methodology of heart examination* (single versus multiple examiners, first hand

review of hearts versus only histology slides or necropsy protocol review) and the *magnitude of the registry* (small case series versus large numbers of patients with wide age ranges) are important varying factors. For this reason, it is useful to combine all of the available medical literature reports rather than relying on a single registry result.

• Previously Reported Subjects – Several previous studies[8-44] have reported exercise-related sudden death in 72 subjects 30 years or younger (Table 1-1). The ages ranged from 11 to 30 years (mean 19); 65 (90%) were males. Clinically relevant data are scant in most of these reports.

The largest series, by Maron and colleagues,[11] reports the causes of sudden and unexpected death in 29 highly conditioned, competitive athletes aged 13 to 30 years. Death occurred during or just after severe exertion on the athletic field in

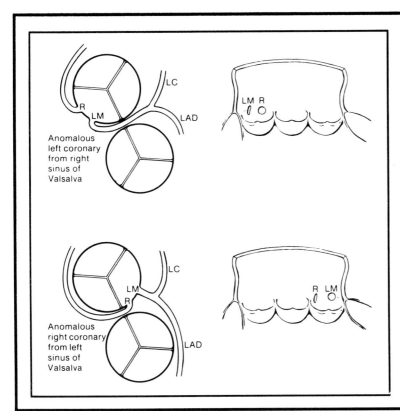

Figure 1-4: Anomalies – The two most frequent congenital coronary artery anomalies associated with exercise-related sudden death: Origin of both arteries from the right or the left sinus of Valsalva. The coronary ostium of the anomalous vessel is slit-like (arrow) compared to the normal oval shape. LAD = left anterior descending, LC = left circumflex, LM = left main, R = right.

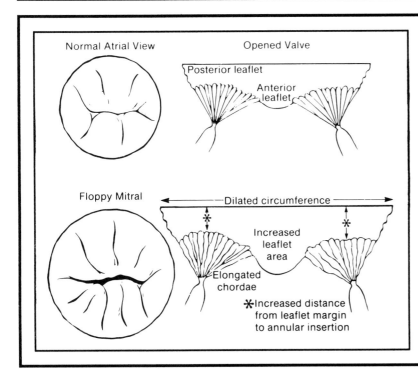

Figure 1-5: Normal vs Floppy – Comparison of features of the normal mitral valve (top) and the floppy mitral valve (bottom). Floppy mitral valves have a dilated circumference, increased leaflet area, and increased distance from the leaflet margin to annular insertion.

22 (76%) of these athletes. Structural cardiovascular abnormalities were identified at necropsy in 28 of the 29 athletes. The most common cause of death was hypertrophic cardiomyopathy, present in 14 (48%). Six (21%) had probable cardiovascular disease, classified as idiopathic left ventricular hypertrophy. Other causes of death identified were congenital coronary disease (3 athletes), and ruptured aorta (2 athletes with Marfan syndrome) (Figure 1-7).

Of eight conditioned subjects aged 11 to 25 years with exercise-related sudden death in another study,[15] the most common structural cardiac abnormality found at necropsy was congenital cardiac anomalies, found in five subjects. One subject had myocarditis, one had discrete subaortic stenosis, and one showed aortic dissection (non-Marfan).

Another study of seven subjects under age 30 with non-traumatic sudden death[9] found one with valvular heart disease (floppy mitral valve) and one with severe coronary atherosclerosis with acute myocardial infarction. The cause of death was uncertain in the other five; no cardiovascular abnormality was identifed.

Of the 72 previously reported conditioned sub-

Table 1-1
Causes of Sudden Death Found at Necropsy on 103 Athletes Age ≤ 30 Years Dying During or Shortly After Exercise

Condition	Indiana University Registry	Previously Reported Studies	Totals
• Congenital Coronary Anomaly	5 (16%)	28 (39%)	33 (32%)
1. Origin of left main artery from sinus of Valsalva	(1)	(20)	(21)
2. Origin of right artery from left sinus of Valsalva	(3)	(3)	(6)
3. Origin of left coronary artery from pulmonary trunk	(0)	(2)	(2)
4. Single coronary artery	(0)	(2)	(2)
5. Hypoplastic right, left or both coronary arteries	(0)	(1)	(1)
6. High takeoff coronary ostia	(1)	(0)	(1)
• Atherosclerotic Coronary Heart Disease	0	4 (6%)	4 (4%)
• Hypertrophic Cardiomyopathy	13 (42%)	16 (22%) †	29 (28%)
• Rupture or Dissection Ascending Aorta	0	3 (4%)	3 (3%)
• Valvular Heart Disease	4 (13%)	2 (3%)	6 (6%)
1. Floppy mitral valve	(3)	(2)	(5)
2. Ebstein's tricuspid valve	(1)		(1)
• Idiopathic Dilated Cardiomyopathy	0	1 (1%)	1 (1%)
• Myocarditis	1 (3%)	1 (1%)	2 (2%)
• Trauma	0	1 (1%)	1 (1%)
• Noncardiac and/or Uncertain	8 (26%)*	16 (23%)**	24 (23%)
Totals	**31 (100%)**	**72 (100%)**	**103 (100%)**

*Of 8 subjects, 6 had idiopathic left ventricular hypertrophy.
**Of 16 subjects, 4 had idiopathic left ventricular hypertrophy.
†Includes one subject with discrete subaortic stenosis.

jects (aged ≤30 years) dying suddenly during exercise, the most common structural cardiac abnormality found at necropsy was a congenital coronary anomaly, found in 28 subjects (39%). Of these, 20 (71%) had origin of the left main coronary artery from the right sinus of Valsalva and passage between the aorta and pulmonary trunk (Figure 1-4), three (11%) had origin of the right coronary artery from the left sinus of Valsalva and

passage between the aorta and pulmonary trunk (Figure 1-4), two had a single epicardial coronary artery, two had origin of the left coronary artery from the pulmonary trunk, and one had hypoplastic epicardial arteries.

The second most common structural cardiac abnormality causing sudden death in these subjects was hypertrophic cardiomyopathy (including discrete subaortic stenosis) (Figure 1-2),

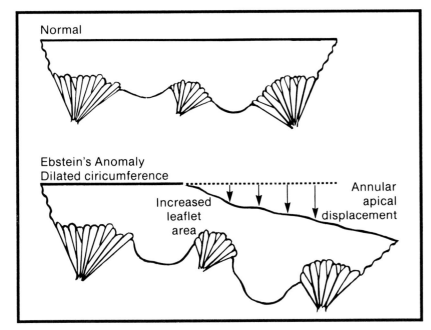

Figure 1-6: Ebstein's anomaly of the tricuspid valve. The normal annular insertion site is displaced apically. In addition, the annulus is dilated and the leaflet area is increased.

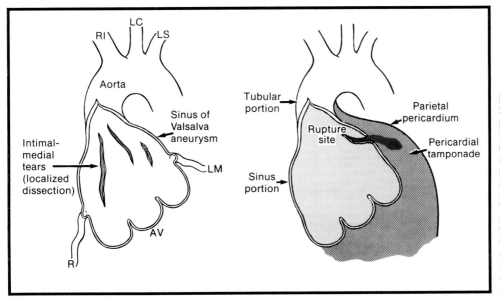

Figure 1-7: Marfan's Syndrome – The morphologic features of the Marfan ascending aorta causing exercise-related sudden death. The sinus portion of the ascending aorta is markedly dilated (aneurysm). In some patients (left) the aorta has multiple intimal-medial tears, and in others (right), the sinus of Valsalva aneurysm ruptures. AV = aortic valve, R = right coronary artery, LM = left main coronary artery.

observed in 22%. Other cardiovascular abnormalities included atherosclerotic heart disease (6%), floppy mitral valve (3%), idiopathic dilated cardiomyopathy, and myocarditis (1% each). The remaining 17 subjects (24%) had traumatic or undetermined causes of exercise-related sudden death.

In another study,[45] of 690 cases of sudden death, 34 were related to sports; eight of these, mean age 24, had hypertrophic cardiomyopathy; seven died playing basketball and one died swimming. Severe atherosclerosis was the etiology in nine athletes, mean age 32.

Sudden Death in Athletes Aged Older Than 30

Morphologic observations in exercise-related sudden deaths of conditioned subjects over age 30 have also received attention.[4, 7, 8, 26-32]

• The St. Vincent Registry Findings – Of the 57 sudden-death victims studied, 26 (46%) were aged 34 to 65 years (mean 47). Of these 26, 25 were males and 8 were competitors. Running was the most common form of exercise (25 subjects), followed by tennis, basketball, baseball, and swimming. The single woman in this age group was a karate belt holder. The runners had run regularly from 1 to 12 years before death. None of the 26 subjects had symptoms suggesting heart disease before they became regular exercisers, but at least one had been advised to stop running because of an abnormal resting and exercise electrocardiogram (obtained for a routine life insurance exam) two months before death.

• Necropsy Findings – Heart weights ranged from 320 to 555 grams (mean 434). Unequivocal structural cardiac disease was identified in all 26 of these subjects, but none had congenital coronary artery anomalies. Instead, 25 (96%) had atherosclerotic coronary artery disease (Figure 1-8), whereas the single female athlete had hypertrophic cardiomyopathy with clean epicardial coronary arteries. Each of the 25 runners had at least one of the three major coronary arteries (left anterior descending, left circumflex, right) narrowed 76% to 100% in cross-sectional area by atherosclerotic plaques. In addition, transmural **healed** myocardial infarcts (clinically "silent" events) were found in 17 of the 25.

• Previously Reported Subjects – Several previous studies[9, 15, 25-29, 32-37] have reported causes of death in conditioned subjects over 30 years of age. Few, however, provide detailed clinical or cardiac morphologic information.

Waller and Roberts[28] reported clinical and necropsy observations in five white males aged 40 to 53 years, who had run 22 to 176 km/wk (mean 53) for 1 to 10 years before they died while running. Two of the five men had been marathoners, and none of them had had clinical evidence of cardiac disease before they became habitual runners. At necropsy, all five had severe atherosclerotic luminal narrowing of all three major epicardial coronary arteries (Figures 1-9, 1-10).

Virmani and colleagues[9] described the sudden, non-traumatic deaths of 23 male runners aged 31 to 57 years. Seven of the 23 had displayed symptoms of coronary heart disease **before** beginning to exercise. The men had run from 7 to 195 miles/ week for six months to 28 years; two had completed at least one marathon. Of the 23 runners, 21 (91%) had severe narrowing by atherosclerotic plaques of at least one major coronary artery, and

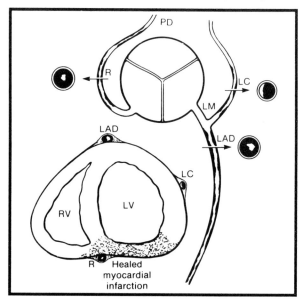

Figure 1-8: Atherosclerosis – The morphologic features of atherosclerotic coronary artery disease in patients with exercise-related sudden death. Usually two or three of the major coronary arteries are narrowed >75% in cross-sectional area by plaque. Some athletes have a healed myocardial infarct. LAD = left anterior descending, LC = left circumflex, LM = left main, PD = posterior descending, R = right.

13 (62%) had transmural myocardial infarcts. All four main epicardial coronary arteries (including the left main) were severely narrowed by plaques in a 38-year-old marathoner who had been running 105 miles per week for 23 years. The cause of death was found to be atherosclerotic coronary artery disease in 22 of the 23 runners; one died with a floppy mitral valve.

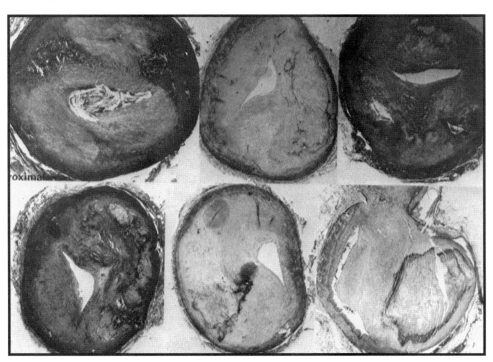

Figure 1-9: Maximal Narrowing – Photomicrograph of coronary artery sections at sites of maximal narrowing. Top panel, left to right: left anterior descending, and left circumflex arteries from the proximal and (lower panel) distal halves of the respective arteries. These arteries are from a competitive 49-year-old runner who had run for 10 years (173 km/wk), including six Boston Marathons. (From Waller and Roberts,[28] with permission).

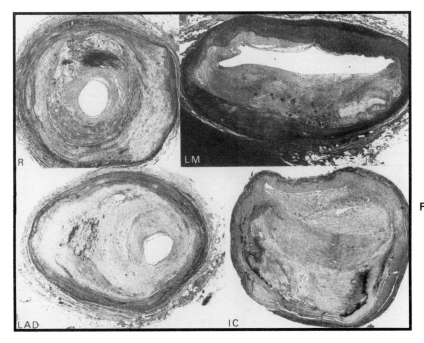

Figure 1-10: A 46-year-old Runner – The right (R), left main (LM), left anterior descending (LAD), and left circumflex (LC) coronary arteries at the sites of maximal narrowing from a 46-year-old runner who had run 67 km/wk for three years and had completed one standard marathon. (From Waller and Roberts,[28] with permission.)

Another study[27] reported the causes of exercise-related death in 18 runners or joggers. Thirteen were men over 40 years of age who died of atherosclerotic coronary heart disease. Although 6 of these 13 had clinical histories relevant to the cardiovascular system, atherosclerotic coronary heart disease had been diagnosed in only one. Two subjects had exercised for less than a month, five had been exercising regularly for at least a year, and nine had exercised for three years or more.

Severe coronary atherosclerosis was also found at necropsy in four of five marathon runners aged 36 to 44 years.[26] The other runner had hypertrophic cardiomyopathy.[34] Only one of these four runners with atherosclerosis experienced exercise-related sudden death, however; one died in the hospital awaiting coronary bypass surgery for unstable coronary angina pectoris, and two had traumatic deaths.

In summary, of 48 conditioned subjects over 30 years of age who died suddenly during or shortly after exercise (described in these and other reports), 46 (98%) died from atherosclerotic coronary heart disease (Table 1-2).

Comparison of Exercise-Related Sudden Deaths in Younger and Older Athletes

In both young (≤30 years) and older (>30 years) conditioned subjects dying suddenly with exercise, the killer of most is congenital or acquired disease of the epicardial coronary arteries (Table 1-3). However, there is a striking difference in the

---

Table 1-2
Causes of Sudden Death Found at Necropsy in 74 Athletes Age > 30 Years Dying During or Shortly After Exercise

Condition	Indiana University Registry	Previously Reported Students	Totals
• Congenital Coronary Anomaly	0	1 (2%)	1 (1%)
1. Hypoplastic coronary arteries[15]		(1)	(1)
• Atherosclerotic Coronary Heart Disease	25 (96%)	46 (96%)	71 (96%)
• Hypertrophic Cardiomyopathy	1 (4%)	1 (2%)[34]	2 (3%)
Totals	**26 (100%)**	**48 (100%)**	**74 (100%)**

Table 1-3
Cardiovascular Causes of Sudden Death in Conditioned Athletes

Abnormal Cardiac Structure	Age at Death		
	≤ 30	> 30	Total
• Coronary Artery	37 (47%)	72 (98%)	109 (72%)
• Myocardium	32 (43%)	2 (2%)	34 (22%)
• Valve	6 (6%)	0	6 (4%)
• Aorta	3 (4%)	0	3 (2%)
Totals	**78 (100%)**	**74 (100%)**	**152 (100%)**

pattern of necropsy findings between the two groups. The leading causes of death in the younger subjects (Table 1-1) were all of congenital origin: congenital coronary artery anomalies (32%), hypertrophic cardiomyopathy (28%), and valvular heart disease (6%). In contrast, among the older subjects (Table 1-2), acquired heart disease was responsible for nearly all the deaths: 96% displayed fatal atherosclerotic coronary heart disease. Only 2 of 74 subjects studied died from hypertrophic cardiomyopathy, and one from a congenital coronary anomaly.

Cardiovascular Structural Abnormalities in Exercise-Related Sudden Deaths

Cardiovascular morphologic abnormalities associated with sudden death during exercise can be grouped into four categories: coronary arterial, myocardial, valvular, and aortic. Of 177 subjects shown in Tables 1-1 and 1-2, 152 (86%) had an identifiable cardiovascular structural abnormality (Table 1-3), of which the majority involved the coronary arteries.

Coronary Arterial Abnormalities

Sudden death from coronary abnormalities is the most frequent cause of all sudden cardiac deaths, both with and without associated physical exertion. Several subgroups of abnormalities can be listed:
• Coronary atherosclerosis
• Congenital coronary anomalies
• Tunneled epicardial coronary arteries
• High take-off of coronary ostia
• Coronary trauma
• Coronary spasm

• **Coronary Atherosclerosis** – The most frequent cause of exercise-related sudden death, coronary atherosclerosis accounted for 42% of the deaths reported in this chapter, including 96% of those involving conditioned subjects over 30 years of age.

• **Anomalous Origin of a Major Coronary Artery** – Anomalous origin of a major coronary artery from the sinuses of Valsalva was the second most frequently found abnormality in these exercise-related sudden deaths, accounting for 19% of all subjects, and 32% of those ≤30 years. Until the

study by Cheitlin and colleagues in 1974,[23] single coronary arteries and the origin of both left and right coronary arteries from the same sinus of Valsalva were regarded as having little clinical significance. Cheitlin's group examined 51 necropsy patients with anomalous coronary origins: 31 (61%) with origin of the left main and right coronary arteries from the right sinus of Valsalva, and 18 (35%) with origin of both arteries from the left sinus (Figure 1-4). Of the 51 patients, 7 (14%) died suddenly on exercising, all of whom had origin of the left main artery from the right sinus.

A study[24] of 21 necropsy patients with anomalous origin of major coronary arteries reported exercise-related sudden death in two patients, both of whom had the left main arising as the first branch of the right coronary artery, with leftward passage between the walls of the aorta and pulmonary trunk. Four other patients with origin of the left main from the right sinus but with passage around the anterior surface of the pulmonary trunk did not have sudden death.

Of 10 necropsy patients[10] in whom the right coronary artery arose from the left coronary sinus and then passed to the right atrioventricular sulcus by coursing between the aorta and pulmonary trunk, three died suddenly, including one during exercise. Thus, origin of the right coronary artery from the left sinus may produce fatal cardiac dysfunction.

The mechanism of sudden death with exercise in subjects with origin of both coronary arteries from a single coronary sinus and passage of one artery between the walls of the aorta and pulmonary trunk is depicted in Figure 1-11. The acute take-off angle of the anomalous artery appears to be an important factor in producing myocardial ischemia.

• **Tunneled Epicardial Coronary Arteries** – Tunneled epicardial coronary arteries ("myocardial bridges") (Figure 1-12) received renewed attention in a report by Morales and colleagues[25] of sudden death during strenuous exercise in three patients in whom a tunneled portion of the left anterior descending coronary artery was present at necropsy. The authors concluded that this finding represented a potentially lethal anatomic variant.

Burke et al[45] reported two of 34 athletes with exercise-related sudden death who had tunneled

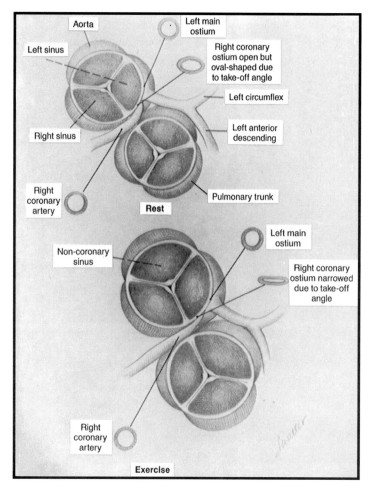

Aorta
Left sinus
Left main ostium
Right coronary ostium open but oval-shaped due to take-off angle
Left circumflex
Left anterior descending
Right sinus
Right coronary artery
Pulmonary trunk
Rest

Non-coronary sinus
Left main ostium
Right coronary ostium narrowed due to take-off angle
Right coronary artery
Exercise

Figure 1-11: Ischemia – The mechanism of coronary ischemia in patients with origin of the right coronary artery from the left sinus of Valsalva. With increased cardiac output (exercise, tachycardia) (bottom), the aorta and pulmonary trunk dilate. The slit-like ostium of the anomalous artery becomes even more narrowed and coronary flow is diminished.

left anterior descending arteries. Tunneled coronary arteries were observed in two (7%) of the 27 subjects in the St. Vincent Hospital registry series (see Table 1-1) and in five (3%) of the 158 previously reported subjects with sudden death and exercise. In view of the wide range (5% to 85%)[25] of tunneled coronary arteries found at autopsy, however, their link to sudden death is open to question.

• **High Take-off of Coronary Ostia** – It has been suggested[38] that high take-off of a coronary artery, defined as an origin of coronary ostia 5 mm or more above the aortic sinotubular junction, may precipitate sudden death. One subject in the Indiana University registry, a 17-year-old basketball player, had the left coronary artery ostium arising about 5 mm above the sinotubular junction, and

also had an anomalous origin of the right coronary artery from the left sinus of Valsalva. This combination appears to be the first such observation in an athlete dying suddenly with exercise.

• **Coronary Arterial Trauma** – Coronary trauma is an infrequently reported cause of sudden death associated with physical trauma. One report[39] concerned the sudden death of a player while walking back to the huddle after having run a pass pattern in a professional football game. The subject had severe coronary atherosclerosis, but the unusual feature was extensive atherosclerosis plaque hemorrhage. It was postulated that rough tackling and blocking caused trauma to the severely narrowed left anterior descending coronary artery, producing atherosclerotic "cracks" with subsequent bleeding into them.

• **Exercise-Induced Coronary Spasm** – Exercise-induced coronary spasm has recently been proposed[30] as a mechanism for sudden death in athletes. Circadian variation has also been reported;[40] of 13 subjects with exercise-induced coronary spasm, all had ST-segment elevation with exercise in the morning, but only two had the same finding in the afternoon. Thus, whereas coronary spasm has not been reported as a real factor in exercise-related sudden death, its potential seems logical. If patients with evidence of coronary spasm desire to participate in regular exercise, exercise testing should be performed to detect the small subgroup of patients with exercised-induced spasm, and these patients should be advised to exercise in the afternoon.

Myocardial Abnormalities

Structural abnormalities of ventricular myocardium are the second most frequently observed morphologic cardiac alteration in conditioned subjects with exercise-related sudden death, affecting 34 (22%) of the subjects reported (Table 1-3). Hypertrophic cardiomyopathy (Figure 1-1, 1-2) was found most often, occurring in 31 of the 34. Of these 31, 29 were aged 30 years or under. The myocardial abnormalities found in the other subjects were myocarditis (two patients), and idiopathic dilated cardiomyopathy (familial) (one patient).[18]

Another report[35] described two joggers (12 to 14 miles/week) who developed dyspnea on exertion that ultimately prevented each from exercising. Both died within a year of discontinuing running (mode of death not provided) and were found at necropsy to have cardiac amyloidosis.

Valvular Abnormalities

Floppy mitral valve appears to be the major valvular abnormality observed at necropsy in conditioned subjects dying suddenly with exercise, present in five of the six subjects reported in this chapter who were found to have valvular abnormalities (Table 1-3). The remaining subject had Ebstein's anomaly of the tricuspid valve (Figure 1-6).

Aortic Abnormalities

Diseases affecting the aorta accounted for the sudden death of three (2%) of the 152 subjects reported. Two of these were male basketball players, 18 and 21 years old, who had rupture of a markedly dilated ascending aorta.[11] At least one had typical physical stigmata of Marfan's syndrome (Figure 1-7). Histologic examination of aortic wall in each disclosed a diminished number of

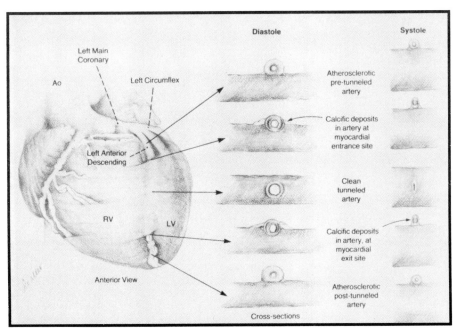

Figure 1-12: Tunneled left anterior descending coronary artery (myocardial bridges). The tunneled segment lies within the myocardium and becomes severely narrowed during ventricular systole.

medial elastic fibers ("cystic medial necrosis"). The third subject was a 15-year-old weight lifter and wrestler[15] who had aortic dissection unassociated with Marfan syndrome.

Conduction System Abnormalities

Occasionally, gross and histologic cardiac examination may fail to find a structural cardiovascular abnormality that provides a reasonable explanation for sudden death in an athlete. Electrocardiographic abnormalities such as bradycardia with sinus pauses, second-degree atrioventricular block, and even atrioventricular dissociation have been reported in highly trained athletes, but no available data suggest that these abnormalities predispose to sudden death.

An examination of the conduction system in two young athletes who died suddenly[13] found striking changes at the level of the sinus node, consisting of medial degeneration, hyperplasia, and intimal proliferation producing luminal narrowing of the sinus node artery. Sudden cardiac death also has been reported in young athletes with congenital partial absence of right ventricular myocardium.[42] Right ventricular dysplasia has been associated by epicardial mapping with life-threatening right ventricular tachycardia, and the term "arrhythmogenic right ventricular dysplasia" has been proposed for this entity.[43]

Conduction system abnormalities have been reported[44] in three other young athletes with exercise-related sudden death. One, an 11-year-old girl, had micro-Ebstein's anomaly of the tricuspid valve associated with a septoseptal Kent fascicle through a wide gap of the central fibrous annulus and upper Mahaim fibers. A 24-year-old football player had focal but severe atherosclerotic narrowing in the proximal left anterior descending coronary artery, but examination also found that upper and lower Mahaim fibers joined the atrioventricular node and the left bundle branch with the crest of the ventricular septum. A 26-year-old cycling champion had an atrial fascicle bypassing the atrioventricular node to anastomose with the His bundle (James accessory atrioventricular pathway). The report[44] concluded that these atrioventricular conduction system abnormalities may have played a fatal arrhythmogenic role in the three athletes, and raised questions regarding the identification and prevention of electrical instabil-

ity in young individuals engaged in competitive sports.

Implications for Screening and Exercise Prescription Based on the Autopsy Findings

One purpose of autopsy examinations is to provide morphologic information that might be useful clinically in the future diagnosis, treatment, and management of disease processes.[5, 7] The information derived from the studies discussed here suggest several points important in prescribing healthful exercise:

1. Screening of the cardiovascular system should be conducted in athletes. Structural cardiac abnormalities account for most exercise-related sudden deaths. Thus, any major medical screening effort in athletes should concentrate on the cardiovascular system.

Editor's Note: Careful screening of athletes is the most important factor in the detection of cardiac conditions that can result in serious complications, including sudden death. This is discussed in detail in the following chapter. – WPH

2. A cardiovascular examination in athletes over age 30 should focus on coronary atherosclerosis. Because coronary atherosclerosis accounts for almost all of the athletic sudden deaths during midlife, examination efforts should focus on the detection and evaluation of this condition. Furthermore, a cardiovascular examination seems warranted for middle-aged persons who are just beginning to exercise on a regular basis.

Editor's Note: I would like to strongly support this wise advice. Too often, we see examples where this screening evaluation has either not been done, or not been done properly, and strenuous exercise has produced a serious complication of heart disease. – WPH

3. Pay attention to new symptoms. For those middle-aged persons who are currently exercising, the appearance of any new symptoms – especially those suggestive of myocardial ischemia, whether directly associated with vigorous exercise or not – should be promptly evaluated. Increasing the duration and intensity of running for the "relief of new-onset chest discomfort" may result in "running to death."

4. A cardiovascular examination in athletes under age 30 should be directed towards detecting congenital heart disease, which includes hypertrophic cardiomyopathy [formerly called idiopathic hypertrophic subaortic stenosis (IHSS) or hypertrophic obstructive cardiomyopathy (HOCM)]. Since the most common of these congenital heart lesions is hypertrophic cardiomyopathy, the echocardiogram would be extremely useful in such an examination.

Editor's Note: In fact, the diagnosis of hypertrophic cardiomyopathy can often be made or suspected in the initial screening examination of the athlete. The echocardiogram can then be done for further documentation, or if there is any question on the screening exam that might suggest this condition. The electrocardiogram, too, is a useful screening test, since a normal ECG almost rules out hypertrophic cardiomyopathy. – WPH

Chapters 2 through 5 will review further the usefulness of various screening tools in detecting the entities found to be associated with exercise-related sudden death.

References

1. Roberts WC: An agent with lipid-lowering, antihypertensive, positive inotropic, negative chronotropic, vasodilating, diuretic, anorexigenic, weight-reducing, cathartic, hypoglycemic, tranquilizing, hypnotic and antidepressive qualities (editorial). *Am J Cardiol* 53:261, 1984.
2. Department of Health, Education, and Welfare: *Healthy people: The Surgeon General's report on health promotion and disease prevention.* PHS Publication No. 79-55071, 1979.
3. Fletcher GF: *The dangers of exercise.* In Hurst, JW (Ed): *The Heart: Update V.* McGraw-Hill Book Company, New York, 1981, p 161.
4. Waller BF: Sudden death in midlife. *Cardiovasc Med* 10:55, 1985.
5. *Perrier Survey of Fitness in America.* Study No. S2813. Louis Harris and Associates, Inc., 1978.
6. Sheehan GA: The case for exercise (editorial): *Am J Cardiol* 53:260, 1984.
7. Waller BF: Sudden death in middle-aged conditioned subjects: Coronary atherosclerosis is the culprit (editorial). *Mayo Clin Proc* 62:634, 1987.
8. Cantwell JD and Fletcher GF: Sudden death and jogging. *Phys Sports Med* 3:94-98, 1978.
9. Virmani R, Robinowitz M, McAllister HA Jr: Nontraumatic death in joggers. A series of 30 patients at autopsy. *Am J Med* 72:874-881, 1982.
10. Roberts WC, Siegel RJ, and Zipes DP: Origin of the right coronary artery from the left sinus of Valsalva and its functional consequences: Analysis of 10 necropsy patients. *Am J Cardiol* 49:863-867, 1982.
11. Maron BJ, Roberts WC, McAllister HA Jr, Rosing DR, and Epstein SE: Sudden death in young athletes. *Circulation* 62:218-229, 1980.
12. Tsung SH, Huang TY, and Chang HH: Sudden death in young athletes. *Arch Pathol Lab Med* 106:168-170, 1982.
13. James TN, Froggatt P, and Marshall TK: Sudden death in young athletes. *Ann Intern Med* 67:1013-1021, 1967.
14. Hanzlick R, Stivers RR: Sudden death in marathon runner with origin of the right coronary artery from the left sinus of Valsalva. *Am J Cardiol* 51:1467, 1983.
15. Jokl E, and McClellan JT: Exercise and cardiac death. *Med and Sport* 5:1-185, 1971.
16. Roberts TJ, and Loube SD: Congenital single coronary artery in man. *Am Heart J* 34:188, 1947.
17. Opie LH: Sudden death and sport. *Lancet i* (7901):263-266, 1975.
18. Rotter W: Uber den abnormen Abgan der liden Herzkranzarterie aus de Lungenschlagader. *Zentralbl Allg Path Anat* 89:160, 1952.
19. Koplan JP: Cardiovascular deaths while running. *JAMA* 242:2578-2579, 1979.
20. Nieod JL: Anomalie coronaire et mort subite. *Cardiologia* 20:172, 1952.
21. Cohen LS, and Shaw LD: Fatal myocardial infarction in an 11-year-old boy associated with a unique coronary artery anomaly. *Am J Cardiol* 19:420, 1967.
22. Benson PA, and Lack AR: Anomalous aortic origin of left coronary artery. *Arch Pathol* 86:214, 1968.
23. Cheitlin MD, DeCastro CM, and McAllister HA: Sudden death as a complication of anomalous left coronary origin from the anterior sinus of Valsalva. A not-so-minor congenital anomaly. *Circulation* 50:780-787, 1974.
24. Liberthson RR, Dinsmore RE, Bharati S, Rubeinstein JJ, Caulfield J, Wheeler EO, Hathorne JW, and Lev M: Aberrant coronary artery origin from the aorta. *Circulation* 50:774-779, 1974.
25. Morale AR, Romanelli R, and Boucek RJ: The mural left anterior descending coronary artery, strenuous exercise and sudden death. *Circulation* 62:230, 1980.
26. Noakes TD, Opie LH, Rose AG, and Kleynhans PHT: Autopsy-proved coronary atherosclerosis in marathon runners. *N Engl J Med* 301:86-89, 1979.
27. Thompson PD, Stern MP, Williams P, Duncan K, Haskell WL, Wood PD: Death during jogging or running. A study of 18 cases. *JAMA* 242:1265-1267, 1979.

28. Waller BF, and Roberts WC: Sudden death while running in conditioned runners aged 40 years or over. *Am J Cardiol* 45:1292-1300, 1980.

29. Waller BF, Csere RS, Baker WP, and Roberts WC: Running to death. *Chest* 79:346, 1981.

30. McManus BM, Waller BF, Grayboys TB, Mitchell JH, Siegel RJ, Miller HS, Froelicher VF, and Roberts WC: Exercise and sudden death – Part 2. *Cur Prob Cardiol* 10:1-57, 1982.

31. McManus BM, Waller BF, Grayboys TB, Mitchell JH, Siegel RJ, Miller HS, Froelicher VF, and Roberts WC: Exercise and sudden death – Part 1. *Cur Prob Cardiol* 9:1-89, 1981.

32. Thompson PD, Funk EJ, Carleton RA, and Sturner WQ: Incidence of death during jogging in Rhode Island from 1975 through 1980. *JAMA* 247:2535-2538, 1982.

33. Green LH, Cohen SI, and Kurland G: Fatal myocardial infarction in marathon racing. *Ann Intern Med* 84:704-706, 1976.

34. Noakes TD, Rose AG, and Opie LH: Hypertrophic cardiomyopathy associated with sudden death during marathon racing. *Br Heart J* 41:624-627, 1979.

35. Siegel RJ, French WJ, and Roberts WC: Spontaneous exercise testing. Running as an early unmasker of underlying cardiac amyloidosis. *Arch Intern Med* 142:345, 1982.

36. Colt E: Coronary-artery disease in marathon runners. *N Engl J Med* 302:57, 1980.

37. Vuori I, Makarainen M, and Jaaskelainen A: Sudden death and physical activity. *Cardiology* 63:287-304, 1978.

38. Vlodaver Z, Amplatz K, Burchell H, and Edwards JE: *Coronary Heart Disease. Clinical, Angiographic and Pathologic Profiles.* Springer-Verlag, New York, 1976.

39. Roberts WC, and Maron BJ: Sudden death while playing professional football. *Am Heart J* 102:1061-1063, 1981.

40. Yasue H, Omote S, Takizaua A, Nagao M, Miwa K, and Tanaka S: Circadian variation of exercise capacity in patients with Prinzmetal's variant angina: Role of exercise-induced coronary arterial spasm. *Circulation* 59:938-948, 1979.

41. Warren SE, Boice JB, Bloor C, and Vieweg WVR: The athletic heart revisited. Sudden death of a 28-year-old athlete. *West J Med* 131:441-447, 1979.

42. Virmani R, Robinowitz M, Clark MA, and McAllister HA: Sudden death and partial absence of the right ventricular myocardium: A report of three cases and a review of literature. *Arch Pathol Lab Med* 106:163-167, 1982.

43. Fontaine G, Guiraudon G, Frank R, Vedel J, Grosgogeat Y, and Cabrol C: Modern concepts of ventricular tachycardia: The value of electrophysiological investigations and delayed potentials in ventricular tachycardia of ischemic and nonischemic etiology (31 operated cases). *Eur J Cardiol* 8:565-580, 1978.

44. Thiene G, Pennelli N, and Rossi L: Cardiac conduction system abnormalities as a possible cause of sudden death in young athletes. *Human Pathol* 14:704-709, 1983.

45. Burke A, Farb A, Virmani R, Goodin J, Smiolek J: Sports-related and non-sports-related sudden cardiac death in young adults. *Am Heart J* Vol 121, No. 2, Part 1, Feb. 1991.

CHAPTER 2

THE MOST COMMON CAUSES OF SUDDEN DEATH IN ATHLETES: CLUES FROM THE PHYSICAL EXAM, PARTICULARLY AUSCULTATION OF THE HEART

W. Proctor Harvey, MD

Professor of Medicine
Division of Cardiology
Georgetown University Medical Center

Editor's Note: This chapter is written by the foremost authority on cardiac auscultation – W. Proctor Harvey. His practical approach to clinical auscultation can be used by all of us in examining athletes. With the information provided in this chapter, life-threatening cardiac conditions can be "spotted" before they produce a tragic outcome. – BFW

Sudden death from cardiac causes occurs in athletes at all levels – high school, college and professional. Can those athletes at risk be spotted? Many believe that, if this can be done at all, it would require extensive specialized tests such as treadmill, echocardiogram, and perhaps even cardiac catheterization. Obviously, such tests are so expensive that they would not be practical for large scale screening. However, we believe that those prone to serious cardiac disease and who have a risk of cardiac complications, including sudden death, can often be suspected and identified by the well-trained physician utilizing a careful history and physical examination. The most important part of the physical exam is detailed auscultation of the heart. This can be accomplished by the well-trained physician when he

performs the screening evaluation of the athletes. If this initial examination discloses any question or suspicion of heart disease, additional studies of the cardiovascular system should be obtained, including an electrocardiogram, chest x-ray, and echocardiogram. Even more sophisticated diagnostic procedures can be done as needed for the individual athlete. As described in the preceding chapter, the following conditions are the most common causes of sudden death in young (under 30) athletes:
- Hypertrophic cardiomyopathy
- Dilated cardiomyopathy
- Myocarditis
- Drugs
- Congenital aortic stenosis/bicuspid aortic valve
- Arrhythmias
- Marfan's syndrome and variants

In patients (including athletes) older than 30, the most common causes of sudden death are:
- Coronary artery disease, including atherosclerosis and congenital coronary artery anomalies
- Marfan's syndrome and variants
- Drugs
- Arrhythmias

Most of the above conditions and other uncommon ones usually can be suspected and even diagnosed in the doctor's office by means of a careful cardiovascular evaluation.

In general, the most important aspect of the complete cardiovascular examination is the history; but, in the case of the athlete who might be at risk of sudden death, it is *the physical examination, particularly auscultation, that is most likely to provide the clue or diagnosis.* The exception to this rule is in the instance of cocaine use. A history of cocaine use by the athlete provides etiologic clues for myocarditis, dilated cardiomyopathy, and coronary artery pathology.

Worthy of emphasis is the fact that the clinical excellence of the examining physician is the most important key in spotting the athlete prone to sudden death. The diagnostic skills of every physician, particularly proficiency in auscultation, can be sharpened to accomplish this. Of great aid in this respect is attending and participating in postgraduate courses that provide special emphasis on improvement of the necessary clinical skills.

Hypertrophic Cardiomyopathy

This condition was formerly termed idiopathic hypertrophic subaortic stenosis (IHSS) in the United States, or hypertrophic obstructive cardiomyopathy (HOCM) in the British Isles. The present internationally accepted designation is hypertrophic cardiomyopathy. (Figure 2-1). It should always be carefully searched for in an athlete, since it is one of the most common causes of sudden death in such individuals, especially those under the age of 30. Unfortunately, it may cause no symptoms until the tragic episode of sudden death occurs. To illustrate this point, recently in the Washington, D.C., area a young teen-aged high school football player, a star of the team, weighing about 250 pounds, died suddenly following a "light scrimmage." The most likely cause in such cases is hypertrophic cardiomyopathy.

This condition can frequently be suspected and diagnosed by the examining physician, even on simple office examination. This applies to the screening exam of the athlete. An early clue as to its presence may come from the arterial pulse. On first greeting and shaking hands with the patient or athlete, palpate his or her radial pulse (Figure 2-2). If you feel a "quick rise" or "flip," suspect the

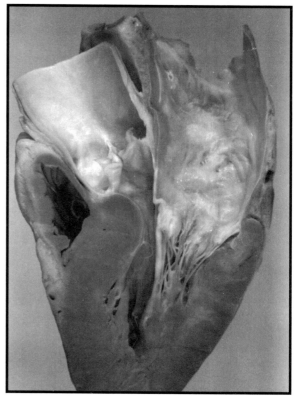

Figure 2-1: **Hypertrophic Cardiomyopathy** – Photograph shows echocardiographic view of hypertrophic cardiomyopathy. The ventricular septum is much thicker than the free wall (asymmetric septal hypertrophy), the left ventricular cavity is small, and the left atrium is dilated.

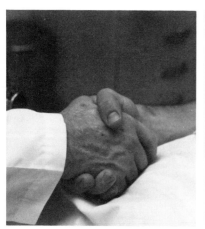
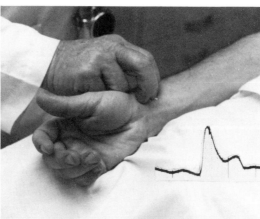

Figure 2-2: Checking for a Quick Rise – When first greeting a patient, shake hands and then move to palpate the radial pulse. If a quick rise or "flip" of the pulse is noted (see arterial pulse tracing – right panel), it could be an early clue to the presence of hypertrophic cardiomyopathy.

possibility of hypertrophic cardiomyopathy. The sensation of a flip is illustrated in Figure 2-3, where the middle finger of one hand strikes the middle finger of the other hand. The flip can vary from slight to strong. All of the following may cause such a quick rise:

• Aortic regurgitation
• Mitral regurgitation
• Ventricular septal defect
• Patent ductus arteriosus
• Hypertrophic cardiomyopathy (the most common cause of sudden death in an athlete under the age of 30).

vents the unsteadiness and lack of concentration of the physician if he or she attempts to squat along with the patient (a simple but important point).

Other maneuvers can help detect the murmurs of hypertrophic cardiomyopathy, such as the Valsalva maneuver (diagnostic increase in the systolic murmur on straining or having the patient blow on his or her finger) (Figure 2-7) and the isometric hand grip; however, the most useful is the squatting maneuver.

Another clinical feature aiding in the diagnosis of hypertrophic cardiomyopathy is the precordial

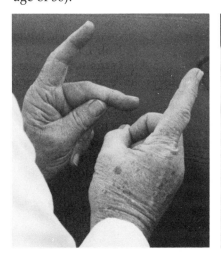
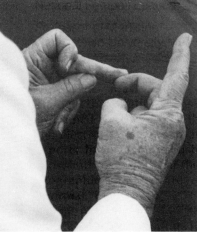

Figure 2-3: **"Flip"** – Illustrating the sensation of a "flip" or quick rise of the arterial pulse. The middle finger of one hand is flipped against the middle finger of the other hand. Either a mild or more intense flip or quick rise can thus be simulated.

Following is what we have termed the 1, 2, 3, 4 diagnosis of hypertrophic cardiomyopathy:

1. A quick rise in the arterial pulse (radial or carotid most frequently used).

2. Aortic regurgitation is suspected as a possibility; however, no aortic diastolic murmur is present.

3. Instead, a systolic murmur is heard (Figure 2-4).

4. Use the squatting maneuver. When the patient squats, the systolic murmur becomes fainter or disappears. On standing, the systolic murmur becomes louder, sometimes even doubling in intensity (Figure 2-5). These findings represent solid evidence of hypertrophic cardiomyopathy. Remember to squat the patient several times, since the diagnostic changes may be best heard only after the first squat.

The squatting maneuver is ideally performed if the physician remains seated and listens while the patient squats and stands (Figure 2-6). This pre-

movement. On palpation of the precordium with the patient turned to the left lateral position and feeling with the index and middle fingers, a presystolic and a double systolic movement may be detected. This has been referred to as the "triple

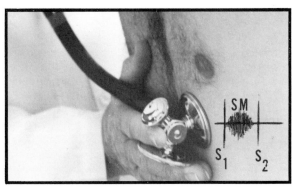

Figure 2-4: **Hypertrophic Cardiomyopathy** – Listening along the left sternal border for an aortic diastolic murmur; instead, a systolic murmur (SM) is heard.

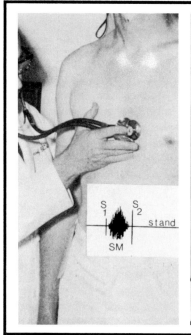
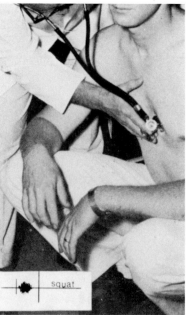

Figure 2-5: The Squatting Manuever – The systolic murmur (SM) heard on standing becomes fainter (sometimes even disappears) on squatting. On standing again, the murmur may become louder again. Remember to repeat this manuever several times, as it may be only on the third or fourth time that the difference in the murmur is best detected. Note that the physician is standing and then squats with the patient.

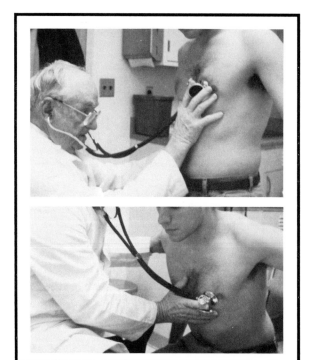

Figure 2-6: A Better Way to Do the Squatting Manuever – The most comfortable and efficient way is for the physician to remain seated and listen as the patient squats.

ripple," a term coined by one of the former Georgetown fellows in cardiology. An atrial (S_4) gallop is heard that correlates with the presystolic movement in addition to the systolic murmur.

The electrocardiogram is also very useful in screening for hypertrophic cardiomyopathy, since a normal electrocardiogram usually rules out this diagnosis. The electrocardiogram may show left axis deviation, left ventricular hypertrophy, abnormal Q-waves, or poor progression of R-waves across the precordium. The electrocardiogram in this condition can thus simulate previous myocardial infarction in an athlete who has never had any symptoms.

Myocarditis

It is clinically apparent that varying degrees of myocarditis can occur, and thus the signs and symptoms will vary. Acute pulmonary edema can accompany severe and acute fulminating myocarditis. Symptoms and signs of heart failure are obvious in these patients and should be easily recognized. Lesser degrees of inflammation of heart muscle can present with more subtle findings and be more difficult to diagnose. A virus infection may be the culprit and symptoms, including dyspnea, fatigue, and occasional palpitations (arrhythmias), may be attributed to the "flu."

However, immediate clues to myocardial involvement and cardiac decompensation include:

- Pulsus alternans (Figure 2-8)
- Alternation of sounds (especially the second sound) (Figure 2-9)
- Alternation of murmur (usually systolic)
- Ventricular (S_3) diastolic gallop (this correlates with the pulsus alternans and alternation of the sounds and murmurs)
- Atrial (S_4) diastolic gallop is also frequently present (Figure 2-10)

These findings may be very subtle and most often must be specifically searched for. Unfortunately, this is too often not done. Not only do we find what we look for, but we have to *know* what we are looking for. Patients with myocarditis can die suddenly due to ventricular arrhythmias, which unfortunately can be the first indication of this serious condition. Physical effort might well trigger this catastrophic event. It is apparent that any athlete could be such a victim. It follows that every patient examined must be carefully screened to make sure there is no pulsus alternans, alternation of sounds and murmur, or gallop rhythm.

Acute pericarditis can also be accompanied by myocarditis. After the pericarditis has subsided, subtle findings of the myocarditis may remain and be overlooked. An example of this is a man in his early 40's, an employee of the U.S. State Department, who was at his post in Africa. He had an acute pericarditis, presumably from a viral infection, that was documented by typical clinical symptoms and signs, including a three component pericardial friction rub and characteristic electrocardiographic changes on ST and T-waves.

At the end of six weeks he was sent back to the United States. Upon his arrival in Washington, D.C., he was now feeling well and other than some residual inverted T-waves on his electrocardiogram, it had been assumed that he had recovered and was now ready to resume normal physical activities and work. He stated, "I can't wait to get back to jogging again."

However, on physical examination he had subtle but definite findings of a myocarditis: weak pulsus alternans, alternation of the second sound, alternation of the Grade 2 systolic murmur, and both an atrial (S_4) and a ventricular (S_3) diastolic gallop (Figures 2-8 and 2-9). These were

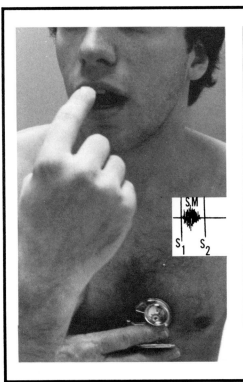
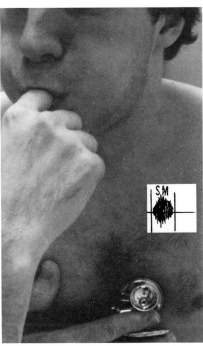

Figure 2-7: Valsalva Manuever – A different and efficient Valsalva Manuever. The patient places his index finger in his mouth (left). He seals his lips around the finger (right) and is instructed to "blow hard." Note the increase in the systolic murmur.

very subtle but definite findings. Jogging and other more strenuous physical activity would be the last thing he should do. Restriction of physical activities was advised, and the patient accepted and followed this advice.

At the end of approximately two months, all previous signs of myocarditis had disappeared. Now, years later, he has no evidence of heart disease and is leading a perfectly normal life. Had he *not* restricted his activities on return to the United States, but instead resumed a strenuous exercise program, he could have progressed from the subtle signs of myocarditis to overt symptoms and signs of cardiac decompensation with irreversible myocardial damage – and a diagnosis of dilated cardiomyopathy, not pericarditis. With early recognition and treatment, a cure can occur, as illustrated by our patient.

The alert physician can detect these subtle signs of alternation of sounds and murmurs, and gallop rhythm in the office or during screening examinations.

Dilated Cardiomyopathy

Dilated cardiomyopathy (Figure 2-11) can cause a spectrum of findings, from mild to severe (Figure 2-12). With moderately severe or severe involvement, reversibility with treatment might not be achievable. On the other hand, with mild to moderate severity, early suspicion, early diagnosis, and early treatment can result in reversibility. Cure is most likely, of course, in the presence of mild cardiomyopathy.

The diagnosis of a dilated cardiomyopathy in an athlete is the same as in a non-athlete. It is similar to acute myocarditis. The signs and symptoms of dilated cardiomyopathy are those of cardiac decompensation (some already discussed under myocarditis); these include dyspnea, arrhythmias, cardiomegaly, pulsus alternans, alternation of the intensity and quality of heart sounds and murmurs, and gallop rhythm. The more advanced physical signs of heart failure (rales in the lung, liver enlargement, and peripheral edema of the lower extremities) would be rarely seen when screening athletes, since their condition would already have been diagnosed at an earlier stage and they would have ceased participation.

However, some athletes who have occult dilated cardiomyopathy with areas of healed and active inflammation of the myocardium have been able to participate in their sport and have died suddenly. Certainly in this group of athletes, the findings of gallop rhythm, probable pulsus alternans, and cardiomegaly are present and will be found if carefully searched for; if detected, appropriate laboratory procedures should be done. If the diagnosis of dilated cardiomyopathy is established, the athlete should not be given medical clearance but should be advised not to participate in highly competitive, strenuous sports.

Congenital Aortic Stenosis – Bicuspid Aortic Valve

The diagnosis of a congenital aortic stenosis (Figure 2-13) can and should be detected during screening evaluation of athletes. The patient may have no symptoms. With more advanced degrees of stenosis, dizziness, near syncope or syncope, dyspnea, and fatigue can occur; a significant aortic systolic murmur also would be present to alert the examining physician to this possibility.

Of absolute importance is to differentiate the murmur of congenital aortic stenosis from the innocent systolic murmur that is so common in athletes. It is, therefore, essential that the physician be able to accurately diagnose the typical characteristics of an innocent systolic murmur, as will be discussed in the next chapter.

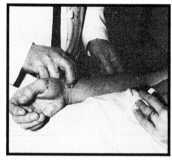

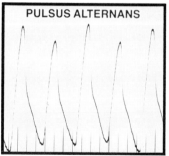

PULSUS ALTERNANS

Figure 2-8: Pulsus Alternans – Pulsus alternans is noted on palpation of the radial pulse. Note that every other beat is weaker than the preceding one. Pulsus alternans can be one of the earliest, most subtle signs of cardiac decompensation. It is also a clue that you should search for alternation of the second sound, alternations of murmurs, and a ventricular (S_3) diastolic gallop.

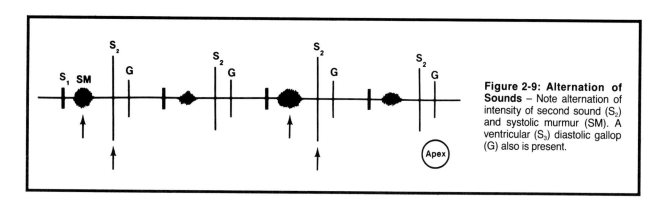

Figure 2-9: Alternation of Sounds – Note alternation of intensity of second sound (S_2) and systolic murmur (SM). A ventricular (S_3) diastolic gallop (G) also is present.

The auscultory findings in a patient with a congenital bicuspid aortic valve can cover a wide spectrum, as shown in Figure 2-13. Most commonly, an early to mid-systolic murmur, of Grade 1 to 3 intensity is present. Frequently it has a harsh quality similar to the sound of clearing one's throat. In some, an early blowing, high frequency aortic diastolic murmur grade 1 to 3 also may be present. Firm pressure on the stethoscope's flat diaphragm chest piece should always be used to best detect this diastolic murmur, listening along the left sternal border, with the patient sitting upright, leaning forward, and breath held in deep expiration (Figure 2-14). Since aortic events are usually well heard at the apex, the systolic murmur of aortic stenosis may be detected from the apex to the aortic area (Figure 2-15). This is also true of the aortic ejection sound that is another key to the diagnosis of this condition (Figure 2-15).

The Systolic Ejection Sound of the Congenital Bicuspid Aortic Valve

The ejection sound is a hallmark of this lesion and occurs with "doming" of the valve in early systole. It, too, as with the systolic murmur, is generally well heard from the apex to the aortic area (Figure 2-15). It does not diminish in intensity with inspiration (as can occur with the ejection sound of congenital pulmonic stenosis) (Figures 2-15 and 2-16).

If severe aortic stenosis is present in athletes, one readily hears a loud (grade 4 to 6) precordial

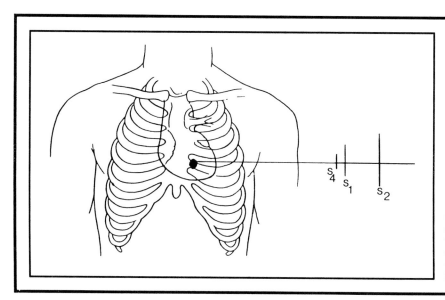

Figure 2-10: Another Sign of Myocardial Involvement – An atrial (S_4) diastolic gallop does not correlate with the pulsus alternans and cardiac decompensation, as does the ventricular (S_3) gallop. However, it is often present in addition to the other findings.

murmur. However, aortic stenosis of a mild to moderate degree can easily be overlooked on a cursory physical examination, especially if the examining physician is not listening specifically for the tell-tale findings of an *ejection sound* and a systolic murmur. It is also worthwhile to remember that an athlete's body build (large frame, heavy weight, and highly developed chest musculature) can diminish the intensity of sounds and murmurs heard with the stethoscope. In contrast, murmurs in children, young people, and athletes with thin chests will be more readily detected.

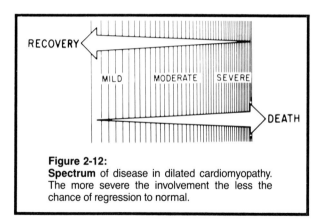

Figure 2-12:
Spectrum of disease in dilated cardiomyopathy. The more severe the involvement the less the chance of regression to normal.

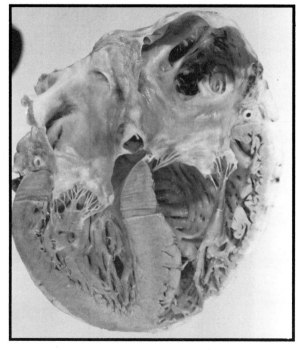

Figure 2-11: Dilated Cardiomyopathy – Photograph shows 4-chamber view of idiopathic dilated cardiomyopathy. All 4 cardiac chambers are dilated, the 4 valves are normal and the coronary arteries are free of otherosclerosis. Note the thrombus (black) in the left atrial appendage.

With increasing severity of stenosis due to a congenital bicuspid aortic valve, the systolic murmur usually becomes louder, harsher, and longer in duration (Figure 2-16). It may be well heard in the neck, supraclavicular area, and over the carotids. An aortic diastolic murmur is not an unexpected finding. It is of interest that, as part of the spectrum of findings in congenital bicuspid aortic valve, aortic regurgitation rather than stenosis may be the dominant lesion and in perhaps 5% of

cases it may be of an advanced severe degree. In some patients, *no* murmur is present, but only the ejection sound giving a clue to the correct diagnosis.

Most athletes who have a congenital bicuspid aortic valve previously undetected would have mild to moderate degrees of stenosis (Figure 2-13). Can such an athlete, asymptomatic and having a moderate degree of aortic stenosis, die suddenly? Yes; for example, I recall a 15-year-old boy personally evaluated who had only a moderate degree of aortic stenosis documented by cardiac catheterization. While playfully wrestling with a friend on a beach, he died suddenly. This also can occur, of course, in strenuous sports such as football, basketball, track, swimming, wrestling, and others. An athlete having this type of congenital bicuspid aortic valve should be spotted during the screening evaluation; the systolic murmur and the typical ejection sound are the clues.

In contrast, an innocent murmur would have no ejection sound, and would be associated with a normal electrocardiogram and chest x-ray.

Even if the athlete with a bicuspid aortic valve is asymptomatic, the electrocardiogram might show abnormalities such as left axis deviation and some increase in voltage over the left ventricle, indicating left ventricular hypertrophy. An x-ray might show some post-stenotic dilatation of the ascending aorta or other variant from normal. Such a patient would then, of course, have additional tests, including an echocardiogram and possibly cardiac catheterization to establish the diagnosis.

The congenital bicuspid aortic valve is the second most common congenital heart lesion seen in adults (the first being mitral valve prolapse).

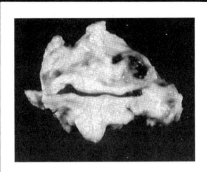
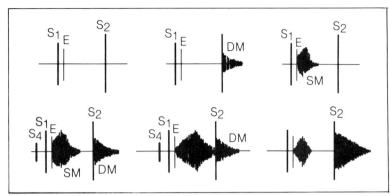

S₁ – First heart sound
S₂ – Second heart sound

Figure 2-13: Bicuspid Aortic Valve – Left, a pathologic specimen. Right, the spectrum of findings on auscultation of a congenital bicuspid aortic valve vary from only an ejection sound (E) (no murmur) to a systolic murmur (SM), or a diastolic murmur (DM), or combinations of both. The murmurs also are variable in intensity. An atrial sound (S_4) is likely to be present with more severe degrees of stenosis.

Marfan's Syndrome or Variant

A patient with a typical Marfan's syndrome is likely to be identified by his or her physical appearance: tall, thin, long arm span, long supple fingers and joints, and a high arched palate (Figures 2-17, 18, and 19). Due to eye defects such as dislocation (subluxation) of the lens, thick glasses may be worn, thereby affording another clue to the presence of this condition. I remember one patient who told me: "People say I look like Abraham Lincoln." The patient did indeed resemble Lincoln and had the classical pathological finding of aortic root pathology with aneurysmal dilatation of the ascending aorta. Associated clinical findings were an aortic diastolic murmur, systolic ejection sound, systolic murmur, and accentuation of the aortic component of the second sound – typical auscultatory findings. Rupture of an aneurysm can result in sudden death in these patients.

Not all patients with Marfan's syndrome have *all* of the typical features. Thus the physician must be alert and use extra care to look for a Marfan's variant where only some of the features are present.

Of course, Marfan's is most likely to be found in basketball or volleyball players rather than in football players. In screening athletes, the typical physical appearance, even in the absence of diagnostic physical and auscultatory findings, should prompt one to order additional laboratory tests.

Marfan's patients can have mitral rather than aortic valve involvement as the predominant lesion. They may have varying degrees of mitral valve regurgitation, the etiology of which may be related to mitral valve prolapse.

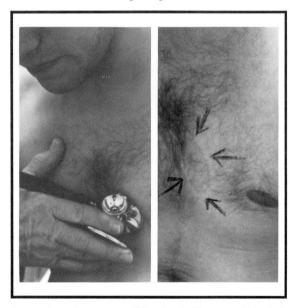

Figure 2-14: Detecting a Faint Aortic Murmur – To detect a faint grade 1-3 aortic diastolic murmur, use firm pressure with the diaphragm of the stethoscope along the mid left sternal border. The patient should be sitting, leaning forward, with breath held in deep expiration. Enough pressure is exerted to leave an imprint of the chest piece on the skin of the chest wall (right photo).

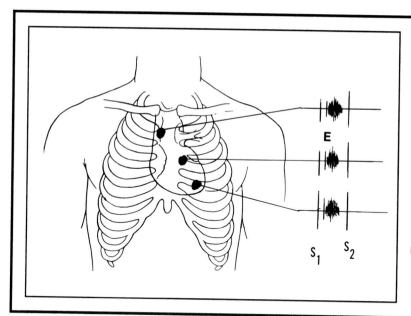

Figure 2-15: Congenital Bicuspid Aortic Valve Stenosis – Aortic events, systolic murmur, and ejection sound (E) are well heard at the apex.

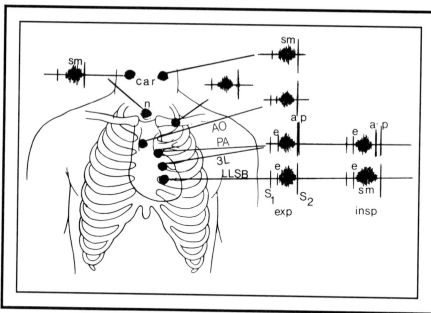

Figure 2-16: Aortic Stenosis – A 56-year-old man who has a congenital bicuspid aortic valve. The ejection sound (e) is unchanged by respiration and is the same over the pulmonic area (PA), third left sternal border (3L), and at the lower left sternal border (LLSB). Murmur and ejection sound are also well heard at the apex. The ejection sound is not eliminated with firm pressure of the stethoscope, as should be the case with an atrial gallop. Note the wide transmission of the systolic murmur (SM) over the precordium and neck areas including carotids (CAR). Normal splitting of the second sound (A-P) is heard over the pulmonic area and third left sternal border.
N = Suprasternal notch.

Osteogenesis Imperfecta (blue sclera, brittle bones)

This is a disease in the same category or "family group" as Marfan's, affecting in a similar fashion the aortic and mitral valve. Blue sclera and the tendency for bone fracture are clues to this possibility. The cardiovascular findings and workup would be similar to that of the Marfan's syndrome patient. This condition is not a problem in the usual athletic programs, particularly at the professional or college levels. It could be rarely encountered at the high school or grammar school level; therefore it is included to remind the physician of the similarity to the Marfan's patient.

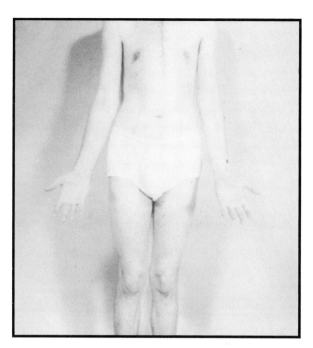

Figure 2-17: Signs of Marfan's Syndrome – Typical body habitus of Marfan's Syndrome: tall, long legs, wide arm span.

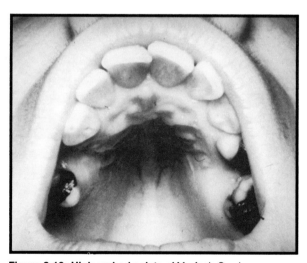

Figure 2-18: High arched palate of Marfan's Syndrome.

Mitral Valve Prolapse

This condition is discussed in detail by Dr. Jeresaty in Chapter 9. Mitral valve prolapse represents the most common congenital cardiac lesion in adults. Probably 15 million Americans have it. The great majority are asymptomatic and usually are unaware of its presence until informed by the physician or some other medical person. While it is not one of the most common causes of sudden death in athletes, it can cause such a tragedy. Probably 90% of patients with mitral valve prolapse need no treatment except education about the condition and reassurance; the other 10% have significant symptoms of chest discomfort, dizziness, palpitation due to various arrhythmias (premature beats, tachycardia, dyspnea, and anxiety). This smaller group may need treatment.

Sudden cardiac death due to ventricular fibrillation can occur in patients with mitral valve prolapse, but in the past the incidence of this catastrophic event has been exaggerated. The diagnosis of mitral valve prolapse is usually made from a spectrum of findings heard on auscultation of the heart. It is important to realize that there are many auscultatory variants of mitral valve prolapse, all of which can be diagnosed with the stethoscope (Figure 2-20). It might be manifested by a systolic click (or clicks) and varying degrees of mitral regurgitation, including acute severe mitral regurgitation with heart failure from ruptured chordae tendineae. Pulmonary edema may immediately ensue, leading to death. However, rupture of smaller or fewer chordae may result in chronic regurgitation and be tolerated without significant symptoms for months to several years. Rupture of a major chorda tendinea produces a characteristic systolic murmur that is holosystolic (pansystolic), peaking in midsystole but decreasing in the latter part of systole (Figure 2-21). Such a murmur configuration is due to significant mitral regurgitation that quickly fills the left atrium (initially of normal size), thereby rapidly building up pressure accompanying the murmur, usually peaking in midsystole; a point is reached in the latter part of systole where the atrium can no longer accommodate additional blood; thus, in the last part of systole, the pressure, along with the intensity of the murmur, decreases. The configuration of this typical murmur is shown in Figure 2-22. With chronic mitral regurgitation associated with a large dilated left atrium, the unobstructed regurgitant leak may continue to fill the atrium throughout all of systole; the murmur, therefore, is holosystolic up to the second heart sound, occasionally continuing beyond the aortic closure component of S_2.

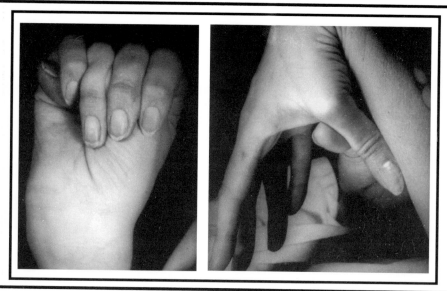

Figure 2-19A and B: More Signs of Marfan's – Note the supple joints and long fingers. Also, note the position of the patient's thumb in both photos (compare to your own hand).

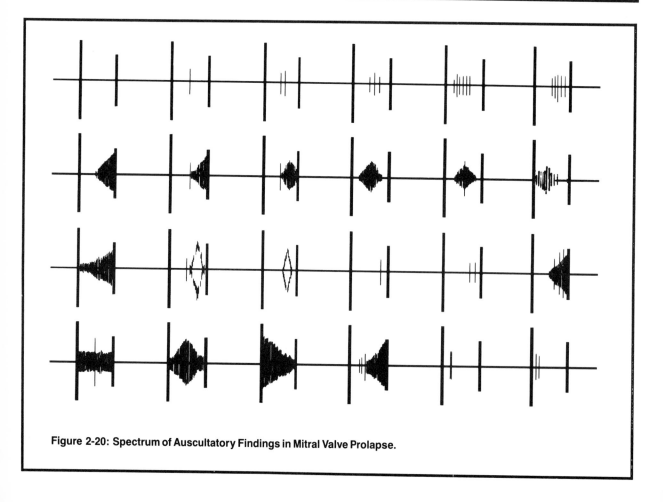

Figure 2-20: Spectrum of Auscultatory Findings in Mitral Valve Prolapse.

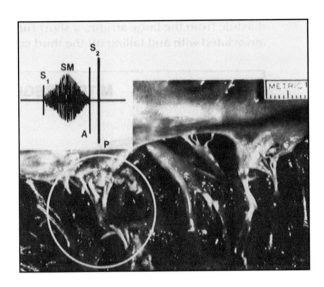

Figure 2-21: **Ruptured chorda tendineae** resulting from infective endocarditis and producing acute severe mitral regurgitation.

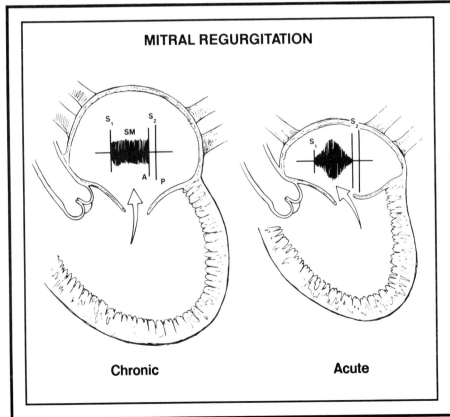

MITRAL REGURGITATION

Chronic

Acute

Figure 2-22: **Mitral Regurgitation** – During left ventricular systole, blood flows into the left atrium as well as the aorta, thereby emptying the left ventricle earlier. Therefore, the aortic valve (A_2) closes earlier, causing a wider split of the second sound (AP). Chronic regurgitation causes more left ventricular hypertrophy and left atrial enlargement, as well as more progressive regurgitation. Holosystolic murmur with chronic regurgitation extends up to A_2 and sometimes beyond. With acute regurgitation, the holosystolic murmur decreases in the latter part of systole because left atrial pressure significantly increases in a normal sized (or slightly enlarged) left atrium to about midsystole and then decreases in late systole.

Coronary Artery Disease

Although coronary artery disease is unusual in the young person or athlete it does occur. As discussed by Dr. Waller, coronary artery disease under the age of 30 is usually due to a congenital coronary anomaly. In athletes over the age of 30, it is usually due to atherosclerosis and is the most common cause of sudden death.

A careful history might suggest the presence of coronary disease. Symptoms of chest pain need careful analysis and might lead to the diagnosis of angina pectoris or an ischemic type of chest pain. Because coronary artery disease is so unexpected in a group of apparently healthy young athletes, it is easy to understand why chest discomfort might be passed off as insignificant and not of coronary origin. However, certainly a family history of coronary disease should provide a caution flag even in young people. This is especially important if death from coronary artery disease occurred at a young age on both paternal and maternal sides. Fortunately such a history is uncommon.

The physical exam might afford a clue, such as detection of an S_4 (atrial) gallop. The most common causes of this gallop are coronary artery disease, systemic hypertension, cardiomyopathy (both hypertrophic and dilated types), and myocarditis.

A systolic murmur might be present and if so would have to be evaluated. The electrocardio-gram could afford a clue, although it may be perfectly normal. Frequent ventricular arrhythmias, even though asymptomatic to the athlete, should lead to more screening procedures of that particular athlete.

Prevention of Sudden Death

Sudden cardiac death in athletes is a tragic event that continues to occur. Can it be prevented? We believe the answer is yes, at least in some, and probably in many.

It is apparent that athletes who harbor a condition which may lead to sudden death should, if at all possible, be detected and screened out of highly competitive athletic programs requiring maximal physical exertion and endurance.

The individual athlete who is denied the opportunity to perform in the activity or sport of his or her choice, is bound to be greatly disappointed. However, avoidance of a possible fatal outcome is, of course, the justification. The situation calls for compassion, empathy, special management, and wisdom on the part of everyone concerned – physicians, coaches, family, and friends.

It is especially important for the physician to take special care to avoid the term "sudden death." Instead, stress the positive side and suggest the individual funnel his (or her) physical activities to those sports and exercises more appropriate to his physical condition.

CHAPTER 3

TECHNIQUES OF CLINICAL CARDIOVASCULAR EVALUATION, WITH SPECIAL EMPHASIS ON EXAMINATION OF ATHLETES

W. Proctor Harvey, M.D.

Professor of Medicine
Division of Cardiology
Georgetown University Medical Center

Donald M. Knowlan, M.D.

Team Physician
Washington Redskins
National Football League
Professor of Medicine
Georgetown University Medical Center

Editor's Note: The next discussion will stress the necessity for a careful, detailed clinical cardiovascular evaluation, which nevertheless can be performed by a well-trained physician in his office. The principles outlined here apply to all patients, but are particularly appropriate in examining young athletes, since we usually do not expect to find pathology in these young, strong men and women. – WPH

Editor's Note: This chapter represents a classic review of general auscultatory "pearls" by a master teacher – W. Proctor Harvey. He and Donald Knowlan set forth basic principles of cardiac auscultation that, if applied to athletic evaluations, will aid in detection of cardiovascular disease and reduce the problem of sudden unexpected death. – BFW

A proper cardiovascular evaluation includes the following general principles:

1. It cannot be emphasized enough that a very careful cardiovascular examination is essential for the detection of heart disease in the athlete. The physical exam, particularly auscultation, is of prime importance. An abbreviated, cursory examination will not suffice. The physician should not be rushed. Too often, too many athletes are scheduled to be examined in a very short time. Nevertheless, with a well-trained physician who has a good understanding of cardiac auscultation, a thorough screening evaluation can be accomplished in a reasonably short time.

2. An examining table should be used, and the patient should be properly attired for the examination. One should not attempt to examine an athlete whose clothing has not been removed down to the underwear. A sheet or "johnny" gown can prevent unnecessary exposure.

3. A quiet area is needed for proper auscultation. Also a good stethoscope – one that is able to detect the faintest low frequency diastolic rumble or gallop and, at the other end of the scale, high frequency murmurs such as the faintest grade 1 or 2 early blowing aortic diastolic murmur.

4. The patient should be examined in various positions – supine, turned to the left lateral position (listening with the bell of the stethoscope over the point of maximal impulse of the left ventricle), sitting, standing, and squatting. Also be sure to listen with the stethoscope over the neck areas, back, and abdomen.

5. Remember that *we find what we look for* – but we must *know what we are looking for*. If we know the most common causes of sudden death and their auscultatory clues, most athletes with suspicious findings can be detected on screening examination. This group can then be referred for more definitive testing.

A complete cardiovascular evaluation of an athlete, as with all patients, must start with the basics – The five finger approach (Figure 3-1):

1. A careful, detailed history

2. A thorough physical examination, especially auscultation

3. An electrocardiogram
4. A chest x-ray
5. Other appropriate tests such as an echocardiogram or exercise treadmill testing.

For the initial screening examination, the history and physical examination are most essential; the electrocardiogram, chest x-ray, and additional, more sophisticated tests are not usually utilized or necessary unless something in the history or physical raises suspicion of a possible problem. In such cases, additional information will be required and the other aspects (fingers) of the cardiovascular evaluation can be utilized.

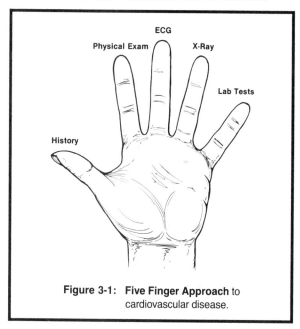

Figure 3-1: Five Finger Approach to cardiovascular disease.

History

A careful, detailed history might elicit clues to symptoms suggesting cardiovascular disease: chest discomfort, unusual dyspnea, fatigue, effort intolerance, dizziness, palpations. It is very unlikely that the athlete to be examined has any type of serious illness or overt symptoms and signs of heart disease. The great majority have no complaints. The final analysis of the history should be the responsibility of the examining physician.

Chest Discomfort

A history of chest discomfort or pain in a trained athlete is unusual, and warrants careful, detailed analysis rather than assuming it is insig-

nificant and noncoronary in origin. Congenital as well as acquired causes of coronary artery disease can occur in young people.

If there is a family history of coronary disease, this provides a caution flag. It is especially important if present in both the maternal and paternal sides of the family and/or if there is a family history of death from coronary artery disease occurring at a young age (premature coronary disease). Any patient, including an athlete, with such a history and who complains of chest discomfort, should have a careful review of the electrocardiogram which may reveal some abnormalities, even in a young patient. If there is any question as to the presence of coronary disease, additional screening studies such as an echocardiogram, exercise treadmill, thallium exercise treadmill, and even coronary angiography may be indicated.

Chest discomfort in an athlete also should alert the physician to the possibility of hypertrophic cardiomyopathy, the leading cause of sudden death in athletes less than 30 years of age. Many patients with hypertrophic cardiomyopathy have no symptoms. However, if symptoms are present, chest discomfort is the most common. It often simulates the type of pain seen in coronary ischemic disease. Some complain of dizziness, while others have both chest discomfort and dizziness.

Murmurs

If a history of a murmur is elicited, it is probable the athlete has previously been told that it is of no significance. However, with such a history, the physician is alerted to look for a murmur, and if found, to determine for himself whether it is significant or innocent. To be emphasized: innocent murmurs are very common, particularly in young people, children, and athletes. It is very important that a physician who screens athletes for participation in sports be able to differentiate innocent from significant murmurs. This can usually be readily accomplished during the office or screening evaluation and without specialized laboratory procedures such as the Doppler echocardiogram.

• **Auscultatory Findings of Mitral Valve Prolapse** (Clicks, Murmurs, Whoops, or Honks) – Proper precordial examination for these findings includes listening to the patient in various positions: lying supine, then with the patient turned to the left lateral position and listening over the point of maximal impulse of the left ventricle, sitting, standing, and squatting. Auscultation is the best way of diagnosing prolapse. Echocardiography is, of course, very useful, but not needed in the great majority of patients, including athletes, to make the diagnosis. If prolapse *is* present, the echocardiogram is useful in some patients to determine the thickness of the mitral valve, its movement characteristics, regurgitation and annulus size; such information can be of help in determining the likelihood of complications of mitral valve prolapse.

The physician who examines and screens athletes should be familiar with the many variants of mitral valve prolapse (Figure 3-2). This can be accomplished by attending postgraduate courses stressing clinical auscultation and also by listening to high fidelity recordings of actual patients who have these variants of mitral valve prolapse. The physician can become very accurate in diagnosis by these methods and develop the expertise needed for office detection of this condition.*

To repeat: *The diagnosis of mitral valve prolapse can be accurately made in the great majority of patients, including athletes, with office evaluation. Routine echocardiography is not absolutely indicated but can be useful in documentation.*

Shortness of Breath and Fatigue

It is rare that recurring shortness of breath or extreme fatigue, other than that with strenuous exertion, is present in the athlete. These symptoms, therefore, would be immediate clues to the presence of cardiac decompensation.

Arrhythmias and Heart Block

Various arrhythmias are known to be present in athletes, from premature beats and tachycardias to first-, second-, or third-degree heart block. Most are of no significance and sophisticated laboratory tests are usually not necessary, but should, of course, be done if there is any doubt in the examining physician's mind.

If a person gives a history of palpitations, one can often gain valuable information as to the exact nature of the palpitation by moving one's hand over one's chest, simulating the arrhythmia (Figure 3-3). This can help the patient more accurately describe the rhythm. For instance, palpitation to one person might mean only an increase of the normal heart rate; to another, premature beats or

*See "Clinical Auscultation of the Cardiovascular System." High fidelity recordings of more than 450 actual patients with companion texts, by W. Proctor Harvey MD and David C. Canfield. Available from Laennec Publishing, 7 Penn Avenue, Newton, NJ 07860.

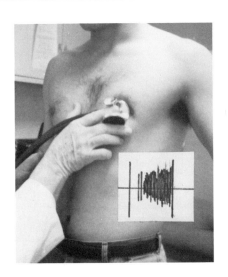 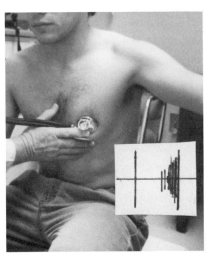

Figure 3-2: Effect of the Squatting Maneuver – The squatting maneuver can be very helpful in diagnosing mitral valve prolapse. On squatting, clicks move toward the second sound and the systolic murmur may get longer. On standing, the clicks move toward the first heart sound and the systolic murmur becomes shorter and also moves toward the first sound. Such changes are strong evidence of mitral valve prolapse.

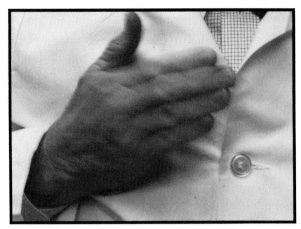

Figure 3-3: Simulation – The physician's hand movements can simulate and illustrate various arrhythmias. The hand is moving up and down rapidly to indicate a tachycardia.

atrial fibrillation; and to still another, it would represent paroxysmal atrial tachycardia, rapid atrial fibrillation, or ventricular tachycardia.

• **A Case in Point** – Recently one of us (WPH) had the opportunity to evaluate a senior on a college swim team who had a history of recurrent tachycardia characterized by sudden onset and just as sudden cessation of a rapid but regular rhythm of 250 beats a minute. Fortunately, the tachycardia never occurred during a competitive swim meet, but did occur during practice sessions of more strenuous and prolonged effort. In fact, his last episode took place while he was playing a strenuous game of handball.

His diagnosis, paroxysmal atrial tachycardia, was readily suggested by the history (sudden onset and just as sudden cessation of a rapid regular tachycardia). The 250 beats per minute were documented. It was fortunate that his episodes of paroxysmal atrial tachycardia never lasted more than one or two minutes. The rhythm was regular and rapid, which could be simulated by wagging one's hand rapidly and regularly over the mid-precordium (readily identified by the patient).

This swimmer's normal heart rate was the typical slow rate of sinus bradycardia so often found in healthy athletes. He also had a typical faint, short, innocent systolic murmur occurring in midsystole and heard over his precordium in several areas but best heard over the aortic area (Figure 3-4).

What advice and treatment would you give to this young man?

Since competitive swimming was so important to him and his episodes of paroxysmal atrial tachycardia were short in duration, did not occur in actual competitive races, and produced no symptoms except for the awareness of a fast heart beat, no medication was necessary. He was given medical clearance to continue as a member of his college swim team. He was told that if longer periods of tachycardia occurred or he devloped other symptoms, then he should be re-evaluated. He was also advised that when the tachycardia took place to report to a medical facility where his rhythm could be documented and treatment given if necessary.

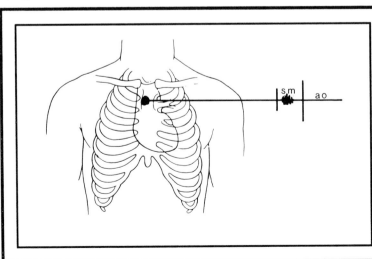

Figure 3-4: The Swimmer's Murmur: – This patient was a 20-year-old man, a member of a college varsity swimming team. He had sinus bradycardia and an innocent systolic murmur (SM) heard from the aortic area (AO) to the apex.

Dizziness or Syncope

A history of dizziness, near syncope, or syncope immediately suggests the possibility of arrhythmia which can occur in the absence of other cardiac pathology, or be a sign of heart conditions such as aortic stenosis, hypertrophic cardiomyopathy, and myocarditis.

A history of rheumatic fever or symptoms of same should be specifically asked for; fortunately today, in most sections of the United States, the incidence of rheumatic heart disease has declined greatly and it would be a very uncommon cause of a murmur. A "cardiac pearl" – if there is a history of rheumatic fever, there is a 50% chance of having a rheumatic heart; another "pearl" – only one-half of patients having rheumatic mitral stenosis have a history of rheumatic fever. (A cardiac pearl is a fact or finding that either makes the diagnosis or provides a clue that leads to the diagnosis. It is unchanged by time. It will be just as good 25 years from now as it is today).

The Physical Examination

Proper evaluation of patients includes auscultation in various positions: lying flat, turned to the left lateral position and listening over the point of maximal impulse, sitting, standing, and squatting.

Innocent Murmurs

A murmur is a frequent finding in athletes. For example, most professional football players, perhaps more than 90%, will be found to have an innocent precordial systolic murmur if it is carefully searched for.

The following are characteristics of innocent precordial murmurs that may be found in any patient, including athletes (Figure 3-5):

1. The murmur is short, occurring in early to midsystole. It is not holosystolic.

2. The murmur is faint – Grade 1 to Grade 3 on a scale of 1 to 6. (A Grade 1 systolic murmur is not heard immediately when the stethoscope is placed over the chest. It takes an adjustment of the stethoscope, making sure the ear tips fit well and comfortably into the ear canals, for a Grade 1 murmur to be heard. Grade 2 is the faintest murmur that can be heard immediately on listening with the stethoscope. Grade 6 is the loudest murmur and may even be heard before the stethoscope actually touches the chest. If we can "see daylight" between the stethoscope and the chest wall and still hear a systolic murmur, it is Grade 6. Grade 5 is the next in intensity to Grade 6, but cannot be heard unless the stethoscope is actually touching the chest. A Grade 3 murmur is easily heard, although it is not loud. A Grade 4 murmur is loud and may be associated with a palpable thrill, as may Grades 5 and 6).

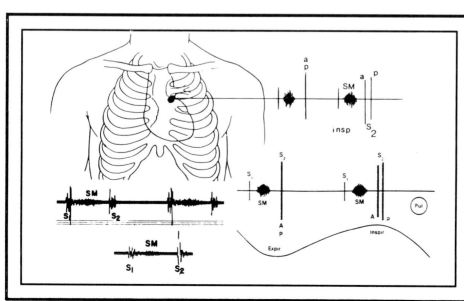

Figure 3-5: Innocent Murmurs – A composite of four patients with innocent murmurs (SM). The murmur is short in duration and occurs in early to mid-systole. Note normal splitting of the second sound (S₂, A-P), single with expiration (expir) and widening with inspiration (insp), shown in top and lower left panels.

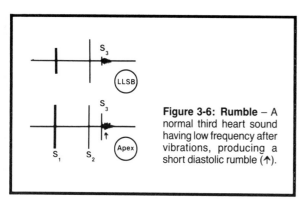

Figure 3-6: Rumble – A normal third heart sound having low frequency after vibrations, producing a short diastolic rumble (↑).

3. The murmur is not associated with an ejection sound or "fixed" wide splitting of the second heart sound.

4. Diastolic murmurs are usually significant murmurs, not innocent. An exception: Occasionally a normal third heart sound has duration, with after-vibrations producing a short rumble murmur heard on auscultation. (Figure 3-6).

Another innocent murmur is the venous hum (Figure 3-7), a continuous murmur with both systolic and diastolic components. It is a very common finding in many athletes; it was detected in more than 90% of the professional football players recently examined by one of the editors of this book (WPH). A venous hum is a continuous murmur that may have a low frequency, a very high frequency, or both. It is best heard over the supraclavicular fossa with the patient's head turned to the opposite direction and the neck on a "stretch"

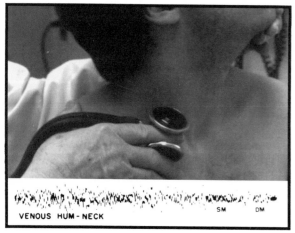

VENOUS HUM - NECK

Figure 3-7: Venous Hum – A venous hum can best be heard by listening with the bell of the stethoscope over the right supraclavicular fossa with the head turned to the opposite direction and "on a stretch."

(Figure 3-7). With professional football players, the venous hum often can be heard even before the head is turned and the neck stretched. We theorize that this might be due to the fact that these athletes have large muscular necks (Figure 3-8) as a result of their weight lifting program. These large neck muscles alter jugular vein position, causing turbulence similar to what happens when the neck is put on a stretch. The venous hum can be eliminated by very gentle pressure with the palpating finger on the vein, or moving the head back to the forward position.

Significant Murmurs

In contrast to innocent murmurs, significant systolic murmurs are holosystolic (or pansystolic) (Figure 3-9). Such a murmur immediately suggests three possible conditions:
- Mitral regurgitation
- Tricuspid regurgitation
- Ventricular septal defect (Figure 3-9)

An innocent systolic murmur may at first simulate an atrial septal defect, mild pulmonic stenosis, idiopathic dilation of the pulmonary artery, or aortic stenosis caused by a bicuspid aortic valve.

The differences are that an ejection sound is usually present with pulmonic stenosis, idiopathic dilatation of the pulmonary artery, and congenital bicuspid aortic valve stenosis. With atrial septic defect, there is a so-called wide "fixed" splitting of the second heart sound. Thus, by associated findings present on cardiac exam, a significant murmur can be distinguished from an innocent murmur.

The Heart Rate in a Trained Athlete

In contrast to non-athletes, the heart rate in a trained athlete is slower, often with normal sinus bradycardia, with rates in the 50s and 60s. This is a consistent and expected finding. This slow heart rate may be a contributing factor to the slightly higher normal systolic blood pressure seen in some athletes. It relates to a forceful contraction during systole; it also may be a factor in causing an innocent murmur.

Heart Sounds: The First Heart Sound

As a rule, the first heart sound is normal in intensity in all patients, including athletes. The

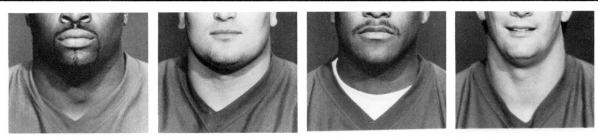

Figure 3-8: Football Players – Their large muscular necks may make a venous hum more easily heard.

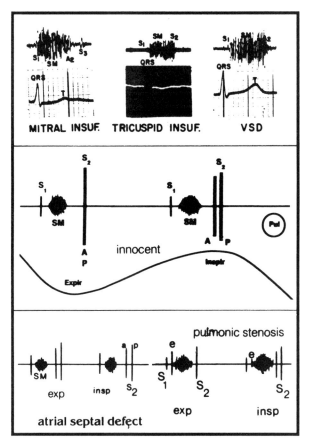

Figure 3-9: Significant Murmurs – Upper panel: Three causes of holosystolic murmurs [mitral insufficiency, tricuspid insufficiency, and ventricular septal defect (VSD)]. Middle panel: An innocent systolic murmur (SM) in early to mid-systole. Note normal splitting of the second sound, single with expiration (expir), and split (S_2, A-P) with inspiration (inspir). Lower Left: With atrial septal defect, the second sound remains wider split with both expiration (expir) and inspiration (inspir). Lower Right: Pulmonic stenosis: Note that the ejection sound (e) on expiration becomes fainter with inspiration.

length of the P-R interval on the electrocardiogram is related to the intensity of the first heart sound. If there is a *short* P-R interval (eg, 0.14 or 0.15 seconds), the first heart sound is accentuated (Figure 3-10). If the P-R interval is prolonged (eg, 0.19 to 0.22 seconds or longer), the first sound is faint. Some athletes have a longer P-R interval (first degree heart block), which may be of no clinical significance and may be related to increased vagal tone; at times, second and third degree heart block has been found in athletes – (see Chapter 4 for more detailed discussion).

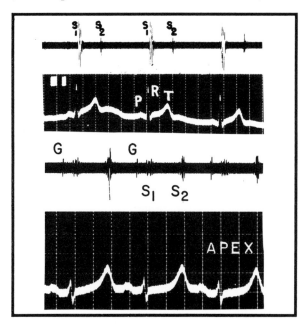

Figure 3-10: First Heart Sounds – Upper panel: Note loud first heart sound (S_1) with a short P-R interval (0.15 seconds). Lower panel: The first sound is faint, with a longer P-R interval (0.20 seconds). An atrial (S_4) sound (G) is also present.

• Splitting of the First Heart Sound – Splitting of the first heart sound is a normal occurrence in all people and is produced by closure of the mitral and tricuspid valves (Figure 3-11). The mitral closure (M-1) occurs before the tricuspid closure (T-1). In athletes, the splitting is often wider than usually seen in normal non-athletes. This is possibly due to the normal slower heart rate associated with increased vagal tone, and an increase in the volume of blood that might be ejected with each systolic contraction.

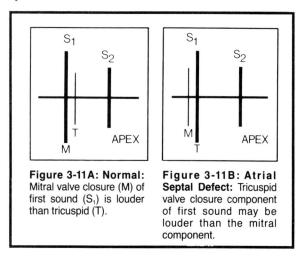

Figure 3-11A: Normal: Mitral valve closure (M) of first sound (S₁) is louder than tricuspid (T).

Figure 3-11B: Atrial Septal Defect: Tricuspid valve closure component of first sound may be louder than the mitral component.

The Second Heart Sound

Following the usual sequence where left-sided events of the heart occur before the right, the aortic valve closure of the second sound (A-2) occurs normally before the pulmonic valve closure (P-2). The second sound is single or closely split with expiration and becomes wider with inspiration (Figure 3-12). However, the second heart sound may not become single in trained athletes; and many have a wider split of the second heart sound on expiration, with further widening on inspiration. This can simulate right bundle branch block, and if an innocent pulmonic systolic murmur is present (also a frequent finding in athletes), it may sound like atrial septal defect. A simple way to distinguish these conditions and make the diagnosis is to listen to the patient in both the sitting and standing positions; if the second heart sound becomes single or closely split on expiration, widening promptly with inspiration, it practically rules out right bundle branch block and/or atrial septal defect (Figure 3-12).

The Normal Third Heart Sound

A third heart sound is an expected finding in youth. Some years ago, the Division of Cardiology at Georgetown examined a large number of school children, the average age being approximately 10 to 12 years. One of us (WPH) personally examined about 100 of these children. A normal physiological third heart sound was detected in almost all of them (Figure 3-13). A normal venous hum was also heard in 100% of these children; an innocent systolic murmur in approximately 65%; a carotid bruit (short systolic murmur) in approximately one third, and a supraclavicular murmur in approximately one third.

The normal physiologic third heart sound in youth is usually best heard with the patient turned to the left lateral position, listening with the bell of the stethoscope held lightly, barely making an air seal over the point of maximal impulse over the left ventricle (Figure 3-14). The normal third heart sound usually disappears in men in their 20s and in women in their 30s, although those continuing in athletic endeavors in later years may retain their normal third sounds. It may be brought out by turning the patient to the left lateral position and listening over the point of maximal impulse. A prominent third sound may then be easily detected. It may, however, become faint or disappear after a few beats. Other maneuvers, such as having the patient cough several times or take a series of rapid deep breaths several times, might also bring out the third sound. (This same technique can be used to uncover the telltale diagnostic rumble of mitral stenosis: Turn the patient to the left lateral position, use the bell of the stethoscope barely making an air seal with the skin of the chest wall, and listen over the point of maximum impulse of the left ventricle).

Elevation of the legs (Figure 3-13) also may bring out the third heart sound in some patients, though this maneuver is usually not necessary. Speeding up the ventricular rate by a brief exercise of sit-ups or a short run-in-place also has been helpful in bringing out the third sound.

At times, low frequency vibrations producing a rumble murmur of short duration can follow the normal third heart sound (Figure 3-6). Occasionally, these normal findings have been mistaken for the opening snap and short rumble of mitral stenosis. This is more likely to happen if the first

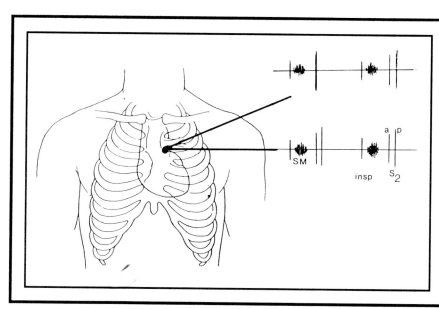

Figure 3-12: Second Sound –
Lower panel: The athlete is lying on his back. Note second sound (S_2, A-P) is more widely split with both inspiration (insp) and expiration. Upper panel: The athlete is standing. The second sound is single with expiration.

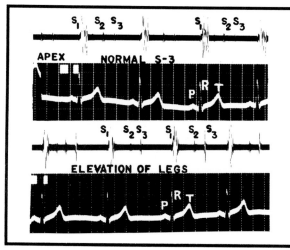

Figure 3-13: **Normal Third Heart Sound** – A patient with a normal physiological third heart sound (S_3, upper panel), which became louder when his legs were elevated (lower panel).

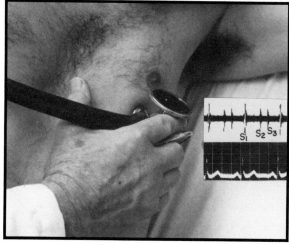

Figure 3-14: **Optimal Detection of a Third Heart Sound** – The patient is turned to the left lateral position. Listen with the bell of the stethoscope held lightly over the point of maximal impulse of the left ventricle. A normal third heart sound (S_3) can become audible or louder in this position.

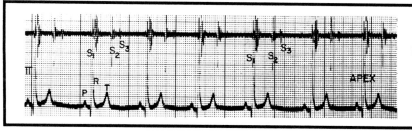

Figure 3-15: Misinterpretation – Note loud first sound (S_1), short P-R interval, and normal third sound (S_3), which was misinterpreted as an opening snap of mitral stenosis.

heart sound is accentuated due to a short P-R interval on the electrocardiogram (Figure 3-15).

The normal third sound is not a surprise finding in swimmers, runners, basketball and baseball players, serious tennis players, and other athletes. An interesting exception is the professional football player, whose third sound is usually *not* heard. This will be discussed later in this chapter.

The term "athlete's heart" is misleading, since there is no specific type of heart disease related to the athlete. In some, the heart may be somewhat enlarged with a degree of hypertrophy of the left and/or right ventricle (Figure 3-16). In the trained athlete these features may be related to physical conditioning, vagal tone, and muscle development. Further discussion of the "athlete's heart" compared to significant, often lethal, hypertrophic cardiomyopathy is found in Chapter 5.

SPECIAL SECTION

Auscultatory Findings in National Football League Players

We have had the unusual opportunity to evaluate and examine approximately 90 professional football players – rookies as well as the regular players. The majority were 22 to 30 years old, tall but of stocky build, weighing between 180 to over 300 pounds. A few, particularly running backs and wide receivers, were of lesser height, 5 feet 8 inches to 5 feet 10 inches, and weighed about 170 to 190 pounds, but most were huge, weighing between 200 and 300 pounds and 6 feet or more in height.

In our careful history and physical examination, we also looked for detailed findings on auscultation of the cardiovascular system. High fidelity tape recordings also were made in various positions: sitting, standing, and lying flat. We listened at the left sternal border, apex, third left sternal border, pulmonic area, and aortic area. With the patient turned to the left lateral position and using the bell of the stethoscope held lightly against the chest wall, we listened at the point of maximum impulse of the left ventricle. The neck areas were also examined and recorded.

Heart Rates

Most ventricular rates were slower than the av-

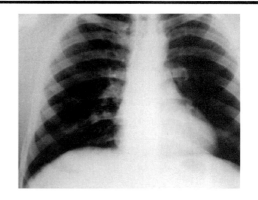
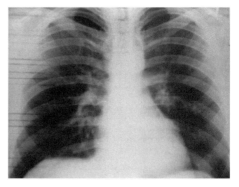
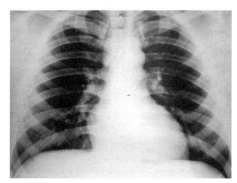

Figure 3-16: Large Hearts – These x-rays of professional football players show that they have large heart silhouettes.

erage person's, frequently in the 50s and 60s due to their conditioning and increased vagal tone.

Rhythm

The rhythm was regular sinus, though some had normal sinus arrhythmia. Premature beats were not common, but occasionally occurred.

The First Heart Sound

The football players had wider splitting of the first heart sound (mitral and tricuspid valve component closures) than the average person. This, however, is a perfectly normal finding (Figure 3-17).

The Second Heart Sound

Wider splitting of the second heart sound was a frequent finding in the football players. Even with expiration, the second heart sound was usually split, not becoming single with expiration. This finding, together with an innocent murmur heard over the pulmonic area, and/or third left sternal border would lead to the impression of possible atrial septal defect. However, on sitting or standing, the second heart sound became single or closely split, indicating the second heart sound splitting was normal (Figure 3-18).

The Third Heart Sound

Although one of us (WPH) had been told that normal third heart sounds are common in these professional football players, careful examination of them failed to reveal a third heart sound (except

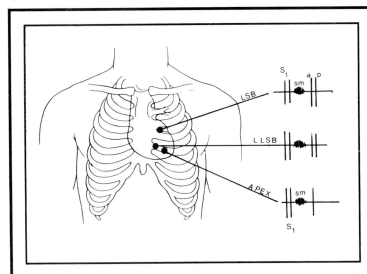

Figure 3-17: Football Player – All-Pro NFL football player lying supine. Note wide split of first sound (S$_1$), innocent systolic murmur (SM), and wide split of S$_2$ (A-P), which did not become single on expiration. However, it did become single on expiration in the sitting position.

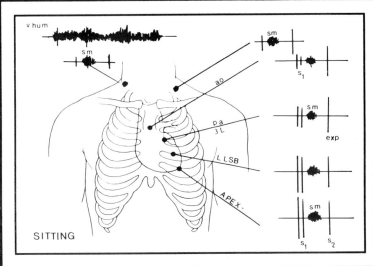

Figure 3-18: Sitting – Same patient as Figure 3-17- sitting. S$_2$ becomes single with expiration (exp). Note innocent systolic murmur (SM) heard from the apex to the aortic area. On auscultation of the neck, note the short innocent systolic murmur (SM) at the left supraclavicular fossa. There is also a venous hum plus a short innocent systolic murmur at the right supraclavicular fossa.

in one); nor were they recorded using high fidelity techniques. The fact that the third heart sound was not detected was unexpected, since in other athletes it is a frequent finding. Absence of the third sound may be due to the thick chest muscular development and increased weight of these players, which provides an insulating effect between the heart and the stethoscope. It is a known fact that obesity, emphysema, and increased anterior/posterior diameter of the chest wall may make auscultation of the heart sounds and murmurs more difficult to hear. The thin chest wall of growing children and the poor muscle development of some adults enables one to more easily hear heart sounds and murmurs.

Systolic Murmur

An innocent systolic murmur was present in more than 90% of the professional football players. The murmur was typical of the innocent type: Grade 1-3 in intensity, occurring in the early to mid-part of systole. It was heard over various areas of the precordium, most commonly the lower left sternal border, apex, pulmonic area, and aortic area (Figure 3-18). A clinical point often not well appreciated is the fact that the innocent murmur, also a normal finding in children, youths, pregnant women, and others, is usually not limited to one specific area such as the pulmonic area. It may be heard over various areas of the precordium, if specifically searched for.

The professional football players had typical innocent murmurs. None were of the Still's type (about 90 years ago, George Frederic Still of London described the vibratory innocent murmur: "Its characteristic feature is a twanging sound, very like that made by twanging a piece of tense string"). None had holosystolic murmurs or those characteristic of mitral valve prolapse. Athletes not having hyperdevelopment of the chest muscles like the football player would be expected to have the normal third sound readily detected.

Venous Hum

More than 90% of the professional football players had a venous hum, which usually was heard in the supraclavicular fossa of the neck even without the head turned to the opposite direction and placed on a "stretch." To explain this, perhaps the thick muscular development of the neck (Figure 3-8) (again related to the weight lifting training program) altered the position of the jugular vein so that the blood flow created turbulence analogous to turning the head on a stretch. The venous hum is a benign finding.

Systolic Murmur of the Carotid Arteries in the Neck

Another common finding in football players was the presence of a normal systolic murmur, Grade 1-3, heard over the supraclavicular and carotid areas. These are also innocent murmurs (bruits) (Figures 3-17 and 18).

CHAPTER 4

THE ELECTROCARDIOGRAM IN THE ATHLETE

Donald M. Knowlan, MD

Team Physician
Washington Redskins
National Football League

Professor of Medicine
Georgetown University Medical Center

Athletes may exhibit electrocardiographic changes that might be considered abnormal in the untrained person. Since the first description of the electrocardiogram in athletes in 1929[1] many reports have been published on the subject.[2-42] Most authors agree that the following electrocardiographic changes are common and usually "normal" in athletes:

• Sinus bradycardia
• Incomplete right bundle branch block
• Rightward QRS axis
• Prominent P waves in lead II
• Ventricular hypertrophy
• Minor ST segment depression or elevation
• Altered T waves

Since the resting electrocardiogram is a common screening test in the evaluation of athletes, this chapter will focus on the interpretation of expected and unexpected changes one might observe.

Electrocardiographic changes observed in the "athletic heart syndrome," are actually a spectrum of findings from "normal" to "abnormal." Changes characteristic of dynamic, isotonic, aerobic, volume-overload sports such as distance running or basketball differ from those characteristic of isometric, anaerobic, pressure-overload sports such as wrestling or weightlifting. The electrocardiogram of an individual athlete, however, may reflect both types of exercise, since swimmers and distance runners may also lift weights, and wrestlers and football players may run for aerobic balance.

Sinus Node

Sinus Bradycardia

Of all the electrocardiographic findings in the athlete, bradycardia is the most common. In general, as the intensity of training increases, the slower the baseline heart rate becomes. There is an inverse correlation between the exercise capacity and the resting heart rate.

• Sinus bradycardia was found in about 25% of a large population of Air Force personnel.[2]
• In another study,[3] sinus bradycardia (<50 beats/min) was found in 65% of athletes, and their heart rates fell below 40 during sleep.
• A third study compared 20 trained athletes with similar but untrained controls using ambulatory electrocardiographic monitoring. The results showed a significantly lower heart rate ($p<0.01$) in the athletes both during sleep and during other activities.[4]
• In 20 long-distance runners,[5] heart rates were 10 beats/minute slower when compared with 50 untrained professional students of similar age,[6] using 24-hour Holter monitoring during normal activity. Average heart rates during sleep in the runners ranged from 31 to 43 beats/minute (average 36 ± 3)[5] compared to 33 to 55 (average 43 ± 5) in the untrained subjects.[6]
• Chapman[7] reported a 16-year-old well-trained wrestler (who experienced occasional lightheadedness) with a resting sinus rate of 25 beats/minute. During exercise he increased his sinus rate to 146 beats/minute.

The degree of bradycardia is most profound in athletes engaged in sports requiring the greatest endurance. One study[8] found average heart rates of 56 beats/minute in 74 runners, 57 beats/minute in 53 cyclists, 62 per minute in 66 swimmers, and 66 beats/minute in 51 wrestlers. At given exercise loads, athletes have lower heart rates than untrained subjects, and the exercise heart rate returns to resting levels more rapidly in trained individuals.[9]

Sinus Arrhythmias

Sinus arrhythmias frequently are present in athletes at rest but usually disappear with exercise.[8, 10-12] One group[13] found sinus arrhythmias in 77% of well conditioned football players. Others[5] found no significant difference in the incidence of sinus arrhythmias in long-distance runners (100%) compared to the normal population (86%).

Editor's Note: Sinus arrhythmia is very common in young people and is an expected normal finding. One would predict that, the younger the athlete, the more likely the presence of sinus arrhythmia. The simple expedient to eliminate this normal type of arrhythmia (the heart rate speeding up and then slowing down) is to have the patient hold his breath. – WPH

Sinus Pause

Researchers[2] have found significantly longer sinus pauses in long-distance runners both while awake (1.35 to 2.55 seconds) and while asleep (1.6 to 2.8 seconds) compared to untrained controls. Another group[14] found that 13 of 35 athletes had sinus pauses greater than 2.0 seconds, whereas only two controls exceeded 2.0 seconds. In another series,[3] 7 out of 37 top athletes had sinus pauses greater than 2.6 seconds during 24-hour Holter monitoring; 51% had pauses of at least 2 seconds.

AV Node

First degree, second degree (Mobitz Type I and Mobitz Type II) and, rarely, third degree or complete heart block have been reported as benign findings in highly trained athletes.

First Degree Block

One group of researchers[14] found first degree heart block in 37% of athletes, compared to 14% of controls. Others[4] found first degree heart block in

3 of 20 male athletes aged 14 to 16 years, compared to only 1 of 20 nonathletic controls. Hiss and Lamb's review[2] of 122,000 electrocardiograms from normal males found that 6.5/1000 (<1%) had first degree AV block (PR>0.20 sec) (Table 4-1).

Editor's Note: A heart block can be accurately detected on auscultation by the presence of a faint first sound and, at times, an atrial sound (Sx) in presystole. – WPH

Editor's Note: If the P-R interval is short, the first sound will be loud. – WPH

Second Degree Block

Second degree AV block may be a sign of organic heart disease, but it is not uncommon as a normal variant in the athlete. Hiss and Lamb[2] found the incidence of Wenckebach AV block (Mobitz I) to be about 0.003%. Others[15] reported a marathon runner who had Wenckebach AV block before, but not after a 100-yard dash. Grimby and Saltin[16, 17] described two middle-aged athletes with Wenckebach periods on the resting ECG which disappeared during exercise. Cullen and Collin[18] observed two men who began long-distance running for the first time at ages 35 and 41, and who developed Wenckebach AV block at rest, which disappeared after exercise. In one man, the AV block was present only during periods of training and disappeared between such periods.

A study comparing athletes to controls[14] found second degree AV block in 8 (23%) of the athletes and 2 (5.7%) of the controls. In another report,[3] 13% had second degree AV block. In a study of 20 athletes,[4] second degree AV block was found in three of them, but in only one untrained control. The authors concluded that various forms of vagally-mediated heart block are seen more commonly in athletes than in nonathletes.

Zeppili and associates[19] studied ten male athletes with second degree Wenckebach block. They used various forms of sympathetic stimulation including exercise, atropine, and isuprel infusion, Valsalva, hyperventilation, and position changes. The results were variable with carotid sinus pres-

Table 4-1
Electrocardiographic Findings in 122,043 Individuals

	Percent	Number
First Degree Heart Block	0.65	802
Second Degree Heart Block	—	4
Wenckebach Phenomenon	—	4
Right Bundle Branch Block	0.2	231
Intraventricular Conduction Defect	0.4	505
Left Bundle Branch Block	—	17
Right Ventricular Hypertrophy	—	1
Left Ventricular Hypertrophy	—	5
Atrial Premature Beats	0.4	534
Ventricular Premature Beats	0.8	952
Supraventricular Tachycardia	—	29
Ventricular Tachycardia	—	6
W.P.W.	0.2	187
Non-Specific T Wave Changes	1.0	1405
Inverted T Waves	—	56

From Roland G. Hiss & Lawrence E. Lamb
Circulation 25:947-961, 1962

sure, Valsalva, and hyperventilation. The studies following insuprel infusion and exercise with increased sinus rates resulted in normalization of AV conduction in 9 of 10 individuals (3 of whom had mitral valve prolapse). The conduction changes were felt to be physiological and thus benign.

Atrioventricular conduction changes in athletes are felt to be related to the intensity and length of training. AV conduction changes were observed in a group that had trained five times per week for three years.[4]

These changes appear to reverse after training is reduced or discontinued. Reversal of electrocardiographic changes (including first and second degree heart block) was observed among 95% of 102 Japanese Olympic athletes four years after they reduced the intensity of training. In another case,[21] a 38-year-old hospital administrator and marathoner had a high degree of Mobitz Type II block, with 2-second pauses and a 6-second pause during sleep, but had a normal coronary angiogram. Five years after decreasing her running to 2 to 5 miles per day, the rhythm had returned to sinus and the AV block disappeared. ST segment elevation also returned to normal.

A report on a five-year followup of 122 intensely active middle-aged cross country skiers[22] concluded that the electrocardiographic changes of the "athletic heart," including first and second degree heart block, are secondary to intense training and not to underlying coronary artery disease.

Editor's Note: Second degree heart block can also be diagnosed by auscultation. A prominent extra sound may be heard when the non-conducted atrial excitation with 2:1 block produces an atrial sound sometimes coinciding with the third sound of the rapid filling phase in ventricular diastole, thereby producing a constant sound in diastole. – WPH

Complete Heart Block

Complete heart block is exceedingly rare in athletes.[23, 24] In a review of 15,000 ECG tracings at a Sports Institute,[24] only one case of congenital heart block was found. This individual increased his ventricular rate to 155 with treadmill exercise, indicating that ventricular acceleration with exercise was unaffected by the heart block. When the heart block failed to disappear after vigorous (maximum) exercise, it was felt to represent either congenital or organic complete heart block.

The same researchers[24] reviewed previous cases of complete heart block in athletes. In 25% to 50% of the cases, there was evidence of an additional cardiac defect. Those individuals with congenital complete heart block but without identified structural cardiac defects usually lead normal lives. If these individuals are without a history of Stokes-Adams attacks and are free of high-grade ectopy at rest and exercise, they can perform strenuous work and participate in sports.[24]

Editor's Note: I would advise an athlete with complete heart block not to participate in competitive sports or any strenuous physical activities. – WPH

Author's Note: I would disagree. This should be individualized, based on other findings. If the above general rule was followed, one of the greatest athletes in sports history would never have played. – DWK

A retrospective study[25] of 160 consecutive patients with symptomatic arrhythmias under age 50 found 14 with unexplained strokes, nine of whom had slow rates. Five of these nine were athletes. All the strokes were typical of cerebral emboli, and the athletes had evidence of valvular heart disease. In the overall group, 12 active athletes were followed up because of syncope or dizzy spells. These individuals became symptom-free after reducing their athletic activity. The authors of this study[25] raise the possibility that the adaptive bradycardia of the athlete can become similar to the sick sinus embolizing syndrome.

Another study[3] of 16 athletes who reported syncope, Stokes-Adams attacks, or both, found life-threatening situations that required pacemaker implantation in seven. In eight of the nine remaining athletes, symptoms cleared after they reduced heavy physical training.

Editor's Note: Again, I would advise these athletes not to participate in such sports. – WPH

Based upon these scattered reports, evidence is accumulating that intensive training of the cardiovascular system may become hazardous to a few. The symptomatic athlete with a slow heart rate, heart block of any degree, or both, deserves further evaluation of his or her cardiovascular system, including an assessment of the intensity of the training program.

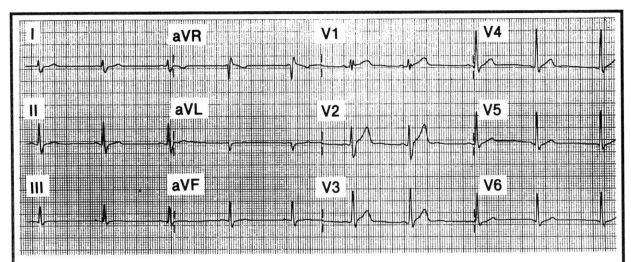

Figure 4-1: Normal Finding in an Athlete – This ECG from a 25-year-old asymptomatic professional football player shows a common "normal" finding on an electrocardiogram of an athlete – vertical axis and RsR1 in V1.

QRS Axis

A summary of several studies[26] reported a QRS frontal plane axis between 0 and +90 degrees in 77.6% of 582 athletes; 74% were between +60 and +90 degrees, and the majority of the remainder were found to have right axis deviation in excess of +90 degrees. A study of 289 professional football players[14] found the mean QRS axis to be 56 degrees, with 5% manifesting right axis deviation. There was only one athlete with left axis deviation. Thus, it appears that vertical and right axis QRS deviations are common findings in highly trained athletes (Figure 4-1: Typical "rightward" normal electrocardiogram in an athlete). Left axis deviation is rare in athletes.

Intraventricular Conduction Delays

Prolongation of intraventricular conduction is commonly seen in athletes, manifesting commonly as incomplete right bundle branch block (Figure 4-1). Of 107 Olympic athletes, 51.1% had incomplete right bundle branch block.[27] Another tabulation of ten studies involving 527 athletes[9] showed 84 (16%) with this finding, which probably represents early right ventricular overload and not a conduction problem per se. Of 289 profes-sional football players, 60% had a QRS duration of 0.10 seconds but only one had complete right bundle branch block.[14] Thus, it can be seen that incomplete right bundle branch block is extremely common in highly trained athletes, but complete right bundle branch block and left bundle branch block are rare.

Ventricular Hypertrophy

Electrocardiographic evidence of right and left ventricular hypertrophy are commonly observed in well trained athletes (Figure 4-2). Criteria vary from study to study, but certain generalizations may be made. On the whole, electrocardiographic evidence for ventricular hypertrophy is more common in endurance-trained than in isometrically trained athletes, but as training programs for each group overlap and become less specialized, these electrocardiographic differences are becoming less noticeable.

Among world-class marathon runners, 76% were found to have voltage criteria for left ventricular hypertrophy,[28] whereas a summary of several studies involving 952 athletes[26] found 32% to have evidence of left ventricular hypertrophy (range 1% to 76%). Among professional football players, 35% displayed voltage criteria for left ventricular hypertrophy.[14] (Figure 4-2).

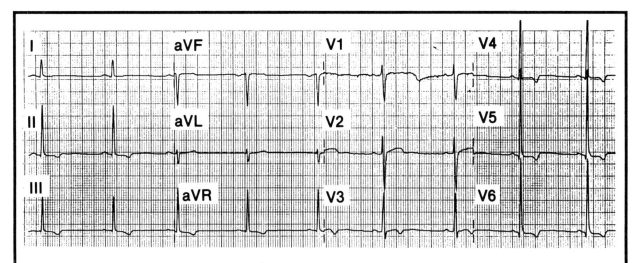

Figure 4-2: "Athletic Heart Syndrome" – This 28-year-old professional athlete was asymptomatic with a typical electrocardiogram of the "Athletic Heart Syndrome" – left ventricular hypertrophy and strain.

A summary of five studies of 669 athletes[26] showed that 19% fulfilled the criteria for right ventricular hypertrophy. Another review of four large studies[29] found criteria for right ventricular hypertrophy to be present in 18% to 69% of athletes, occurring more often in those with dynamic rather than static training. In one study,[26] right ventricular hypertrophy was present equally in statically-trained athletes and in non-athletic, sedentary controls.

Sequential increases in QRS voltage have been shown to occur as training continues. The increase in QRS voltage parallels the intensity and type of training. With cessation of athletic training, the electrocardiographic changes of ventricular hypertrophy revert toward normal in some instances, but may take years to do so.

Editor's Note: It is a known clinical fact that the ECG findings of hypertrophy can regress toward normal (presumably in patients with milder, early changes). – WPH

ST Segment Repolarization Abnormalities and Juvenile Patterns

Changes in the ST segment, T wave, or both have been reported to occur with increased frequency in both endurance and isometrically trained athletes.[14, 30, 31] The ST segment changes resemble the pattern commonly called early repolarization. J point elevation commonly occurs in the anterior lateral leads (V_3 through V_6). (Figure 4-3 shows three different patterns in four normal athletes A - D). These changes may be seen in the inferior (II, III, AVF) leads, as well. Such changes have been reported in up to 50% of highly trained athletes. They were found in the electrocardiogram of 13% of professional football players studied.[14] The ST changes can be mistaken for the changes of acute pericarditis, but the clinical setting and findings are absent.

T wave changes in highly trained athletes are common and variable. The T wave may be tall and peaked, flattened, notched, slightly or significantly inverted in the precordial leads. The changes may be confused with ischemic changes but are similar to the benign juvenile pattern seen

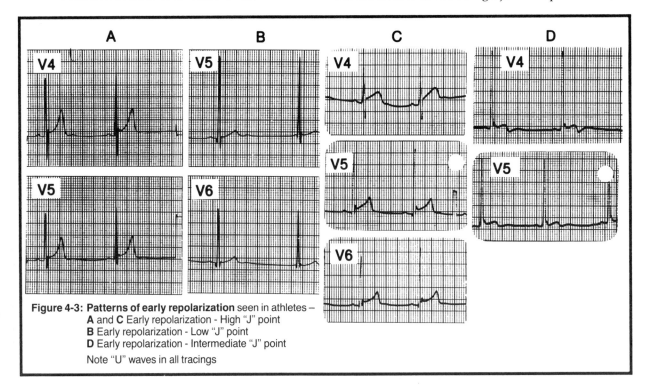

Figure 4-3: Patterns of early repolarization seen in athletes –
A and **C** Early repolarization - High "J" point
B Early repolarization - Low "J" point
D Early repolarization - Intermediate "J" point

Note "U" waves in all tracings

in young adults. Four examples of the juvenile pattern in highly trained athletes are shown in Figure 4-4.

Inversion of the T wave in the anterior precordial leads in a highly trained athlete that was mistaken for acute ischemic changes is shown in Figure 4-5. One one occasion, this electrocardiogram caused surgery to be delayed, and on another, he was admitted to an I.C.C.U. for observation from an emergency room, where he had been seen for an unrelated problem and an electrocardiogram was taken. Ten years later, his electrocardiogram remains unchanged, and he is free of symptoms, fully active and without evidence for cardiac disease.

Small Q waves in the inferior leads can be seen in highly trained athletes as a normal variant (Figure 4-6). At a recent meeting where top college football players were medically evaluated,[32] a small number had electrocardiograms that were reported consistent with diaphragmatic wall infarction because of small Q waves in leads II, III, and AVF.

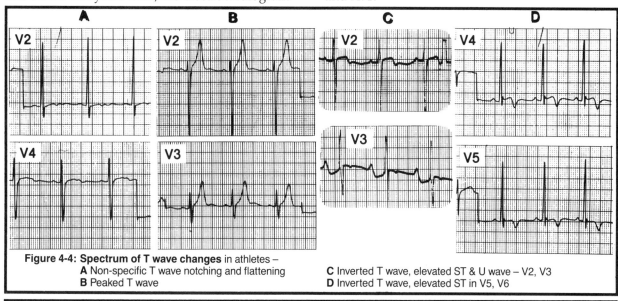

Figure 4-4: **Spectrum of T wave changes** in athletes –
A Non-specific T wave notching and flattening
B Peaked T wave
C Inverted T wave, elevated ST & U wave – V2, V3
D Inverted T wave, elevated ST in V5, V6

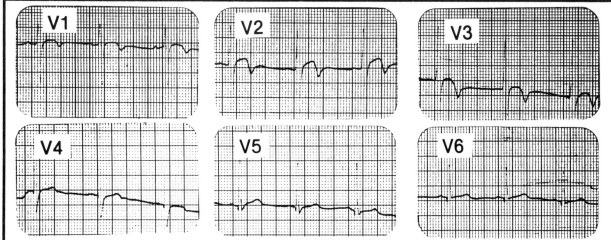

Figure 4-5: **Inverted T Waves** – This ECG is from a 29-year-old professional athlete. It shows inverted T waves in leads VI through V4. He was temporarily admitted to the ICCU on one occasion and on another had surgery cancelled because of these findings. This ECG was taken in 1979. Ten years later, the electrocardiogram is unchanged.

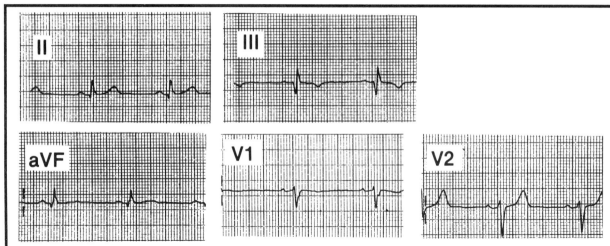

Figure 4-6: Small Q Waves – This ECG is from a 32-year-old professional football player. It shows common small Q waves in diaphragmatic leads, which occasionally are mistaken for more serious pathology. His electrocardiogram has remained unchanged for 13 years!

Arrhythmias

Both supraventricular and ventricular ectopic beats and tachyarrhythmias have been reported in highly trained athletes.

Supraventricular Arrhythmias

One hundred percent of 20 long-distance runners had premature atrial beats on 24-hour continuous ECG recordings,[5] but only one had more than 100 premature atrial beats in 24 hours. The presence of these beats did not correlate with the presence of a wandering pacemaker, marked sinus arrhythmia, sinus bradycardia, prolonged PR interval, or the echocardiographic determination of atrial size.[5]

Another study of 80 healthy runners[33] found ectopic supraventricular complexes in 33 (41%), but again only one athlete had more than 100 ectopics per 24 hours. A team of researchers led by Coelho[34] also reported tachyarrhythmias in young athletes. They found 10 athletes with supraventricular arrhythmias, all of whom had a documented underlying cause. Five had paroxysmal atrial fibrillation, and five had paroxysmal supraventricular tachycardia. Three had underlying Wolff-Parkinson-White (WPW) syndrome, five had mitral valve prolapse, and two had a concealed Kent bundle.

Editor's Note: I recall a Redskin professional football player (guard or tackle) who occasionally had PAT (paroxysmal atrial tachycardia) that would suddenly occur during a football game, causing him some dizziness and muscular weakness. He would take himself out of the game at that point. The tachycardia was short in duration and he could resume playing when normal sinus rhythm took place. – WPH

An unusual case has been reported[35] of an athlete documented to have had a brief run of supraventricular tachycardia in the recovery phase of maximum exercise testing, in which the heart rate reached almost 500 beats/minute.

Athletes with supraventricular tachycardias, whether exercise-induced or not, should be evaluated and managed in the same way as would be done in non-athletes. The individual should undergo a complete history and physical examination in an effort to discover underlying heart disease. Supraventricular tachycardias generally are not incapacitating in athletic competition, so athletic participation is a function of the ability to control the arrhythmia and the etiology of the arrhythmia.

Editor's Note: Recently, I examined a college swimmer. He had had several episodes of PAT, but only during ultra exertion, and never during a competitive swimming match. He continued to compete for his team without any problem (and without any prophylactic medication). – WPH

Author's Note: For another example, one 29-year-old male professional athlete had bouts of sudden supraventricular tachycardia (PAT) precipitated by exercise (sprints), but had no known heart disease. The attacks were aborted easily by either a Valsalva maneuver, carotid sinus pressure, or both. They occurred three times in eight years, and prophylactic medicine was not felt to be indicated. – DMK

Junctional Rhythm

There appears to be an increase in AV junctional rhythms in athletes. In one study,[15] seven of 35 highly trained athletes had junctional rhythm during Holter recordings. The junctional rhythm was intermittent and appeared to occur when the sinus rate slowed to less than 56 beats per minute.

One 31-year-old white male professional athlete had junctional rhythm at rest. When the sinus rate reached 90 beats/minute, normal conduction resumed. An extensive cardiac evaluation including electrophysiological studies failed to detect any underlying cardiac pathology. The rhythm was found to be present for eight years without change.

Wolff-Parkinson-White Syndrome

Whether or not the incidence of WPW is increased in athletes is debatable. One group[36] has reported a higher incidence in athletes, but fewer episodes of arrhythmias. Others who have observed professional athletes estimate the incidence to be close to the 1.5/1000 reported in a large study of the normal population. It's difficult not to think the incidence of WPW is higher in athletes than non-athletes when one professional football team had three individuals with this conduction pattern on its 45-man roster at one time. Two of the three were not symptomatic and hence were not studied. The third had vague symptoms and was studied and found to go into normal conduction with exercise (Figure 4-7). None of the three were treated. There are highly trained athletes participating in competitive sports who have documented WPW on their electrocardiogram.

WPW in the athlete should be approached in a similar manner to WPW in non-athletes. The general approach has been to evaluate completely any symptomatic individual with WPW, beyond the routine history and physical examination with tests including Holter monitoring, maximum stress testing and echocardiography. Electrophysiological studies should then be considered.

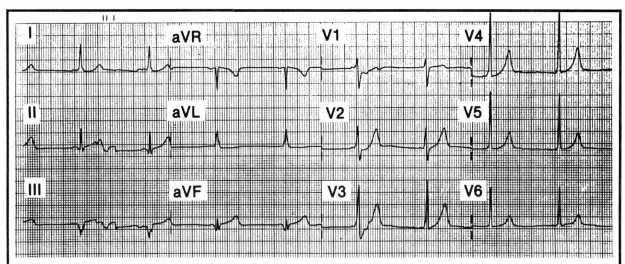

Figure 4-7: WPW – This ECG is from a 25-year-old professional football player with asymptomatic Wolff-Parkinson-White syndrome, one of three players on the team in one year who had WPW!

Ventricular Arrhythmias

Premature ventricular contractions and ventricular tachycardias have been reported in athletes during exercise and in the immediate post-exercise period. During treadmill testing of 60 well-conditioned runners,[37] 27% had ventricular arrhythmias, but only 3% had higher-grade ectopy. In contrast, 60% of the runners had ventricular arrhythmias during a monitored long-distance run: 10% bigeminal, 10% couplets, and 5% multifocal. Treadmill testing significantly underestimated the incidence of arrhythmias, since 57% of the runners who had ventricular arrhythmias while running had none on the treadmill.

In a study of 20 highly trained marathon runners,[38] only one exhibited high-grade arrhythmias (polymorphic ventricular arrhythmias). Six months later, this individual developed angina, leading the researchers to conclude that any high-grade ventricular arrhythmias should be considered abnormal in highly trained athletes.

Another study of 80 healthy runners[33] found ectopic ventricular couplets in 41 and ectopic supraventricular beats in 33. No relationship was found between the frequency of ventricular ectopy and the amount of weekly running.

A third study[39] used 24-hour continuous ECG monitoring to compare 20 runners, 20 cyclists, and 40 nonathletic controls for the frequency of ventricular ectopy. A slightly higher frequency of premature ventricular beats (70% vs 55%, $p > .05$) was found in the athletes. Complex forms of ectopy also were more common in the athletic groups (25% vs 5%, $p > .05$). Other researchers,[40] however, reported a frequency of ventricular ectopy of 33.9% in 165 highly trained athletes, but only a 3.6% incidence of complex ventricular arrhythmias. Thus, there remains a difference of opinion about the frequency of complex ventricular arrhythmias in the athlete.

Ventricular Tachycardia

Among 19 athletes evaluated because of symptomatic tachyarrhythmias,[34] paroxysmal ventricular tachycardia occurred in eight (sustained in five), and ventricular fibrillation occurred in one. All the arrhythmias developed during strenuous exercise. Abnormalities of the heart were found in 15 (79%) of the 19 evaluated. Of the nine athletes with ventricular arrhythmias, four had mitral valve prolapse and one had cardiomyopathy.

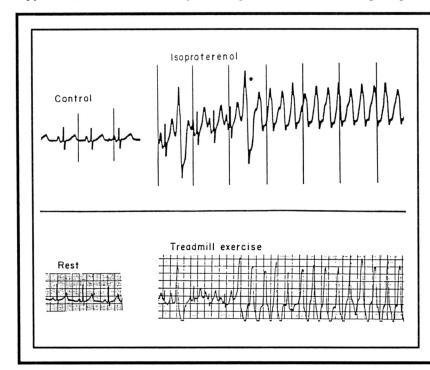

Figure 4-8:
Ventricular Tachycardia – Electrocardiographic rhythm strips from one patient with documented sustained ventricular tachycardia. The top panel shows sinus rhythm during the control period (left) and onset of ventricular tachycardia during infusion of isoproterenol at 5µg/min (right). Note that the first beat of tachycardia (*) does not resemble subsequent beats. Time lines are at intervals of one second. The bottom panel shows sinus rhythm during rest (left) and onset of ventricular tachycardia during treadmill exercise (8 METs) (right). Dark lines are at intervals of 200ms. (From Coehlo et al,[34] p 240. Reprinted with permission from the American College of Cardiology).

Several different varieties of symptomatic ventricular tachycardia have been described in the athlete. One variety can be induced and terminated by programmed ventricular stimulation and probably usually reflects reentry.[41, 42] This variety of tachycardia usually occurs in the setting of severe chronic ischemic heart disease and generally arises from the left ventricle or the interventricular septum.[43] Attacks of this variety of tachycardia are usually unrelated to exercise, and treadmill exercise or infusion of isoproterenol rarely provokes the arrhythmia.[44]

Another variety of symptomatic ventricular tachycardia, however, *is* exercise-provoked. Two groups of researchers[45, 46] first recognized this remarkably homogeneous group of patients (Figure 4-8). The patients were young, sometimes athletic, and had a paucity of heart disease. Their tachycardias originated in the outflow tract of the right ventricle and could not be induced by programmed ventricular stimulation, but could be reproducibly provoked by treadmill exercise or infusion of isoproterenol. Administration of propranolol or verapamil prevented the occurrence of ventricular tachycardia with exercise, whereas Class I antiarrhythmic drugs usually were ineffective. Other groups[47, 48] have subsequently reported similar patients. It has been suggested that this variety of symptomatic ventricular tachycardia may reflect catecholamine-enhanced automaticity or be triggered by delayed afterdepolarizations.[45, 46]

Editor's Note: If I had the responsibility of giving the medical O.K. for an athlete who has had documented ventricular tachycardia, to compete in strenuous sports such as football, basketball, wrestling, etc., I would not do so. Of course, despite this, a number of athletes may elect to continue their physical activities. The physician would be wise, in such a case, to record his advice in writing and have witnesses to this discussion with the athlete and preferably with a responsible member of his family. – WPH

Summary

The effects of training in the athlete may lead to a number of adaptive changes in the electrocardiogram that are not pathologic. Intensive training may cause changes in the conduction system, particularly at the sinus and atrioventricular nodes. Repolarization changes may be intensified, resulting in abnormalities of the ST-T waves resembling pathological entities.

A slow sinus rate, first or second degree heart block, or both are common in the highly trained athlete and they should be considered normal variants unless the individual is symptomatic or other findings are present. Symptomatic bradyarrhythmias may need further evaluation. A decrease in the intensity of the athletic training alone may be sufficient to eliminate any symptoms. However, complete heart block should be approached as it would be in the nonathlete.

A vertical, rightward, or right axis deviation of QRS forces is so common that by itself it may be considered normal in the athlete. Similarly, early repolarization abnormalities, juvenile patterns, and certain precordial ST and T wave changes are so common in the highly trained athlete that their presence alone should not be considered abnormal. Left axis deviation, complete right bundle branch block, left bundle branch block, and the Wolff-Parkinson-White syndrome should be approached as for the nonathlete. None of these arrhythmias should disqualify athletes from sports participation, but further studies may be needed to determine the presence of associated cardiac pathology.

Electrocardiographic changes of ventricular hypertrophy (either right or left) are not considered abnormal in the absence of other clinical findings.

Supraventricular arrhythmias, high-grade ventricular premature contractions (Grade 4 or above), and ventricular tachycardia require a complete cardiac evaluation in an attempt to uncover underlying cardiac disease to determine eligibility for sports participation.

Selected recommendations of the 16th Bethesda Conference regarding eligibility for competition of athletes with findings of cardiac arrhythmias and blocks are summarized in Table 4-2.

Table 4-2
Electrocardiographic Findings in Athletes:
Recommendations Regarding Eligibility for Competition
Based on the Sixteenth Bethesda Conference

1. **Disturbances of Sinus Node Function**
   (Sinus tachycardia, sinus bradycardia with/without junctional escape beats, sinus arrhythmia, sinus pause, sinus arrest, sinoatrial exit block, wandering pacemaker, sick sinus syndrome):
   ▪ Inappropriately slow rates with wandering pacemaker probably need further testing (24-hour ambulatory monitoring, exercise test).
   ▪ Sinus pause, sinus arrest, sinoatrial exit block, and sick sinus syndrome are considered abnormal and require further testing.
   ▪ Patients with syncope or presyncope should not participate in sports until the cause is determined.
   ▪ Symptomatic arrhythmias need treatment. If the patient is asymptomatic for six months, then he or she may participate in sports.
   ▪ Patients treated with pacemakers should not engage in competitive contact sports.

2. **Premature Atrial Complexes**
   ▪ In the absence of structural heart disease, participation in all competitive sports is permitted.

3. **Atrial Flutter, Fibrillation**
   ▪ Further evaluation for underlying heart disease is needed (24-hour ambulatory monitoring, echocardiogram). Full participation in all competitive sports should not be allowed until the patient has had no episode of atrial flutter for six months (with/without treatment).

4. **AV Junctional Escape Rhythm**
   ▪ Recommendations same as for sick sinus syndrome (above).

5. **Supraventricular Tachycardia** (including AV nodal re-entry tachycardia):
   ▪ Patients need 24-hour ambulatory monitoring during athletic activity, exercise testing, and an echocardiogram. It is important to know ventricular response rate with exercise.
   ▪ Symptoms produced by the arrhythmia require treatment. The patient must be symptom free for six months before competitive sports are permitted.

6. **Ventricular Pre-Excitation**
   ▪ Patients need 24-hour ambulatory monitoring during athletic activity, exercise testing, and an echocardiogram. If asymptomatic with no underlying cardiac abnormalities, no further evaluation is needed and patients may participate in all competitive sports.
   ▪ Untreated patients with WPW syndrome should not participate in competitive sports.

7. **Premature Ventricular Complexes**
   ■ Patients should have 24-hour ambulatory monitoring and an echocardiogram if there is any evidence suggesting structural cardiac disease. If premature complexes disappear during exercise, or at least do not increase in frequency, the patient may participate in all competitive sports.
   ■ If the frequency of premature beats increases with exercise, but there is no recognized structural heart disease, participation should be limited to low-intensity competitive sports.
   ■ Patients with premature complexes associated with prolonged QT intervals should not participate in competitive sports.

8. **Ventricular Tachycardia**
   ■ Further testing and monitoring required. Patients with nonsustained ventricular tachycardia ≤150 beats/minute may participate in all competitive sports with caution.
   ■ Patients with symptoms, tachycardia >150 beats/minute, or tachycardia associated with prolonged QT interval should not engage in competitive sports.

9. **First Degree AV Block, Type I Second Degree Block (Wenckebach)**
   ■ Asymptomatic patients with no underlying cardiac disease and no worsening block with exercise can participate in all competitive sports.

10. **Complete Right Bundle Branch Block**
    ■ Asymptomatic patients who have no ventricular arrhythmias on a 24-hour ambulatory recording and who have no known heart disease can participate in all competitive sports.

11. **Complete Left Bundle Branch Block**
    ■ Because of the rarity of acquired left bundle branch block in children and its association with syncope, an electrophysiologic study is suggested. Acquired block in older patients can be considered as right bundle branch block.
    ■ Patients with normal conduction response to pacing can participate in all competitive sports.

12. **Congenital Complete Heart Block**
    ■ This diagnosis requires 24-hour ambulatory monitoring, an exercise test, and an echocardiogram.
    ■ Patients with a normal heart, no history of syncope or presyncope, a narrow QRS complex, ventricular rates >40 beats/minute increasing with exertion, and no ventricular ectopic activity during exercise can participate in all competitive sports.

Adapted from Zipes et al.[49] The full description of the above entities as well as other categories should be consulted.

References

1. Hoogerwerf S: Elektrokardiographische Untersuchungen der Amsterdammer Olympiakampfer. Julius Springer, Berlin, 1929.

2. Hiss RG and Lamb LE: Electrocardiographic findings in 122,043 individuals. *Circulation* 25:947-961, 1962.

3. Ector H, Verlinder M, Vanden Eynde E, Bourgois J, Herman L, Fagard R and DeGeest H: Bradycardia, ventricular pauses, syncope, and sports. *The Lancet* 591-594, 1984.

4. Kala R and Viitasalo MT: Atrioventricular block, including Mobitz II-like pattern, during ambulatory ECG recording in young athletes aged 14 to 16 years. *Annals of Clinical Research* 14:53-56, 1982.

5. Talan DA, Bauernfeind RA, Ashley WW, Kanakis C Jr, and Rosen KM: Twenty-four hour continuous ECG recordings in long distance runners. *Chest* 82:19-24, 1982.

6. Brodsky M, Wu D, Denes P, Kanakis C and Rosen KM: Arrhythmias documented by 24 hour continuous electrocardiographic monitoring in 50 male medical students without apparent heart disease. *Am J Cardiolog* 39:389-395, 1977.

7. Chapman JH: Profound sinus bradycardia in the athletic heart syndrome. *J Sports Med* 22:45-48, 1982.

8. Klemola E: Electrocardiographic observations on 650 Finnish athletes. *Annales Medicinae Internal Fenniae* 41:121, 1951.

9. Lichtman J, O'Rourke RA, Klein A, Kailener JS: Electrocardiogram of the athlete. *Arch Intern Med* 132:763-770, 1973.

10. Beswick FW, Jordan RC: Cardiological observations at the sixth British Empire and Commonwealth Games. *Br Heart J* 23:113-129, 1961.

11. Hantzschel K, Dohrn K: The electrocardiogram before and after a marathon-race. *J Sports Med Phys Fitness* 6:29-32, 1966.

12. Hunt BPE: Electrocardiographic study of 20 champion swimmers before and after 100 yard sprint swimming competition. *Can Med Assoc J* 88:1251-1253, 1963.

13. Balady J, Cadigan JB and Ryan T: Electrocardiogram of the athlete: An analysis of 289 professional football players. *Am J Cardiol* 53:1339-1343, 1984.

14. Viitasalo MT, Kala R and Eissalo A: Ambulatory electrocardiographic recordings in endurance athletes. *Br Heart J* 47:213-220, 1982.

15. Sargin O, et al: Wenckebach phenomenon with nodal and ventricular escape in marathon runners. *Chest* 57:102-105, 1970.

16. Grimby G and Saltin B: Physiological analysis of physically well-trained middle-aged and old athletes. *Acta Med Scand* 179:513-526, 1986.

17. Grimby G, Saltin S: Daily running causing Wenckebach heart block. *Lancet* 2:962-963, 1964.

18. Cullen KJ, Collin R: Daily running causing Wenckebach heart block. *Lancet* 2:729-730, 1964.

19. Zeppili P, Fenici R, Sassara M, Pirrami MM, and Caselli G: Wenckebach second degree AV block in top-ranking athletes: An old problem revisited. *Am Heart J* 100:281-294, 1980.

20. Murayama M, and Kuruda Y: Cardiovascular future of athletes. In Lubich T and Venerando A (eds): Sports Cardiology. Bologna, Aulo Gaggi: 401-413, 1980.

21. DiNardo-Ekery D and Abedin Zainul: High degree atrioventricular block in a marathoner with 5-year follow-up. *Am Heart J* 113:834-837, 1987.

22. Lie H and Erikssen J: Five-year follow-up of ECG aberrations, latent coronary disease and cardiopulmonary fitness in various age groups of Norwegian cross-country skiers. *Acta Med Scand* 216:377-383, 1984.

23. Torkelson L and Jokl E: Complete congenital heart block in an athlete. *Arch Phys Med Rehabil* 21:54, 1967.

24. Hanne-Paparo N, Drory Y and Kellerman JJ: Complete heart block and physical performance. *Int J Sports Med* 3:9-13, 1983.

25. Nils-Johan A, Landin K and Johansson BW: Athletic bradycardia as an embolizing disorder? Symptomatic arrhythmias in patients aged less than 50. *Br Heart J* 52:660-666, 1984.

26. Ferst JA and Chaitman BR: The electrocardiogram and the athlete: *Sports Medicine* 1:390-403, 1984.

27. Venerando A and Rulli V: Frequency, morphology, and meaning of the electrocardiographic anomalies found in Olympic marathon runners and walkers. *J Sports Med Phys Fitness* 4:135-141, 1964.

28. Smith WG, Cullen KJ, and Thorburn IO: Electrocardiograms of marathon runners in 1962 Commonwealth Games. *Br Heart J* 26:469-476, 1964.

29. Huston TP, Puffer JC and Rodney WM: The athletic heart syndrome. *New Engl J Med* 313:24-32, 1985.

30. Zeppili P, Pirrami MM, Sassara M, and Fenici R: T-wave abnormalities in top-ranking athletes: Effects of isoproterenol, atropine, and physical exercise. *Am Heart J* 100:213-222, 1980.

31. Nishimura T, Kambara H, Chen CH, Yamada Y, Kawai C: Noninvasive assessment of T-wave abnormalities on precordial electrocardiograms in middle-aged professional bicyclists. *Electrocardiology* 14:357, 1981.

32. Hanne-Paparo N, Wnedkos MH, Brunner D: T wave abnormalities in the electrocardiograms of top-ranking athletes without demonstrable organic heart disease.

33. Pilcher GF, Cook J, Johnson BL and Fletcher GF: Twenty-four-hour continuous electrocardiography during exercise and free activity in 80 apparently healthy runners. *Am J Cardiol* 52:859-861, 1983.

34. Coelho A, Paleleo E, Ashley W, Swiryn S, Petropoulos T, Welch WJ and Bauernfeind RA: Tachyarrhythmias in young athletes. *J Am Coll Cardiol* 7:237-243, 1986.

35. Medved R and Bavisic-Medved V: A rare case of paroxysmal tachycardia during load testing a top-ranking athlete. *J Sports Med* 25:211-214, 1985.

36. S'Jongers JJ, Dirix A, Jolie P, et al: Wolff-Parkinson-White Syndrome and sports aptitude. *J Sports Med Phys Fitness* 16:6, 1976.

37. Patano JA and Oriel RJ: Prevalence and nature of cardiac arrhythmias in apparently normal well-trained runners. *Am Heart J* 104:762-768, 1982.

38. Palatini P, Marraglino G, Sperti G, Calzauara A, Libardoni M, Pessina AC and DalPalo C: Prevalence and possible mechanisms of ventricular arrhythmias in athletes. *Am Heart J* 110:560-67, 1985.

39. Biffi A, Pelliccia A and Caselli G: Letter to the editor. *Am Heart J* 112:1349-51, 1986.

40. Wellens HJJ, Duren DR, and Lie KI: Observations on mechanisms of ventricular tachycardia in man. *Circulation* 54:237-44, 1976.

41. Josephson ME, et al: Recurrent sustained ventricular tachycardia: 1. mechanisms. *Circulation* 57:431-40, 1978.

42. Josephson ME, et al: Recurrent sustained ventricular tachycardia: 2. Endocardial mapping. *Circulation* 57:440-7, 1978.

43. Coelho A, et al: Treadmill testing in patients with sustained ventricular tachycardia (abstr). *Circulation 64* (suppl IV):1-13, 1981.

44. Wu D Kou H and Hung J: Exercise-triggered paroxysmal ventricular tachycardia. *Annals of Internal Medicine* 95:410-414, 1981.

45. Palileo EV, et al: Exercise provocable right ventricular outflow tract tachycardia. *Am Heart J* 104:185-93, 1982.

46. Buxton AE, et al: Right ventricular tachycardia: clinical and electrophysiologic characteristics. *Circulation* 68:917-27, 1983.

47. Vlay SC: Catecholamine-sensitive ventricular tachycardia. *Am Heart J* 114:455-461, 1987.

48. Zipes DP, Cobb LA, Garson A, et al: Task force VI: Arrhythmias. 16th Bethesda Conference. Cardiovascular abnormalities in the athlete: Recommendations regarding eligibility for competition. *J Am Coll Cardiol* 6:1225, 1985.

CHAPTER 5

ECHOCARDIOGRAPHIC EVALUATION OF ATHLETES

Charles Presti, MD

Fort Wayne Cardiology
Fort Wayne, Indiana

Michael H. Crawford, MD

Department of Medicine (Cardiology)
University of New Mexico
Albuquerque

Editor's Note: The echocardiogram is not necessary in the routine screening of all athletes in high school, college, or at the professional level. The cost, of course, would be prohibitive and it would be time consuming. However, when the screening evaluation raises any question as to the presence of heart disease in the athlete, then this valuable procedure can be utilized as necessary. This next informative discussion outlines the echocardiographic findings in healthy athletes, those athletes with known heart disease, and those suspected of having it. – WPH

Evaluation of cardiac chamber dimensions, wall thickness and ventricular function is of fundamental importance in the study of cardiovascular capacity as well as in the diagnosis of cardiac disease. The "athletic heart syndrome*" encompasses a number of cardiac changes, including chamber enlargement and increases in wall thickness. Henschen, at the end of the nineteenth century, was the first to describe enlarged hearts in endurance-trained athletes.[1] Using only thoracic percussion, he ascribed the cardiac enlargement found in cross-country skiers to a combination of chamber dilation and hypertrophy, both of which he believed to be a physiologic result of training. Since then, the evolution of non-invasive techniques has allowed for a more exact study of cardiac anatomy and function in athletes.

Chest roentgenography has confirmed the presence of cardiomegaly in endurance trained athletes,[2] but radiographic investigation of the athlete's heart is limited by its ability to evaluate only one phase of the cardiac cycle at a time, as well as by its inability to measure individual chamber sizes and wall thickness.[3] Similarly, although electrocardiographic criteria for left and right ventricular hypertrophy are frequently observed in athletes,[4] the correlation between electrocardiographic findings and data derived from postmortem measurements of myocardial mass is known to be poor.[5]

With the development of echocardiography, it became possible to perform accurate, direct, reproducible, and quantitative noninvasive measurements of cardiac chamber dimensions and wall thickness in athletes. From these direct measurements, it is possible to calculate left ventricular volumes and mass and to quantitate left ventricular function. Most of the existing studies utilizing echocardiography to evaluate the athlete's heart have employed M-mode echocardiography. More recently, studies using two-dimensional and Doppler echocardiography also have been done to assess anatomic and functional changes in the athlete's heart. Although all of these techniques have certain limitations,[6-8] echocardiography has provided useful information and valuable insights into the structure and function of the athlete's heart.

Normal Echocardiographic Findings in Athletes

A large number of studies utilizing echocardiography to investigate the heart of the athlete have been performed since 1975, encompassing the evaluation of over 1700 athletes.[9-56] The most common form of exercise training investigated has

---

*Athletic heart syndrome refers to the physiologic and structural cardiovascular changes that occur as the result of long-term conditioning in highly trained athletes.

been long-distance running, but a wide variety of other athletic activities have been studied, ranging from field hockey to world-class weight lifting. The majority of these studies have involved the comparison of cardiac dimensions of small groups of athletes with age- and sex-matched non-athletic control subjects. Several of these studies also have investigated the relationship of the type of athletic conditioning (isotonic or dynamic vs isometric or static) to specific alterations in cardiac structure.

The preceding studies utilized a cross-sectional assessment of athletes and controls in comparing cardiac dimensions. Longitudinal studies of the effects of chronic exercise on cardiac dimensions also have been performed.[33, 57-74] Both athletes and non-athletes participating in short-term training programs have been investigated with echocardiography to determine the effects of training and detraining on cardiac dimensions. Other echocardiographic studies have investigated left ventricular systolic and diastolic function in the heart of the athlete, while still others have evaluated the role that age may play in training-induced changes in cardiac dimensions.

Left Ventricular Chamber Size

Echocardiographic studies of athletes have demonstrated an increase in left ventricular end-diastolic cavity diameter when compared to non-athletic control subjects. The increase in cavity dimension is generally small, averaging 10% over the value of the control population[9-56] (Figure 5-1 and 5-2). Furthermore, the degree of dilatation is generally within the accepted range of normal values for adults.[77] Although an occasional subject has been reported to have marked left ventricular dilatation, with the largest being 70 mm in a world champion professional cyclist,[36] the average values for left ventricular end-diastolic dimension in athletes have ranged from 43 to 57 mm. These values are significantly lower than those found in patients with either primary myocardial disease or valvular heart disease producing left ventricular dilatation.[42]

The increase in left ventricular diastolic dimension appears to be most pronounced in athletes who perform primarily isotonic (or dynamic) exercise training (Table 5-1). Studies that have compared cardiac dimensions in isotonically trained athletes (primarily endurance runners) with iso-

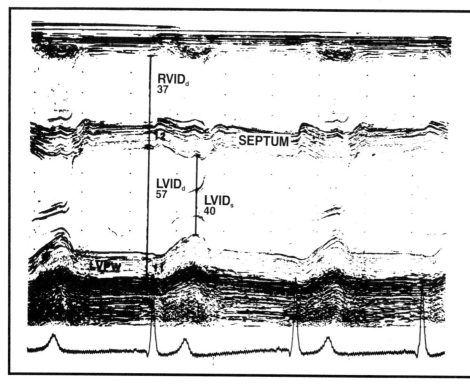

RVID_d
37

SEPTUM
12

LVID_d
57

LVID_s
40

LVPW

Figure 5-1: M-mode Echocardiogram Showing Cardiac Dimensions in a World-Class Oarsman – The left ventricular end-diastolic dimension (LVID_d) is slightly increased (57 mm) and the interventricular septum (12 mm) and left ventricular posterior wall (LVPW) (11 mm) are also mildly thickened. Right ventricular end-diastolic dimension (RVID_d) is also increased (37 mm). (Reproduced with permission from Wieling et al.[33])

metrically trained athletes (primarily weight lifters) have generally found larger left ventricular end-diastolic dimensions in the endurance-trained athletes.[9, 24, 28, 37, 42, 45, 46, 54] Only the studies of Shapiro[45] and Colan and associates[54] demonstrated smaller left ventricular diastolic dimensions in endurance-trained athletes than in isometrically trained athletes.

Some disagreement persists over these results in view of the fact that well-conditioned athletes generally demonstrate slower resting heart rates than non-conditioned subjects and this effect is most pronounced in endurance-trained athletes.[4] Although large changes in heart rate can result in significant changes in left ventricular dimensions,[78] Hirshleifer and colleagues demonstrated only a 2 mm change in left ventricular cavity dimension when a 55% increase in heart rate was induced with atropine.[79] More recently, a study[80] using two-dimensional echocardiography found no relationship between left ventricular end-diastolic volume and heart rate in endurance-trained athletes (Figure 5-3). Hence, it is unlikely that the modest reduction in resting heart rate could by itself account for the consistently observed increase in left ventricular dimensions in trained athletes.

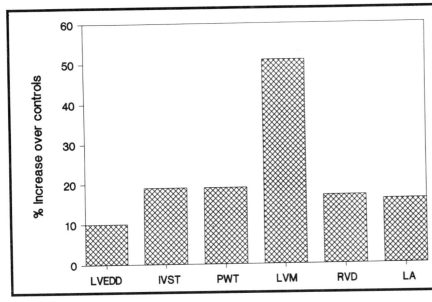

Figure 5-2: Percent Increase of Cardiac Dimensions in Athletes in comparison to nonathletic control Subjects – (Data taken from references 9-56.) LVEDD = left ventricular end-diastolic dimension; IVST = interventricular septal thickness; PWT = posterior wall thickness; LVM = left ventricular mass; RVD = right ventricular end-diastolic dimension; LA = left atrial transverse dimension.

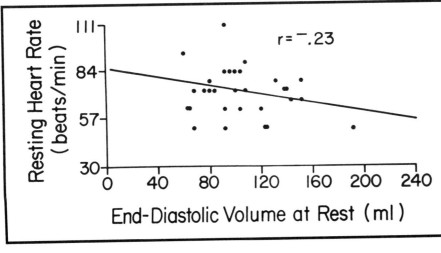

Figure 5-3: End-Diastolic Volume and Resting Heart Rate – Relationship between two-dimensional echocardiographically determined end-diastolic volume and resting heart rate in endurance-trained athletes. No significant relationship is present. Data from Crawford et al.[80]

Left Ventricular Wall Thickness

Along with the change in left ventricular internal diameter, the thickness of both the interventricular septum and the posterior left ventricular free wall are often increased in athletes when compared to age- and sex-matched sedentary control subjects. However, as with the changes in left ventricular dimension, the increases in both septal and posterior wall thickness are generally small, averaging 15 to 20% greater than the control subjects, and are usually still within the normal range. Values for both the interventricular septal and left ventricular free wall thickness tend to be greater in strength-trained athletes as compared to endurance-trained athletes,[9, 28, 42, 45, 46, 54] although not all studies have found this to be true.[24, 37] Indeed, one of the highest values for posterior wall thickness (19 mm) has been reported in an ultraendurance athlete (triathlete).[50] Thus, as with left ventricular cavity dimension, a clear-cut correlation between the type of exercise training and changes in cardiac dimensions cannot be made, although certain trends are apparent (Table 5-1).

Along with the increase in septal and posterior wall thickness in athletes, several studies[11,14, 34, 45, 81, 82] have noted a septal-to-free-wall ratio greater than 1.3, one of the echocardiographic criteria proposed for hypertrophic cardiomyopathy.[83] However, asymmetric septal hypertrophy has been shown to occur in forms of left ventricular hypertrophy other than hypertrophic cardiomyopthy.[84] Roeske et al[11] found septal-to-free-wall ratios greater than 1.3 in 4 of 10 athletes, but also in 5 of 10 control subjects. They postulated that one reason for the high incidence of asymmetric septal hypertrophy was an oblique passage of the M-mode beam through the interventricular septum in their tall thin subjects, resulting in a spuriously high value for interventricular septal thickness.

More importantly, although athletes may demonstrate a high ratio of septal to posterior wall thickness, systolic anterior motion of the mitral valve and early aortic valve closure, findings associated with obstructive hypertrophic cardiomyopathy, are not seen. Furthermore, the increase in ventricular wall thickness seen in athletes does not occur at the expense of the left ventricular cavity, suggesting a mass-to-volume ratio that remains near normal.[34, 42, 85] In contrast, hypertrophic cardiomyopathy is characterized by asymmetric ventricular hypertrophy in conjunction with a small left ventricular cavity, often resulting in cavity obliteration at end-systole.[42] *Thus, in the trained athlete who demonstrates only an increased septal-to-free-wall ratio, a diagnosis of hypertrophic cardiomyopathy is not warranted.*

Table 5-1
Changes in Echocardiographic Parameters in Isotonic and Isometric Athletes

Parameter	Isotonic	Isometric
Left ventricular end-diastolic diameter	†† or no change	† or no change
Left ventricular posterior wall thickness	† or no change	†† or no change
Interventricular septal thickness	† or no change	†† or no change
Interventricular septum/posterior wall ratio	† or normal	† or normal
Left ventricular mass	††	††
Left ventricular mass/lean body mass	†	no change
Left atrial diameter	† or no change	—
Right ventricular diameter	† or no change	—
Fractional shortening	no change	no change
Ejection fraction	no change	no change
Velocity of circumferential fiber shortening	no change	no change

† = slight increase; †† = moderate increase

Left Ventricular Mass

By using the values for left ventricular end-diastolic dimension and septal and posterior wall thickness obtained with M-mode echocardiography, it is possible to calculate left ventricular mass.[86, 87] Since both left ventricular diameter and wall thickness tend to be increased in athletes, left ventricular mass must also increase. Indeed, significant increases in left ventricular mass in athletes were found in 30 of the 32 studies in which this determination was compared between athletes and control subjects.[9-56, 88] The increase in left ventricular mass in trained athletes averages 51% in these comparative studies (Figure 5-2). The study of Snoeck et al[37] found a significant increase in left ventricular mass in endurance trained athletes and although left ventricular mass was increased 31% in weight lifters, this value was not statistically significantly different from the control group. Wolfe et al[49] found increases in left ventricular mass in some, but not all, college basketball players when compared to a group of non-sedentary control subjects.

Since athletes may differ in body size from unconditioned persons, one possible explanation for the increase in left ventricular mass seen in the athlete's heart is an increase in total body mass. However, measurement of left ventricular mass normalized with respect to body surface area has confirmed left ventricular hypertrophy in athletes as compared to controls. In fact, in the studies that determined both values, the mean increase in left ventricular mass was 49% when the absolute value was used versus 45% when the value normalized for body surface area was used.[13, 20, 23, 24, 26, 41, 45, 49, 53, 54, 88] Hence, it is unlikely that the increase in left ventricular mass in the athlete's heart is solely related to a larger body mass.

On the other hand, athletes may differ not only in body size, but also in body composition, with lower percentages of body fat and higher percentages of lean mass than sedentary controls with similar body surface areas.[89] Along these lines, other researchers[24] normalized values for left ventricular mass with respect to lean body mass and demonstrated that athletes trained with static exercise showed no significant difference compared to matched controls, while endurance-trained athletes still showed an increased normalized left ventricular mass. This suggests that the ventricular hypertrophy in endurance-trained athletes is proportionately greater than the increase in skeletal muscle mass.

Left Atrial and Right Ventricular Size

Although left atrial size has been assessed in fewer studies than left ventricular size, there has generally been a trend for an increase in left atrial dimension in athletes. Of the 15 studies that compared athletes to control subjects, 11 found a significant increase in left atrial dimension.[9, 12-15, 17, 20-22, 25, 26, 31, 33, 37, 48, 51] The mean increase in athletes was approximately 16% (Figure 5-2), and as with the changes in left ventricular internal dimension, the increased left atrial dimension in the athlete's heart usually has not exceeded the accepted normal limits for adults.[77] Although some authors have suggested that the increase in left atrial size in athletes is due to abnormal ventricular compliance secondary to left ventricular hypertrophy,[14, 20] this is unlikely, based on more precise evaluations of diastolic function using digitized M-mode and Doppler echocardiography.

A relatively small number of studies have evaluated right ventricular dimension in athletes.[11-15, 17, 22, 23, 29, 33, 48, 51] Assessment of right ventricular size with M-mode echocardiography is generally more difficult than evaluation of left ventricular size due to the more complex geometry of the right ventricle.[90] In addition, due to its substernal location in normal subjects, measurement of right ventricular dimension is very dependent on the position of the subject at the time of the echocardiographic examination. Nevertheless, in the studies that have compared values in athletes to control subjects, a 17% increase in right ventricular diastolic dimension was found in athletes (Figure 5-2). Using two-dimensional echocardiography, Hauser and associates[48] were able to confirm significant increases (16%) in right ventricular transverse axis and right ventricular chamber area (26%) in athletes compared to control subjects. Interestingly, no difference in right ventricular dimension was found between groups in this study. A significant increase in right atrial dimension in athletes was also demonstrated in the same study. However, the greater right atrial and right ventricular dimensions in athletes were proportional to their larger left atrial and left ventricular dimensions, and the ratios of right-to-left atrial area and right-to-left ventricular area were similar between athletes and control subjects.[48] This indicates that the physiologic influences affecting the athlete's heart appear to affect all cardiac chambers equally.

Left Ventricular Systolic Function

Many techniques are available for the assessment of left ventricular systolic performance. The most commonly used echocardiographic variables are fractional shortening, ejection fraction, and velocity of circumferential fiber shortening.[6] These derived values have been used by several investigators to assess ventricular contractility in the trained athlete.[9-56] These studies have generally demonstrated normal indexes of systolic function in athletes under resting conditions. However, one group[22] found that 9 of 20 endurance-trained athletes had reduced fractional shortening, but normal velocity of circumferential shortening. Similarly, another study[13] found a significant reduction in fractional shortening and a small, but not significant, reduction in velocity of circumferential shortening in endurance runners when compared to control subjects.

Other researchers[25] found normal indexes of left ventricular systolic function in professional bicyclists aged 20 to 39 years, but mildly depressed indexes in those aged 40 to 49 years. They postu-

lated that strenuous exercise training over many years may result in depression of left ventricular function.

These reports of reduced left ventricular systolic function may be partially explained by the fact that the traditional indexes used to assess myocardial contractility are not completely load-independent. Indeed, a recent study[54] used non-invasive load-independent indexes of myocardial contractility to study left ventricular systolic function in both endurance and strength-trained athletes. When these load-independent indexes were used, all athletes were found to have normal contractile states despite significant increases in left ventricular mass in both types of athletes and a significant decrease in fractional shortening in the endurance-trained athletes. Hence, it appears that intrinsic myocardial contractility remains normal in athletes despite significant changes in cavity dimension and wall thickness.

Left Ventricular Diastolic Function

Diastolic function of the heart represents a complex interaction of several factors including left ventricular wall thickness and geometry, left ventricular filling pressure, systolic blood pressure, heart rate, myocardial perfusion, and compliance of the left ventricle.[91] Echocardiographic tech-

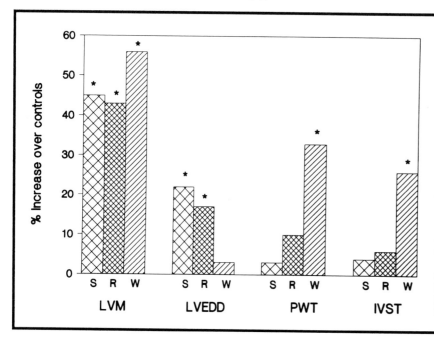

Figure 5-4: Cardiac Dimensions in Athletes vs Non-Athletes – Percent increase of cardiac dimensions in athletes participating in a variety of sports as compared to nonathletic control subjects. Swimmers (S), runners (R), and wrestlers (W) all had statistically significant increases in left ventricular mass (LVM) as compared to controls, whereas only swimmers and runners had an increased left ventricular end-diastolic dimension (LVEDD). Wrestlers had significantly increased thickness of both the interventricular septum (IVST) and the posterior wall (PWT). * = p<0.001. Data from Morganroth et al.[9]

niques used to assess diastolic function include digitized M-mode echocardiography[92] and Doppler echocardiography.[93] Abnormalities in diastolic function have been demonstrated with these techniques in patients with left ventricular hypertrophy due to hypertension, valvular aortic stenosis, and primary myocardial disease.[94-98]

Because exercise training results in the development of left ventricular hypertrophy, several studies have investigated diastolic function in trained athletes.[47, 50, 53, 55, 99, 100] These studies, performed in both endurance-trained and strength-trained athletes, have uniformly demonstrated normal indexes of diastolic function despite significant increases in left ventricular wall thickness and left ventricular mass. Some studies have even shown enhanced early diastolic filling in athletes.[47, 53, 99] Although one study[53] found abnormalities in Doppler-derived indexes of diastolic function in a small subset of weight lifters who were heavy users of steroids, the role that steroids may play in the cardiac hypertrophy process in athletes remains controversial.[82, 101]

The normal diastolic function in athletes as assessed with echocardiography has also been documented using radionuclide angiography.[88] This study demonstrated no impairment of left ventricular filling in endurance-trained athletes despite a 43% increase in left ventricular mass as compared to control subjects. In contrast to the direct relationship noted between the degree of left ventricular hypertrophy and impaired diastolic filling in patients with pathologic hypertrophy,[102, 103] no correlation between left ventricular mass and diastolic parameters has been found in athletes.[53, 55, 88] Thus, although exercise training may result in a substantial increase in myocardial mass, it does not appear to result in any impairment of diastolic function. This concept is in agreement with experimental data suggesting that there are fundamental biochemical and ultrastructural differences between physiologic and pathologic hypertrophy of the heart.[104]

Relationship Between the Type of Exercise Training and Cardiac Changes

Echocardiography also has been used to assess whether the cardiac structural changes seen in athletes are related to the specific type of exercise training. The concept that different patterns of left ventricular hypertrophy develop in response to different types of athletic training was first proposed by Morganroth and colleagues,[9] who found increases in left ventricular mass in both isotonic or endurance-trained athletes and isometric or strength-trained athletes. The increase in calculated left ventricular mass observed in the endurance-trained athletes (swimmers and runners) was associated with a significant increase in left ventricular end-diastolic dimension, but normal wall thickness. In contrast, the increase in left ventricular mass observed in strength-trained athletes (weight lifters) was associated with an increase in left ventricular wall thickness, but normal end-diastolic dimension (Figure 5-4). Hemodynamically, these patterns of left ventricular hypertrophy correlated with the predominant volume load of endurance training and the predominant pressure load of strength training. Several subsequent studies confirmed these differences.[24, 28, 37, 42, 44, 54]

On the other hand, other investigators have not found significant differences in cardiac structure between athletes participating in different forms of exercise training.[36, 45] In contrast to the data of Morganroth et al,[9] Rost[36] found that the greatest increase in left ventricular wall thickness occurred in the hearts with the largest cavity dimensions.

The issue of whether different types of exercise training produce different cardiac morphologic changes is complicated by several factors. First, only rarely does an athletic training program involve purely isotonic or isometric exercise. More commonly, there is substantial overlap between programs, with some component of both isotonic and isometric training present in both. This is illustrated by a study of endurance runners and competitive cyclists,[44] which found that, in runners, there was an increase in left ventricular internal dimension and a proportionate increase in wall thickness. In contrast, whereas the cyclists also demonstrated increases in both left ventricular dimension and wall thickness, the increase in wall thickness was out of proportion to the increase in left ventricular dimension. The authors postulated that this was due to the varying degrees of isometric exercise performed with the upper extremities during cycling.

A second problem in studying the relationship between the type of training program and morphologic cardiac changes is the relationship of cardiac size to total body size. As discussed earlier, it was found that the changes in left ventricular mass induced by exercise training involved changes in lean body mass, with only endurance-trained athletes demonstrating an increased myocardial mass when normalized with respect to lean body mass.[24]

Finally, the development of left ventricular dilation alone or an increase in wall thickness alone would appear to be non-physiologic and, in the case of the former, lead to an inappropriate increase in wall stress. Although these isolated changes may occur at the extremes of the spectrum of physiologic hypertrophy, most athletes seem to develop a combination of dilation and increase in wall thickness. However, even though both isometric and isotonic exercise lead to increases in left ventricular mass, it appears that ventricular dilation predominates in the endurance group, whereas increases in wall thickness predominate in the isometric group (Table 5-1).

Effects of Age and Sex on the Training Effect

A small number of studies have investigated the effects of exercise training on cardiac morphologic changes in children.[12, 21, 51] A team led by Allen[12] compared echocardiographic variables in 77 championship child swimmers (5 to 17 years of age) to previously reported echocardiographic norms for children.[105] The athletes had left ventricular wall, right ventricular wall, and septal thickness greater than normal, but the mean left ventricular diastolic dimension was at the 50th percentile of the normal group with a wide range of variability (28 to 55 mm).

These findings were confirmed in another study,[21] which also found significant increases in left ventricular wall and septal thickness and left ventricular mass but no significant increase in left ventricular diastolic dimension in swimmers 14 years of age when compared to controls.

A study of 72 swimmers[51] (8 to 14 years of age) found significant increases in left ventricular diastolic dimension when compared to controls of similar body surface area. Thus, it appears that

systematic training results in cardiac morphologic changes not only in adult athletes, but also in children. Therefore, when interpreting an echocardiogram in a child, it is important to inquire as to whether the child is a serious athlete.

There have been fewer studies of cardiac morphologic changes in female athletes than in male athletes. Several studies have investigated female athletes alone or a mixture of male and female athletes.[17, 23, 29, 31, 36, 45, 50, 52, 71, 106] In those studies that separate the echocardiographic data of male and female athletes, similar changes in left ventricular mass have been found in both sexes. However, the absolute values may be slightly greater in males.[29, 52, 106]

Longitudinal Echocardiographic Studies

Cardiac Structural Changes Associated with Conditioning

One of the most scientific methods of evaluating structural changes in the heart in response to exercise training is the longitudinal approach. This method uses a patient as his or her own control and involves examination before and after a period of physical training. The usefulness of this approach is that many of the other variables involved in the cross-sectional studies are eliminated. Studies utilizing the longitudinal approach have evaluated the effect of training both in non-athletes and in subjects who were athletically conditioned at the outset.

Several studies have evaluated changes in cardiac morphology with echocardiography following short-term exercise programs in previously sedentary or normally active adults.[57-69] Most of these studies involved endurance-type training (running or cycling) for periods of 6 to 26 weeks. Three studies utilized isometric strength training.

The study by DeMaria and associates,[57] involving echocardiographic evaluation of 24 young normal subjects before and after an 11-week walk-run training program for one hour a day, four days a week, is representative of many of the longitudinal studies. Following the training period, the subjects exhibited small but statistically significant increases in left ventricular end-diastolic dimension, wall thickness, and left ventricular mass (Figure 5-5 and 5-6). The average change for left ventricular diastolic dimension for all of the longitudinal studies involving short-term endurance training was only a 4.4% increase. Similarly, the average increases for interventricular septal thickness, posterior wall thickness, and left ventricular mass were 2.4%, 5% and 16% respectively. These changes are considerably less than those observed in highly trained athletes compared to controls (Figure 5-2) and would correspond to the modest increase in maximal oxygen consumption (average increase 19%) demonstrated in the short-term studies. Three of these longitudinal studies[58, 59, 62] found no significant changes in any

of the variables measured by echocardiography. Even in the studies in which significant changes were noted, the absolute values for cardiac dimensions were generally within normal limits. Similar results were found in the studies utilizing short-term isometric training.[61, 66, 69]

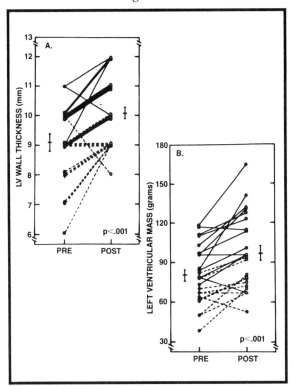

Figure 5-6: **Wall Thickness and Mass** – Changes in (A) left ventricular (LV) wall thickness and (B) left ventricular mass in response to exercise training. (From DeMaria AN, et al.[57] By permission of the American Heart Association, Inc.)

A smaller number of studies have investigated the effects of vigorous exercise training on cardiac structure in subjects who were already either participating in organized training programs or who had done so in the recent past. Ehsani and colleagues[70] studied eight competitive swimmers who had not been involved in any regular exercise activity for two to seven months. During and following a nine-week period of endurance training, echocardiographically determined cardiac dimensions were obtained. Mean left ventricular end-diastolic dimension increased by 5.2 mm (11%) after only one week of training and remained elevated throughout the remainder of the training

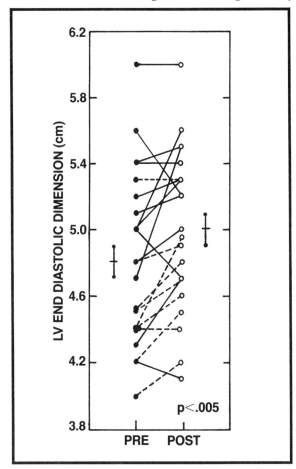

Figure 5-5: **Before and After Exercise Training** – Changes in left ventricular (LV) end-diastolic dimension in response to an 11-week exercise program. Values are demonstrated for both the pre-training and post-training periods. Side bars indicate the mean value and standard error of the mean for the group of 24 subjects. (From DeMaria AN, et al.[57] By permission of the American Heart Association, Inc.)

period (Figure 5-7). Mean left ventricular posterior wall thickness increased by 0.7 mm (7%) by the end of the training period, but unlike left ventricular dimension, did not display the rapid increase during the initial stages of training (Figure 5-7).

Similar results were reported in another study[71] of 11 female swimmers who underwent M-mode echocardiography before and 13 weeks into the swimming season. Small but statistically significant increases in left ventricular end-diastolic dimension, posterior wall thickness, and left ventricular mass were observed following the training period. These effects were observed even though the subjects were physically active prior to the start of their training.

Studies in oarsmen during training[33] have confirmed the rapidity with which changes in cardiac dimensions may occur. However, not all studies have found changes in cardiac dimensions following short-term training. In a group of 12 young women studied before and after participation in an endurance running program, no changes were found in left ventricular chamber size, wall thickness, or left ventricular mass following training.[72] There was also no change in maximal oxygen consumption, indicating a relatively high level of fitness at the beginning of the study.

Effects of Age

The influence of age on the training effect has been investigated in a small number of longitudinal studies. Increases in left ventricular posterior wall thickness and left ventricular mass were found in six- and seven-year-old children following an eight-month aerobic exercise program.[73] A study of 13-year-old canoeist boys[74] demonstrated significant increases in left ventricular end-diastolic dimension, wall thickness, and left ventricular mass when compared to control subjects over a three-year period.

Conversely, short-term training studies in older subjects (mean ages 37 years[58] and 40 years[59, 64]) did not demonstrate any changes in cardiac dimensions following training. These observations suggest that the ability of the left ventricle to adapt to the hemodynamic changes produced by training decreases with advancing age. Such an interaction between age and the effects of training on the heart is supported by animal experiments demon-

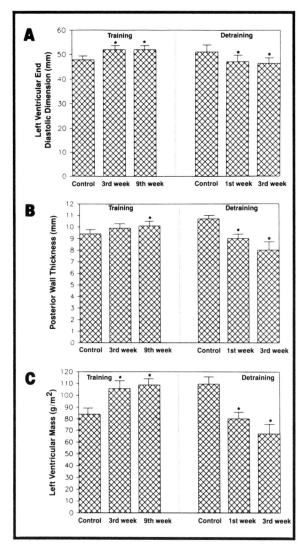

Figure 5-7: Response to Training and Detraining – Serial changes in (A) left ventricular end-diastolic dimension, (B) posterior wall thickness, and (C) left ventricular mass in response to training and detraining. Bars and vertical slashes indicate mean ± standard error. * = p<0.01 (control versus training and detraining period). Reproduced with permission from Ehsani et al.[70]

strating training-induced increases in ventricular weight to be more readily observed in younger rats than in older rats subjected to the same training program.[107]

In summary, several studies have demonstrated increases in cardiac dimensions following short-term training programs. These changes appear to occur rapidly, are small, and generally do not exceed the upper limits of normal. It is likely that the degree of the training effects on echocardiographic dimensions is influenced by the age of the subject, the intensity and duration of the training program, and the physiological state of the subject at the time of beginning training.

Studies of Deconditioning

Athletic conditioning appears to have a small but definite effect on changes in cardiac morphology as assessed with echocardiography. The effect of deconditioning or the cessation of regular athletic training activities has also been investigated. In six competitive runners who stopped training for three weeks,[70] progressive decreases in left ventricular end-diastolic dimension (10%), posterior wall thickness (25%) and left ventricular mass (39%) occurred by the end of the detraining period. As demonstrated with the training effects in this study, the detraining effects also occurred rapidly, with significant decreases in all parameters by the end of the first week of detraining (Figure 5-7).

Similar data were demonstrated in another study[67] of 15 nonathletic subjects before and after a six-week running program. At the end of the six-week period, 10 of the subjects stopped training, while five continued to run. Those who continued to train showed no change in left ventricular diastolic dimension, septal and posterior wall thickness, and left ventricular mass, whereas those subjects who stopped running showed a decline in these values to pre-exercise levels. Reductions in septal and posterior wall thickness were also found in competitive cyclists during the resting season as compared to the competitive season.[39] These changes occurred despite the fact that the cyclists continued to be physically active during the resting season.

Finally, Hickson and associates[65] demonstrated that continued training at reduced levels can prevent the regression of training effects on cardiac dimensions. They studied normally active subjects before and after a 10-week cycling program. All subjects had significant increases in left ventricular diastolic dimension, wall thickness, and left ventricular mass at the end of the training period. Following a subsequent 15-week period during which training was reduced by two-thirds, no significant regression in the echocardiographic

variables was observed. Interestingly, maximal oxygen uptake also remained at the same level following the reduced training period. This suggests that cardiac manifestations of the training effect may be maintained with relatively low levels of exercise.

Effects of Long-Term Exercise Training

Many athletes engage in long-term training programs that may span from early childhood or adolescence well into the adult years. Whether this particularly prolonged exercise training has cumulative effects on cardiac structure has been assessed in a small number of studies using echocardiography. One group[25] studied professional bicyclists in three different age groups: 20 to 29 years (average of five years training), 30 to 39 years (average of 14 years training), and 40 to 49 years (average of 27 years training). Compared to age-matched sedentary controls, all athletes had similar increases in left ventricular end-diastolic dimension; however, only the bicyclists in the 40 to 49-year-old group demonstrated significant increases in interventricular septal and left ventricular posterior wall thickness.

Other researchers[33] studied 14 senior oarsmen who had completed at least one prior rowing season, and nine freshman oarsmen beginning their first season of competition. At the beginning of the seven-month rowing season, the senior oarsmen demonstrated significantly larger left ventricular end-diastolic dimension, interventricular septal thickness, and posterior wall thickness than the freshman oarsmen and nonathletic controls. By the end of the rowing season, both freshman and senior oarsmen demonstrated greater left ventricular dimensions and wall thickness than controls, but the senior oarsmen still had a greater left ventricular dimension and septal thickness than the freshmen.

Another study[108] compared echocardiographic findings in 14 junior (average age 17 years) and 15 senior (average age 25 years) basketball players. Although the duration of training was not stated, the senior players were found to have larger left ventricular end-diastolic dimensions, but no difference in wall thickness as compared to the junior players. Similar findings were demonstrated in a comparison of older endurance athletes (average age 59 years) with younger athletes (average

age 22 years).[27] The findings of these studies suggest that the effects of many years of athletic competition may have a cumulative effect on alterations in cardiac structure.

Acute Effects of Exercise in the Athlete

The cardiac response to exercise in normal subjects has been well characterized. The general response to all types of exercise consists of an increase in heart rate, blood pressure, and cardiac output. Changes in left ventricular end-diastolic volume in response to *isotonic* exercise are variable, but usually there is an increase or no change in this parameter. There is a consistently significant decrease in left ventricular end-systolic volume, with a resultant increase in left ventricular ejection fraction.[109, 110] Both the Frank-Starling mechanism and increased contractility appear to play roles in augmenting cardiac output during exercise. In contrast, hemodynamic changes produced by *isometric* exercise consist primarily of increases in heart rate and blood pressure. Left ventricular end-diastolic volume and ejection fraction are unchanged or slightly decreased.[109, 111, 112]

As has been previously discussed, long-term exercise training results in cardiac structural changes as defined by echocardiography. Whether or not the larger left ventricular dimensions and left ventricular mass present in endurance-trained athletes allow for further changes in cardiac dimension in response to exercise has been investigated as well.[18, 46, 60, 80] A group led by Cahill[18] studied 14 endurance-trained athletes and 7 controls with M-mode echocardiography before and immediately after submaximal upright bicycle ergometry. The athletes had slightly, but not significantly, larger left ventricular end-diastolic dimensions at rest when compared to sedentary controls. However, following exercise, the athletes had significantly larger end-diastolic dimensions than controls, resulting in larger stroke volumes in the athlete group.

Another study,[80] using two-dimensional echocardiographic imaging during upright bicycle exercise in endurance-trained athletes, confirmed that the trained athlete was able to augment stroke volume during exercise by increasing left ventricular end-diastolic volume. Furthermore, the study demonstrated that this effect was most pro-

nounced in the highly trained competitive athlete. Thus, it appears that even though endurance-training results in an increase in left ventricular end-diastolic volume at rest, the highly trained athlete is capable of further increasing end-diastolic volume to augment exercise performance.

Extreme Exercise

The effects of extremely exhaustive exercise on left ventricular performance in the athlete have been investigated in four studies.[56, 113-115] Niemela and colleagues[113] studied 13 ultraendurance athletes before and after participation in a competitive 24-hour run and found a decrease in echocardiographic parameters of left ventricular systolic function after the race. Fractional shortening and mean velocity of circumferential shortening fell by 16% and 9%, respectively, from pre-race values. These changes occurred despite a lower post-race systolic blood pressure. Even though the left ventricular end-diastolic dimension was reduced by 7% after the race and hence may have contributed to the reduction in fractional shortening, the decrease in shortening was not correlated with decreases in end-diastolic dimension, but was correlated with increases in end-systolic dimension, suggesting a true depression of myocardial contractility. Furthermore, the abnormalities of systolic function returned to pre-race levels within two to three days.

Another study[114] of 21 athletes participating in a triathlon competition confirmed these findings of a reversible depression of systolic function following an ultraendurance athletic performance. Athletes participating in the triathlon event were found to have a 10% reduction in fractional shortening at race finish. As in the study by Niemela's group[113] the reduction in fractional shortening correlated with increases in end-systolic dimension, but not with decreases in end-diastolic dimension and returned to normal within one to two days despite a persistent reduction in end-diastolic dimension. Other researchers[115] studied echocardiographic variables in competitive runners before and after a marathon run of 2.5 to 4 hours duration and did not find changes in fractional shortening. The relatively short exercise duration compared to the studies of ultraendurance athletes[113, 114] may explain the inability to demonstrate changes. Indeed, Niemela's study[113] demonstrated a negative correlation between the velocity of circumferential shortening and the distance completed, suggesting an association between depression of myocardial contractility and the distance run.

The effect of exhaustive exercise on diastolic function also has been studied with echocardiography. Studies using digitized M-mode echocardiography[56] and Doppler echocardiography[114] both demonstrated abnormalities in left ventricular diastolic function following extremely exhaustive exercise. As with the changes in systolic function indexes, the depression of diastolic function indexes returned to baseline within one to two days of recovery. Thus, it appears that prolonged, extremely exhaustive exercise, even in highly trained athletes, results in reversible abnormalities of both systolic and diastolic left ventricular performance. The clinical implications of this "cardiac fatigue" over many years of such competition remain to be established.

Significance of Changes in the Athletic Heart: Differentiation from Pathologic Conditions

As discussed previously, the structural changes noted by echocardiography in the athlete's heart are relatively small in comparison to those seen in patients with significant valvular disease or primary myocardial disease. However, occasionally, confusion may arise in the differentiation of "physiologic" changes associated with athletic training from "pathologic" changes seen in a variety of disease states. The most common form of heart disease with which this occurs is hypertrophic cardiomyopathy. When this problem arises, additional information such as family history[116] or the response of left ventricular hypertrophy to a period of deconditioning[117] may be helpful. Nevertheless, sometimes a definite distinction between physiologic and pathologic changes cannot be made and continued follow-up is necessary.

The relationship of the changes in cardiac morphology in athletes to other cardiac abnormalities has also been investigated. An abnormal S-T segment response to exercise was found in 7 of 75 isometrically trained athletes.[41] All of these subjects were less than 30 years of age and asymptomatic. Five of the seven athletes who had positive electrocardiographic changes underwent exercise radionuclide angiography, which demonstrated normal global and regional left ventricular function. Hence, the possibility of coronary artery disease as a cause of the exercise electrocardiographic changes was very unlikely. However, a relationship *was* found between the presence of increased left ventricular mass in the athletes and the electrocardiographic changes seen with exercise, suggesting that the increased left ventricular mass may contribute to the electrocardiographic changes. Similar results were found in a study of older endurance athletes (mean age of 56 years).[118]

Another group[119] studied the occurrence of ventricular ectopic activity in 40 endurance athletes using 24-hour continuous electrocardiographic monitoring. No relation was found between any echocardiographic parameter, including left ventricular mass, and the presence of ventricular ectopy. This is in contrast to findings in patients with left ventricular hypertrophy secondary to hypertension[120] or hypertrophic cardiomyopathy,[121] in which the occurrence of complex ventricular arrhythmias is strongly associated with the magnitude of left ventricular hypertrophy. Thus, it appears that the "physiologic" hypertrophy associated with athletic conditioning does not necessarily predispose the athlete to any adverse consequence.

Implications for Screening in the Competitive Athlete

Although uncommon, sudden death in the seemingly healthy athlete does occur. Previous studies have determined that underlying cardiovascular disease, usually unsuspected, is responsible for the vast majority of these sudden, unexpected deaths.[122, 123] In the young athlete, the most common cause of sudden death appears to be hypertrophic cardiomyopathy, while in the older athlete (>35 years) sudden death is usually due to atherosclerotic coronary artery disease (Table 5-2). However, other abnormalities, including congenital abnormalities of the coronary arteries, Marfan's syndrome with aortic dilation, mitral valve prolapse, and aortic valve stenosis are also potential causes for sudden cardiac death in the athlete. Many of these abnormalities can be detected with echocardiographic techniques and therefore it is appropriate to discuss the role that echocardiography may play as a tool in preventing sudden death in the athlete.

Table 5-2
Causes of Sudden Death in Competitive Athletes

Less than 35 years old	
Hypertrophic cardiomyopathy	48%
Idiopathic left ventricular hypertrophy	18%
Coronary artery anomalies	14%
Coronary heart disease	10%
Aortic rupture	7%
Unexplained	3%
More than 35 years old	
Coronary heart disease	>80%

Data from Maron et al.[122,123]

• Hypertrophic cardiomyopathy is one of the most common cardiovascular diseases causing sudden death in young athletes.[122, 123] M-mode,[124] and especially two-dimensional, echocardiography[125] is very sensitive and specific in detecting hypertrophic cardiomyopathy when the classic features of an asymmetrically hypertrophied and nondilated left ventricle are present.

Editor's Note: Using a single parasternal long-axis view as a "screening" tool would be very easy to perform by well-trained technicians. – BFW

• Aortic rupture associated with Marfan's syndrome or cystic medial necrosis is an occasional cause of sudden death in young athletes. Echocardiography, especially two-dimensional imaging, is very sensitive in detecting the abnormally dilated aortic root present in this condition.[126]
• Similarly, two-dimensional and Doppler echocardiographic techniques are extremely sensitive in detecting significant aortic valve stenosis,[127, 128] which has the potential of causing sudden cardiac death. However, this condition has not been found to be a significant cause of sudden death in athletes,[122, 123] probably because it is easily detected by cardiac auscultation, so that such subjects are excluded from participation in competitive athletics by physical exam alone.
• Mitral valve prolapse is a common abnormality in the general population, affecting approximately 5% of otherwise healthy subjects.[129] Although echocardiography can detect prolapse of the mitral valve and any associated structural abnormalities such as valve thickening or redundancy, mitral valve prolapse is an extremely rare cause of sudden death in the athletic population.[122, 123]
• Congenital coronary artery anomalies may be detected with two-dimensional echocardiography,[130] but its sensitivity as a screening tool for this disease has not been defined.
• Other causes of sudden death in the athlete, such as primary cardiac electrical abnormalities, are not detectable with echocardiography.

Role in Examining Competitive Athletes

Echocardiography is capable of detecting many of the cardiovascular abnormalities responsible for sudden death in the athlete. Hence, it could conceivably be an excellent screening test in evaluating competitive and noncompetitive athletes. However, the extremely large number of athletes at all levels of competition make the use of echocardiography prohibitively expensive as a general screening tool. Anderson[131] estimated that the cost of echocardiographic screening of all adolescents involved in competitive high school athletics would be in excess of two billion dollars, involve more than 2200 work *years* of technician time, and more than 700 work years of physician time. Furthermore, Epstein and Maron[132] estimated that to identify 10 athletes who have cardiovascular disease capable of causing sudden death, 200,000 athletes would have to be screened with a battery of noninvasive tests, including echocardiography. They also estimated that if 10% of these athletes with cardiovascular disease did indeed die suddenly during or following sports participation, then the screening of 200,000 competitive athletes would result in the identification – and presumably the prevention – of *one* sudden death.[132] Thus, echocardiography is impractical to use as a screening examination in the general athlete population.

On the other hand, echocardiography could potentially serve a useful role in *further* evaluation of selected athletes suspected to be at a higher risk for cardiovascular disease, based on information derived from the initial history and physical examination. Maron and associates[133] addressed this issue by using a screening study consisting of personal and family history, physical examination, and 12 lead electrocardiography to evaluate 501 collegiate athletes in an attempt to determine the feasibility of detecting cardiovascular disease. Of the 501 study subjects, 102 had at least one positive finding on the initial screening studies and 90 of these underwent further evaluation with echocardiography. Fourteen (15%) of the 90 athletes had echocardiographically mild mitral valve prolapse without mitral regurgitation, and three athletes had mildly increased thickness of the anterior interventricular septum without systolic anterior motion of the mitral valve or end-systolic cavity obliteration. In addition, one subject was found to have mild systemic hypertension. Thus, using a systematic preparticipation screening program, these authors were unable to identify any athlete who had the cardiac morphologic substrate to pose a significant risk of sudden death.

What then is the role of echocardiography in the screening of athletes for cardiovascular disease? Due to the large number of subjects participating in athletics and the low prevalence of significant cardiac disease in this population, routine echocardiographic screening is impractical. When historical clues (chest discomfort, presyncope or syncope, palpitations, dyspnea, family history of sudden death or unexplained heart disease) or abnormal physical findings (heart murmur, irregular rhythm, oculoskeletal manifestations of Marfan's syndrome) are present, then further noninvasive evaluation is indicated.

However, even this approach is not perfect, as the use of the history and physical examination as an initial screening tool has the potential to miss some potentially important cardiac problems. For example, patients with nonobstructive hypertrophic cardiomyopathy often have no or only a soft murmur[134] and thus would not necessarily be detected by physical examination. Furthermore, declaring a subject as being at "low risk" of sudden death, even after noninvasive evaluation, refers only to a low probability of sudden death and cannot entirely exclude its possibility.[132] Despite these problems, when cardiac disease is suspected, further investigation is warranted prior to participation in athletics.

Summary and Recommendations

Echocardiography has provided a unique tool for investigation of the effects of exercise training on the cardiovascular system. Results of echocardiographic studies have demonstrated that long-term athletic training produces small, but predictable changes in ventricular mass. The structural changes accompanying exercise training are generally still within the normal range and do not appear to have a deleterious effect on left ventricular systolic or diastolic function at rest or during exercise. The cardiac morphologic changes depend somewhat on the type of athletic training, with ventricular dilation predominating in endurance-trained athletes and increases in wall thickness predominating in strength-trained athletes.

These effects of exercise on cardiac structure appear to occur rapidly after a period of intensive training and to reverse rapidly after a period of deconditioning. The effect of vigorous exercise training over many years or of repeated episodes of prolonged exhaustive exercise on cardiac structure and function are incompletely defined, but to date there is no evidence of a permanent deleterious effect to the athlete. Knowledge of the "physiologic" effects of exercise training on cardiac structure and function is important for interpreting the results of the examination and for avoiding labeling an athlete as "abnormal" based on echocardiography alone.

References

1. Henschen S: Skilauf und Skiwettlauf. Eine medizinische. Mitt Med Klink Uppsala 2:15, 1899.

2. Beckner GL, Winsor T: Cardiovascular adaptions to prolonged physical effort. *Circulation* 9:835, 1954.

3. Stein PD, Lewinson H, Potts KH: Cardiac size and left ventricular performance. Lack of correlation with silhouette measurement. *JAMA* 229: 1614, 1974.

4. Lichtman J, et al: Electrocardiogram of the athlete. Alterations simulating those of organic heart disease. *Arch Intern Med* 132:763, 1973.

5. Reicheck N, Devereux RB: Left ventricular hypertrophy: Relationship of anatomic, echocardiographic and electrocardiographic findings. *Circulation* 63:1391, 1981.

6. Popp RL: M-mode echocardiographic assessment of left ventricular function. *Am J Cardiol* 49:1312, 1982.

7. Henry WL: Evaluation of ventricular function using two dimensional echocardiography. *Am J Cardiol* 49:1319, 1982.

8. Pearlman, AS: Evaluation of ventricular function using doppler echocardiography. *Am J Cardiol* 49:1324, 1982.

9. Morganroth J, et al: Comparative left ventricular dimensions in trained athletes. *Ann Int Med.* 82:521, 1975.

10. Raskoff WJ, Goldman S, Cohn K: The "athletic heart." Prevalence and physiological significance of left ventricular enlargement in distance runners. *JAMA* 236:158, 1976.

11. Roeske WR, et al: Noninvasive evaluation of ventricular hypertrophy in professional athletes. *Circulation* 53:286, 1976.

12. Allen HD, et al: A quantitative echocardiographic study of champion childhood swimmers. *Circulation* 55:142, 1977.

13. Gilbert CA, et al: Echocardiographic study of cardiac dimensions and function in the endurance-trained athlete. *Am J Cardiol* 40:528, 1977.

14. Underwood RH, Schwade JL: Noninvasive analysis of cardiac function of elite distance runners – echocardiography, vectorcardiography, and cardiac intervals. *Ann NY Acad Sci* 301:297, 1977.

15. Zoneraich S, et al: Assessment of cardiac function in marathon runners by graphic noninvasive techniques. *Ann NY Acad Sci* 301:900, 1977.

16. Parker BM, et al: The noninvasive cardiac evaluation of long-distance runners. *Chest* 73:376, 1978.

17. Zeldis SM, Morganroth J, Rubler S: Cardiac hypertrophy in response to dynamic conditioning in female athletes. *J Appl Physiol* 44:849, 1978.

18. Cahill NS, et al: A pilot study on left ventricular dimensions and wall stress before and after submaximal exercise. *Br J Sports Med* 13:122, 1979.

19. Grayevskaya ND et al: Echocardiographic study of sportsmen's hearts. *J Sports Med* 19:365, 1979.

20. Ikäheimo MJ, Palatsi IJ, Takkunen JT: Noninvasive evaluation of the athletic heart: Sprinters versus endurance runners. *Am J Cardiol* 44:24, 1979.

21. Lengyel M, Gyárfás I: The importance of echocardiography in the assessment of left ventricular hypertrophy in trained and untrained schoolchildren. *Acta Cardiol* 34:63, 1979.

22. Blair NL, et al: Echocardiographic assessment of cardiac chamber size and left ventricular function in aerobically trained athletes. *Aust NZ J Med* 10:540, 1980.

23. Cohen JL, et al: The heart of a dancer: Noninvasive cardiac evaluation of professional ballet dancers. *Am J Cardiol* 45:959, 1980.

24. Longhurst JC, et al: Echocardiographic left ventricular masses in distance runners and weight lifters. *J Appl Physiol* 48:154, 1980.

25. Nishimura T, Yamada Y, Kawai C: Echocardiographic evaluation of long-term effects of exercise on left ventricular hypertrophy and function in professional bicyclists. *Circulation* 61:832, 1980.

26. Bekaert I, et al: Non-invasive evaluation of cardiac function in professional cyclists. *Br Heart J* 45:213, 1981.

27. Heath, GW, et al: A physiological comparison of young and older endurance athletes. *J Appl Physiol* 51:634, 1981.

28. Keul J, et al: Effect of static and dynamic exercise on heart volume, contractility, and left ventricular dimensions. *Circ Res* 48 (Suppl 1): I-162, 1981.

29. Mumford M, Prakash R: Electrocardiographic and echocardiographic characteristics of long distance runners. Comparison of left ventricular function with age- and sex-matched controls. *Am J Sports Med* 9:23, 1981.

30. Paulsen W, et al: Left ventricular function in marathon runners: echocardiographic assessment. *J Appl Physiol* 51:881, 1981.

31. Rubal BJ, Rosentswieg J, Hamerly B: Echocardiographic examination of women collegiate softball champions. *Med Sci Sports Exercise* 13:176, 1981.

32. Serra Grima Jr, Doxandabaratz J, Ventura JL: The veteran athlete. An exercise testing electrocardiographic, thorax x-ray, and echocardiography study. *J Sports Med* 21:122, 1981.

33. Wieling W, et al: Echocardiographic dimensions and maximal oxygen uptake in oarsmen during training. *Br Heart J* 46:190, 1981.

34. Menapace FJ, et al: Left ventricular size in competitive weight lifters: an echocardiographic study. *Med Sci Sports Exercise* 14:72, 1982.

35. Purfürst WD, et al: The relationship of left ventricular function and mass in arterial hypertension. An echo and apexcardiographic comparison with sportsmen and controls. *Eur Heart J* 3 (Suppl A):119, 1982.

36. Rost R: The athlete's heart. *Eur Heart J* 3 (Suppl A):193, 1982.

37. Snoeck LHEH, et al: Echocardiographic dimensions in athletes in relation to their training programs. *Med Sci Sports Exercise* 14:428, 1982.

38. Dickhuth HH, et al: Two-dimensional echocardiographic measurements of left ventricular volume and stroke volume of endurance-trained athletes and untrained subjects. *Int J Sports Med* 4:21, 1983.

39. Fagard R, et al: Noninvasive assessment of seasonal variations in cardiac structure and function in cyclists. *Circulation* 67:896, 1983.

40. Karvonen J, et al: Abnormal ECG findings and heart function examined by non-invasive methods in a group of athletes. *J Sports Med* 23:364, 1983.

41. Spirito P, et al: Prevalence and significance of an abnormal S-T segment response to exercise in young athletic population. *Am J Cardiol* 51:1663, 1983.

42. Sugishita Y, et al: Myocardial mechanics of athletic hearts in comparison with diseased hearts. *Am Heart J* 105:273, 1983.

43. Child JS, Barnard RJ, Taw R: Cardiac hypertrophy and function in master endurance runners and sprinters. *J Appl Physiol* 57:176, 1984.

44. Fagard R, et al: Cardiac structure and function in cyclists and runners. Comparative echocardiography study. *Br Heart J* 52:124, 1984.

45. Shapiro LM: Physiological left ventricular hypertrophy. *Br Heart J* 52:130, 1984.

46. Cohen JL, Segal KR: Left ventricular hypertrophy in athletes: an exercise-echocardiographic study. *Med Sci Sports Exercise* 17:695, 1985.

47. Colan SD, et al: Left ventricular diastolic function in elite athletes with physiologic cardiac hypertrophy. *J Am Coll Cardiol* 6:545, 1985.

48. Hauser AM, et al: Symmetric cardiac enlargement in highly trained endurance athletes: A two-dimensional echocardiographic study. *Am Heart J* 109:1038, 1985.

49. Wolfe LA, Martin RP, Seip RL: Absence of left ventricular hypertrophy in elite college basketball players. *Can J Appl Spt Sci* 10:116, 1985.

50. Douglas PS, et al: Left ventricular structure and function by echocardiography in ultraendurance athletes. *Am J Cardiol* 58:805, 1986.

51. Medved R, Fabečić-Sabadi V, Medved V: Echocardiographic findings in children participating in swimming training. *Int J Sports Med* 7:94, 1986.

52. Mickelson JK, et al: Left ventricular dimension and mechanics in distance runners. *Am Heart J* 112:1251, 1986.

53. Pearson, AC et al: Left ventricular diastolic function in weight lifters. *Am J Cardiol* 58:1254, 1986.

54. Colan SD, Sanders SP, Borow KM: Physiologic hypertrophy: Effects on left ventricular systolic mechanics in athletes. *J Am Coll Cardiol* 9:776, 1987.

55. Fagard R, et al: Assessment of stiffness of the hypertrophied left ventricle of bicyclists using left ventricular inflow doppler velocimetry. *J Am Coll Cardiol* 9:1250, 1987.

56. Niemelä K, et al: Impaired left ventricular diastolic function in athletes after utterly strenuous prolonged exercise. *Int J Sports Med* 8:61, 1987.

57. DeMaria AN, et al: Alterations in ventricular mass and performance induced by exercise training in man evaluated by echocardiography. *Circulation* 57:237, 1978.

58. Wolfe LA, et al: Effects of endurance training on left ventricular dimensions in healthy men. *J Appl Physiol* 47:207, 1979.

59. Péronnet F, et al: Electro- and echocardiographic study of the left ventricle in man after training. *Eur J Appl Physiol* 45:125, 1980.

60. Stein RA, et al: The cardiac response to exercise training: Echocardiographic analysis at rest and during exercise. *Am J Cardiol* 46:219, 1980.

61. Kanakis C, Hickson RC: Left ventricular response to a program of lower-limb strength training. *Chest* 78:618, 1980.

62. Thompson PD, et al: Cardiac dimensions and performance after either arm or leg endurance training. *Med Sci Sports Exercise* 13:303, 1981.

63. Adams TD, et al: Noninvasive evaluation of exercise training in college-age men. *Circulation* 64:958, 1981.

64. Perrault H: Left ventricular dimensions following training in young and middle-aged men. *Int J Sports Med* 3:141, 1982.

65. Hickson RC: Reduced training duration effects on aerobic power, endurance, and cardiac growth. *J Appl Physiol* 53:225, 1982.

66. Ricci G, et al: Left ventricular size following endurance, sprint, and strength training. *Med Sci Sports Exercise* 14:344, 1982.

67. Shapiro LM, Smith RG: Effect of training on left ventricular structure and function. An echocardiographic study. *Br Heart J* 50:534, 1983.

68. Landry F, Bouchard C, Dumesnil J: Cardiac dimension changes with endurance training. *JAMA* 254:77, 1985.

69. Lusiani L, et al: Echocardiographic evaluation of the dimensions and systolic properties of the left ventricle in freshman athletes during physical training. *Eur Heart J* 7:196, 1986.

70. Ehsani AA, Hagberg JM, Hickson RC: Rapid changes in left ventricular dimensions and mass in response to physical conditioning and deconditioning. *Am J Cardiol* 42:52, 1978.

71. Lamont LS: Effects of training on echocardiographic dimensions and systolic time intervals in women swimmers. *J Sports Med* 20:397, 1980.

72. Marsh R, et al: Effects of chronic, moderate endurance running on body composition and cardiac structure in women. *J Cardiac Rehab* 3:208, 1983.

73. Geenen DL, et al: Echocardiographic measures in 6 to 7 year old children after an 8 month exercise program. *Am J Cardiol* 49:1990, 1982.

74. Csanády M, et al: Three-year echocardiographic follow-up study on canoeist boys. *Acta Cardiol* 41:413, 1986.

75. Feigenbaum H: Echocardiography, ed 4. Lea and Febiger, Philadelphia, 1986, p 134.

76. Ibid., p 30.

77. Henry WL, Gardin JM, Ware JH: Echocardiographic measurements in normal subjects from infancy to old age. *Circulation* 62:1054, 1980.

78. DeMaria AN, et al: Systematic correlation of cardiac chamber size and ventricular performance determined with echocardiography and alterations in heart rate in normal persons. *Am J Cardiol* 43:1, 1979.

79. Hirshleifer J, et al: Influence of acute alterations in heart rate and systemic arterial pressure on echocardiographic measures of left ventricular performance in normal human subjects. *Circulation* 52:835, 1975.

80. Crawford MH, Petru MA, Rabinowitz C: Effect of isotonic exercise training on left ventricular volume during upright exercise. *Circulation* 72:1237, 1985.

81. Oakley DG, Oakley CM: Significance of abnormal electrocardiograms in highly trained athletes. *Am J Cardiol* 50:985, 1982.

82. Salke RC, Rowland TW, Burke EJ: Left ventricular size and function in body builders using anabolic steroids. *Med Sci Sports Exercise* 17:701, 1985.

83. Henry WL, Clark CE, Epstein SE: Asymmetric septal hypertrophy. Echocardiographic identification of the pathognomonic anatomic abnormality of IHSS. *Circulation* 47:225, 1973.

84. Gibson DG, et al: Echocardiographic features of secondary left ventricular hypertrophy. *Br Heart J* 41:54, 1979.

85. Shapiro LM, Kleinebenne A, McKenna WJ: The distribution of left ventricular hypertrophy in hypertrophic cardiomyopathy: comparison of athletes and hypertensives. *Eur Heart J* 6:967, 1985.

86. Troy BL, Pombo J, Rackley CE: Measurement of left ventricular wall thickness and mass by echocardiography. *Circulation* 45:602, 1972.

87. Devereux RB, Reicheck N: Echocardiographic determination of left ventricular mass in man: Anatomic validation of the method. *Circulation* 55:613, 1977.

88. Granger CB, et al: Rapid ventricular filling in left ventricular hypertrophy: I. Physiologic hypertrophy. *J Am Coll Cardiol* 5:862, 1985.

89. Wolfe LA, Cunningham DA, Boughner DR: Physical conditioning effects on cardiac dimensions: A review of echocardiographic studies. *Can J Appl Spt Sci* 11:66, 1986.

90. Sahn DJ, et al: Recommendations regarding quantitation in M-mode echocardiography: Results of a survey of echocardiographic measurements. *Circulation* 58:1072, 1978.

91. Grossman W, McLaurin LP: Diastolic properties of the left ventricle. *Ann Int Med* 84:316, 1976.

92. Gibson DG and Brown D: Measurement of instantaneous left ventricular dimension and filling rate in man using echocardiography. *Br Heart J* 35:1141, 1973.

93. Rokey R, et al: Determination of parameters of left ventricular diastolic filling with pulsed Doppler echocardiography: comparisons with cineangiography. *Circulation* 71:543, 1985.

94. Snider AR, et al: Doppler evaluation of left ventricular diastolic filling in children with systemic hypertension. *Am J Cardiol* 56:921, 1985.

95. Phillips RA, et al: Doppler echocardiographic analysis of left ventricular filling in treated hypertensive patients. *J Am Coll Cardiol* 9:317, 1987.

96. Maron BJ, et al: Noninvasive assessment of left ventricular diastolic function by pulsed Doppler echocardiography in patients with hypertrophic cardiomyopathy. *J Am Coll Cardiol* 10:733, 1987.

97. Hanrath P, et al: Left ventricular relaxation and filling pattern in different forms of left ventricular hypertrophy: An echocardiography study. *Am J Cardiol* 45:15, 1980.

98. Fifer MA, et al: Early diastolic left ventricular function in children and adults with aortic stenosis. *J Am Coll Cardiol* 5:1147, 1985.

99. Matsuda M, et al: Effect of exercise on left ventricular diastolic filling in athletes and nonathletes. *J Appl Physiol* 55:323, 1983.

100. Shapiro LM, McKenna WJ: Left ventricular hypertrophy: Relation of structure to diastolic function in hypertension. *Br Heart J* 51:637, 1984.

101. McKillop G, Todd IC, Ballantyne D: Increased left ventricular mass in a bodybuilder using anabolic steroids. *Brit J Sports Med* 20:151, 1986.

102. Spirito P, et al: Diastolic abnormalities in patients with hypertrophic cardiomyopathy: relation to magnitude of left ventricular hypertrophy. *Circulation* 72:310, 1985.

103. Fouad FM, Slominski JM, Tarazi RC: Left ventricular diastolic function in hypertension: Relation to left ventricular mass and systolic function. *J Am Coll Cardiol* 3:1500, 1984.

104. Wikman-Coffelt J, Parmley WW, Mason DT: The cardiac hypertrophy process. Analysis of factors determining pathological vs. physiological development. *Circ Res* 45:697, 1979.

105. Epstein M, et al: Great vessel, cardiac chamber, and wall growth patterns in normal children. *Circulation* 51:1124, 1975.

106. Falsetti H, et al: Noninvasive evaluation of left ventricular function in trained bicyclists. *J Sports Med* 22:199, 1982.

107. Bloor CM, Pasyk S, Leon AS: Interaction of age and exercise on organ and cellular development. *Am J Pathol* 58:185, 1970.

108. Csanády M, Forster T, Hogye M: Comparative echocardiographic study of junior and senior basketball players. *Int J Sports Med* 7:128, 1986.

109. Crawford MH, White DH, Amon KW: Echocardiographic evaluation of left ventricular size and performance during handgrip and supine and upright bicycle exercise. *Circulation* 59:1188, 1979.

110. Poliner LR, et al: Left ventricular performance in normal subjects: A comparison of the responses to exercise in the upright and supine positions. *Circulation* 62:528, 1980.

111. Laird WP, Fixler DE, Huffines FD: Cardiovascular response to isometric exercise in normal adolescents. *Circulation* 59:651, 1979.

112. Paulsen WJ, et al: Ventricular response to isometric and isotonic exercise: Echocardiographic assessment. *Br Heart J* 42:521, 1979.

113. Niemelä KO, et al: Evidence of impaired left ventricular performance after an uninterrupted competitive 24 hour run. *Circulation* 70:350, 1984.

114. Douglas PS, et al: Cardiac fatigue after prolonged exercise. *Circulation* 6:1206, 1987.

115. Perrault H, et al: Echocardiographic assessment of left ventricular performance before and after marathon running. *Am Heart J* 112:1026, 1986.

116. Maron BJ: Structural features of the athlete heart as defined by echocardiography. *J Am Coll Cardiol* 7:190, 1986.

117. Perna GP, et al: Hypertrophic cardiomyopathy and inadequate septal hypertrophy in athletes. *J Sports Cardiol* 1:96, 1984.

118. Lie H, Ihlen H, Rootwelt K: Significance of a positive exercise ECG in middle-aged and old athletes as judged by echocardiographic, radionuclide and follow-up findings. *Eur Heart J* 6:615, 1985.

119. Palatini P, et al: Prevalence and possible mechanisms of ventricular arrhythmias in athletes. *Am Heart J* 110:560, 1985.

120. McLenachan JM, et al: Ventricular arrhythmias in patients with hypertensive left ventricular hypertrophy. *N Engl J Med* 317:787, 1987.

121. Spirito P, Watson RM, Maron BJ: Relation between extent of left ventricular hypertrophy and occurrence of ventricular tachycardia in hypertrophic cardiomyopathy. *Am J Cardiol* 60:1137, 1987.

122. Maron BJ, et al: Sudden death in young athletes. *Circulation* 62:218, 1980.

123. Maron BJ, Epstein SE, Roberts WC: Causes of sudden death in competitive athletes. *J Am Coll Cardiol* 7:204, 1986.

124. Maron BJ, Epstein SE: Hypertrophic cardiomyopathy: Recent observations regarding the specificity of three hallmarks of the disease: Asymmetric septal hypertrophy, septal disorganization and systolic anterior motion of the anterior mitral leaflet. *Am J Cardiol* 45:141, 1980.

125. Maron BJ, et al: Hypertrophic cardiomyopathy with unusual locations of left ventricular hypertrophy undetectable by M-mode echocardiography: Identification by wide-angle two-dimensional echocardiography. *Circulation* 63:409, 1981.

126. Come PC, et al: Echocardiographic assessment of cardiovascular abnormalities in the Marfan syndrome. *Am J Med* 74:465, 1983.

127. Weyman AE, et al: Cross-sectional echocardiographic assessment of the severity of aortic stenosis in children. *Circulation* 55:773, 1977.

128. Hatle L, Angelsen BA, Tromsdal A: Non-invasive assessment of aortic stenosis by Doppler ultrasound. *Br Heart J* 43:284, 1980.

129. Jeresaty RM: Mitral valve prolapse: Definition and implications in athletes. *J Am Coll Cardiol* 7:231, 1986.

130. Caldwell RL, et al: Two-dimensional echocardiographic differentiation of anomalous left coronary artery from congestive cardiomyopathy. *Am Heart J* 106:710, 1983.

131. Anderson TM: Echocardiographic screening of the athletic adolescent. *Pediatrician* 13:165, 1986.

132. Epstein SE, Maron BJ: Sudden death and the competitive athlete: Perspectives on preparticipation screening studies. *J Am Coll Cardiol* 7:220, 1986.

133. Maron BJ, et al: Results of screening a large group of intercollegiate competitive athletes for cardiovascular disease. *J Am Coll Cardiol* 10:1214, 1987.

134. Epstein SE, et al: Asymmetric septal hypertrophy. *Ann Int Med* 81:650, 1974.

CHAPTER 6

EXERCISE TREADMILL TESTING IN ATHLETES

Lawrence D. Rink, MD

Clinical Professor of Medicine
Indiana University School of Medicine
Team Physician, Indiana University Basketball
Team Physician, United States Olympic Team

Donald M. Knowlan, MD

Team Physician
Washington Redskins
National Football League
Professor of Medicine, Georgetown University
Medical Center

Editor's Note: The following chapter on exercise testing authored by Drs. Rink and Knowlan is not designed for routine screening of high school, college, or professional athletes, but simply outlines the authors' views and experience in reference to athletes. It includes suggestions of how exercise testing can be done, even in those athletes who have binary heart disease. – WPH

Exercise testing as a screening procedure in athletes has been limited by lack of adequate personnel to monitor the test, lack of appropriate facilities, the cost of the procedure, and lack of knowledge concerning the need and benefits. The American College of Cardiology released guidelines for exercise testing in September of 1986,[1] and there was no specific mention of indications for testing athletes. In fact, they described exercise testing to evaluate asymptomatic, apparently healthy men or women with no risk factors for coronary artery disease as a Class III procedure, with Class III defined as "conditions for which there is general agreement that exercise testing is of little or no value, inappropriate or contraindicated by risk." In spite of this, there is general agreement among coaches, exercise physiolo-

gists, athletes, and many physicians that exercise testing can be valuable and does have a role in evaluating athletes, which we will outline in this chapter.[2-5] The majority of articles written about exercise testing in athletes have involved research in the area of aerobic and anaerobic metabolism.

Editor's Note: Exercise testing is not necessary in the great majority of athletes of high school, college and professional levels. However, if in the initial screening there is any question or indication of underlying heart disease, exercise testing can then be employed as appropriate for further workup. Of course, exercise testing is a prerogative of the physician or staff of a particular team or organization. Thus, for some athletic organizations, it may be routine. – WPH

General Considerations in Exercise Testing

Evaluation of Athletes Prior to Exercise Testing

Appropriate pre-test evaluation is essential for proper design, performance, and overall evaluation of an exercise test in an athlete. It is mandatory that the physician understand the type of exercise and intensity of exercise that the athlete will be performing in his or her sport. The exact purpose of the exercise test must also be understood. A history of family health problems, previous cardiopulmonary symptoms, musculoskeletal abnormalities, medications, recent infections, and use of caffeine and tobacco are important. Some estimation of the athlete's exercise history and, if possible, an estimation of the athlete's maximum oxygen comsumption (VO_2 max) should be made, based on his exercise pattern and sport.

Editor's Note: Probably the most difficult serious cardiac pathology to diagnose on routine screening is coro-

nary artery disease, either congenital or acquired, especially in athletes 30 years of age or younger. Symptoms of chest discomfort, dizziness, or palpitations would certainly justify exercise testing. A routine electrocardiogram, which can be obtained at a minimal expense and effort, also might show abnormalities that would justify exercise testing. – WPH

Informed Consent

Like any other patient, athletes should sign an informed consent prior to exercise testing, though the risk is small. If all exercise tests in varied populations are taken into consideration, the risk is approximately one death per 10,000 tests. The risk in athletes is surely much less. In fact, no case of sudden death in athletes during exercise testing has been reported in the literature. Even more important is taking time to explain to the athlete the purpose of the test and the testing protocol. Although athletes are almost always healthy and usually agile, they are often very apprehensive. Considerable demonstration and explanation time is needed to get a maximum test from the athlete.

Contraindications to Exercise Testing

The same contraindications for exercise testing of the general population apply to symptomatic athletes:

1. Severe aortic stenosis.
2. Uncontrolled ventricular dysrhythmia
3. Uncontrolled atrial dysrhythmia (which compromises cardiac function)
4. Suspected or known dissecting aneurysm
5. Active or strongly suspected myocarditis
6. Thrombophlebitis
7. Acute infection
8. Third-degree heart block

Personnel Required for Monitoring the Tests

The ideal exercise test performed on an athlete utilizes the team trainer, team physician, and a knowledgeable exercise testing technician and physician. If a maximal test is to be performed, an experienced physician should always be present. The American College of Sports Medicine states that maximal testing done for individuals at age 35 or above with no symptoms or risk factors should be done under a physician's supervision.[7] Submaximal testing in apparently healthy individuals of any age can be done without physician attendance, if the testing is carried out by well trained individuals who are experienced in monitoring exercise tests and in handling emergencies.

Instructions to Athletes

1. The athlete should be fasting for two to three hours before the test.
2. The athlete should wear shoes and clothes similar to what he or she would wear in competition (when practical).
3. If the athlete is taking a medication that would alter the blood pressure or heart rate response to exercise, it is preferable to withhold that medication for 48 hours. The athlete should discuss this with his personal physician.
4. The athlete should be encouraged to ask questions prior to the testing.
5. If a mouthpiece is used in an effort to measure pulmonary function or gas exchange, a simple list of hand signals should be provided so the athlete can communicate during the examination.

Electrocardiographic Monitoring Leads

Although a single lead, V5, may be adequate for monitoring most athletes, monitoring three leads continuously will allow for a more accurate evaluation for ischemia and arrhythmias. One method involves monitoring lead II to look at the inferior wall, lead V1 or V2 to look at the anterior septal area, and lead V5, which lies over the anterior lateral portion of the heart. A complete resting 12-lead electrocardiogram should be obtained prior to testing the athlete and preferably would be available to be consulted at any time during the test.

Indications for Exercise Testing of Athletes

Evaluation of Symptoms

Electrocardiographically monitored exercise tests of athletes to evaluate their symptoms of chest pain, syncope, pre-syncope, dyspnea, palpitations, and fatigue are the same as those of the general population. The exercise test, which

+---+
| **Table 6-1** |
| **Indications for Stopping an Exercise Test** |
| |
| 1. Athlete requests to stop |
| 2. Failure of the monitoring system |
| 3. Progressive angina |
| 4. Sustained supraventricular tachycardia |
| 5. Ventricular tachycardia |
| 6. Exercise-induced left or right bundle branch block, unless you are aware this is present in the athlete and have evaluated this in the past |
| 7. A significant drop (>10 mmHg) of the systolic blood pressure |
| 8. Light-headedness, confusion, ataxia, pallor, cyanosis, nausea, or signs of severe peripheral circulatory insufficiency |
| 9. Unexplained, inappropriate bradycardia |
| 10. Onset of second- or third-degree heart block |
| 11. Inability to keep up with the exercise protocol |
+---+

should be maximal, is terminated for the same reasons as a test on any other person would be discontinued. (Table 6-1).

Criteria for Positive Treadmill Test

Both clinical and laboratory studies confirm the high degree of reserve in the normal coronary artery blood flow capacity. These studies indicate that coronary atherosclerosis that obstructs the coronary artery lumen ≤ 50% is unlikely to be responsible for ischemia, even during moderate exertion. Thus, exercise testing to detect moderate coronary atherosclerosis is relatively insensitive. It is important to enhance this test by the use of multiple modes of observation (blood pressure and heart rate response, exercise tolerance, symptoms) and evaluation of multiple high-quality electrocardiographic leads.[8]

• **Chest Discomfort** – Chest discomfort is not as sensitive an indicator of myocardial ischemia as ST segment depression,[9] occurring only half as frequently as ST segment depression when ischemia is present. However, when typical angina pectoris does occur during testing, it is a valuable finding and definitely increases the likelihood that significant coronary artery disease is present. In our experience, athletes often have chest wall pain during strenuous exercise. This pain clearly must be differentiated from ischemic pain.

• **ST Segment** – The occurrence and disappearance of a negative displacement of a flat or downward sloping ST segment corresponding to the increase in exercise have been a hallmark of ischemia since the introduction of exercise tests. The theory is that myocardial perfusion is inadequate to meet the increased oxygen requirements during exercise. The subendocardial area becomes ischemic and a diastolic electrical potential is produced, characterized by a vector that is opposite in direction to the major QRS vector.

Hence, there is ST segment depression in leads with dominant R waves.[8] The most common type of ST segment displacement begins at the J point (QRS-ST junction) and the ST segment is flat for the first 80 milliseconds of its duration. It is common for this initially to be up-sloping before it becomes flat, and then may eventually even be down-sloping. As an interpretive criterion, the development of .1 millivolt (1 mm) or more of flat ST segment displacement in a standard electrocardiographic lead is considered positive for ischemia. This ST segment depression returns to baseline shortly after exercise, making it imperative for continuous electrocardiographic measurement if ischemia detection is one of the goals of the exercise test.

J point depression with an up-sloping ST segment may be a normal response to exercise in athletes. However, J point depression >2 mm during exercise usually signifies ischemia.[10] Also, the earlier the ST segment depression occurs in the exercise protocol and the longer that it persists post-exercise, the more likely it will be associated with more severe coronary artery disease and the less likely it will be a false-positive test.[11]

It might be assumed that since increased left ventricular mass has been associated with ST-T wave changes on the electrocardiogram,[12] athletes with increased left ventricular mass would be more likely to have an abnormal ST segment response to exercise. Spirito and colleagues looked at this exact problem.[13] Seven of 75 isometrically trained (more likely to have increased left ventricular (LV) mass) athletes without evidence of heart disease had a positive exercise treadmill test. This was defined as an ST segment depression ≥1 mm from the J point, with horizontal or negative slope for a duration of ≥0.08 seconds during or immediately after exercise. Five of these seven athletes had radionuclide angiography at rest and with exercise, each of which was normal. They concluded that the prevalence of "false-positive" exercise tests in their athletic population was slightly higher, but did not differ significantly, from those in a nonathletic youthful control group.

They also noted that the mean left ventricular mass in athletes with a positive ST segment response to exercise was greater but not significantly different from the left ventricular mass in athletes with normal exercise test results.

Several investigators have described ST-T wave abnormalitites in athletes' resting electrocardiograms, which would become normal with maximal exertion or sympathetic maneuvers.[14, 15] In general, athletes with abnormal baseline electrocardiograms should have less reliable tests for detection of ischemia.

Although the classic ST segment depression of ischemia is the most reliable predictor of coronary artery disease, other factors, such as intensity of cardiac work where ischemia occurs, blood pressure response, heart rate response, and maximal work capacity, are all parameters that should be considered when interpreting the exercise stress test in an athlete. However, generally all athletes tested will have average or above-average exercise tolerance, normal heart rate response to exercise, and normal blood pressure response to exercise. These parameters should be compared to other similarly trained athletes to determine a normal response.

• **Blood Pressure Response** – The normal blood pressure response to exercise in athletes and nonathletes alike is a progressive rise in systolic pressure with increase in exercise intensity and very little change in the diastolic pressure. A pathological fall in systolic blood pressure (>10 mm Hg) during exercise is a highly specific sign of severe coronary artery disease;[16] however, this change is insensitive and unlikely to be found in athletes.

• **Heart Rate Response** – The normal heart rate response of an athlete to exercise is similar to that of other individuals (gradual increased rate proportional to work intensity). The resting heart rate may be as low as 40 beats per minute. Normal resting heart rates in endurance trained athletes are significantly lower than average for age and may be in the low 40's per minute. However, one should not be surprised if well-conditioned athletes have a resting heart rate in the 70s or 80s prior to a treadmill test, since they are usually anxious about the impending exam. Maximal exercise heart rates are slightly less in trained athletes, averaging 5 to 7 beats per minute lower than that of sedentary individuals in each age range.[6] Maximal heart rates for male and female college basketball players have averaged 188 +/− 6.8 and 186.9 +/− 7.1, respectively. Another study found the mean maximal heart rate of female collegiate field hockey, volleyball, and basketball players and swimmers to be 195 beats/minute. In one laboratory, all male college athletes tested over 10 years had maximal heart rates above 170 beats per minute; any maximal heart rate less than that should be considered significantly abnormal.

Statistical Analysis of Exercise Tests

An exercise test interpreted as abnormal in a person who is found not to have disease is called a false-positive test. The most likely cause for this occurrence in athletes is an increase in left ventricular mass, as already mentioned.[13] There are multiple other causes of false-positive tests. The probability of a false-positive test is related to the *specificity* of the test. For example, if 100 people are free of disease and an exercise test is normal in 90 of the 100, then the specificity of the test is 90%. The other 10% are false-positives. Specificity is the percentage of times a test gives a normal response when those without disease are tested.

On the other hand, a false-negative test result will relate to the *sensitivity* of the test. For example, if there are 100 people with disease and the test correctly identifies 90 of those people by their having an abnormal test, the sensitivity of the test is 90% and there are 10% false-negatives. Sensitivity is the percentage of times a test gives an abnormal response when those with disease are tested.

Sensitivity and specificity are inversely related. In general, a positive exercise test in a college athlete is relatively specific, but would have a low sensitivity and very low predictive value. The predictive value of an abnormal test is the percentage of individuals with an abnormal test who have disease. The relative risk of an abnormal test response is the chance of having disease if the test is abnormal, compared to having disease if the test is normal. It has been well established that the predictive value and the relative risk in electrocardiographically monitored treadmill testing of athletes should be very low.

The Athlete with a Positive Test

An athlete with a definitely positive treadmill test for ischemia (identified by ≥1 mm of ST segment depression lasting longer than 30 seconds post-exercise) should be evaluated as any other patient. Before being allowed to participate in competitive athletics, he or she must have a complete history and physical examination, echocardiographic evaluation, and blood tests (CBC, T4, potassium, cholesterol, and fasting blood sugar). He also needs an indirect or direct evaluation of his coronary anatomy, i.e., thallium treadmill testing, exercise echocardiography, and/or coronary angiography. There have not been any long-term follow-up studies of athletes with a positive treadmill test, but a young, asymptomatic, average male with a positive treadmill exam has a 10 times greater probability of developing symptomatic coronary artery disease than such a male with a negative exercise test.[17]

Arrhythmias in Athletes

Palpitations described by the athlete at rest, during normal activity, or competing require further evaluation. The starting point, of course, is the history, physical exam, and resting electrocardiogram.

It is clear that certain arrhythmias are the result of the physiologic response to training, such as sinus bradycardia, sinus arrhythmia, and first-degree AV block.[18] These rhythms, which most likely are due to increased vagal tone, disappear during exercise and do not require further evaluation. Athletes with frequent premature ventricular contractions should have treadmill testing, along with Holter monitor evaluation – preferably during their event. If the exercise test, which should resemble the athlete's type and intensity of work, causes a significant increase in the number of premature ventricular beats or results in more complex dysrhythmias such as ventricular tachycardia, the athlete should be withheld from all sports

except those with low dynamic and low static demands. Then a thorough evaluation can be undertaken.

Exercise testing should be performed as part of the evaluation of the following arrhythmias in athletes: atrial fibrillation, atrial flutter, supraventricular tachycardia, Wolff-Parkinson-White syndrome, ventricular tachycardia, second- and third-degree AV block, right bundle branch block, left bundle branch block or congenital long Q-T syndrome.[19]

Two studies[20, 21] using maximal treadmill tests found that the treadmill test failed to predict the frequency and grade of arrhythmias present on 24-hour monitors or during competition. From a review[20] of 10 studies of arrhythmia detection, six with 24-hour Holter monitors, two with treadmill testing, and two during games, it appears that the 24-hour Holter monitor is the most reliable way to find supraventricular and ventricular arrhythmias. Although an electrocardiographically monitored exercise test is not as good as the Holter monitor to detect arrhythmias or to quantitate them, it appears to be the best method of evaluating whether an athlete with arrhythmias can continue to compete safely.

Evaluating Athletes with Known Cardiovascular Disease

Exercise testing can play a major role in determining whether an athlete with a congenital or acquired valvular heart disease, repaired or unrepaired, should participate in competitive sports. The exercise treadmill test, by defining the athlete's maximum oxygen consumption (VO_2 max), may also be able to help categorize which sport and at what competitive level the athlete should be participating.

Mitral valve prolapse is a common problem in the general population[24] and in the collegiate athletic population, and has been reported to be a cause for false-positive exercise tests.[7, 8] Seven of 42 men's varsity basketball players at Indiana University who were evaluated over a period of nine years had mitral valve prolapse, documented by two-dimensional and M-mode echocardiogram. All of these athletes had normal maximal exercise treadmill tests with no significant difference from the other athletes in ST segment change, heart rate and blood pressure response, maximal oxygen consumption (VO_2 max), anaerobic threshold, or frequency of arrhythmias.[25] Musante reported on 80 athletes with mitral valve prolapse, evaluated by ergometric studies, and found no change from matched controls.[26]

• **Hypertension** – The exact role of exercise testing in athletes with hypertension has not been fully defined. It is, of course, mandatory that the blood pressure be controlled prior to allowing an athlete to participate in competitive sports.[27] If an exercise test is undertaken to evaluate the athlete with hypertension, it is important to design a protocol that is likely to simulate the work intensity involved in the athlete's sport. Sports that require a high to moderate static demand are most likely to dramatically increase the athlete's blood pressure.

Prevention of Sudden Death

Sudden death in healthy athletes is uncommon, but when it occurs the primary mechanism is cardiovascular. The most common causes of sudden death in college-age athletes are hypertrophic cardiomyopathy, aortic rupture due to cystic medial necrosis, and congenital coronary artery abnormality.[28] In athletes over 30 years of age, coronary artery disease is the most common cause of sudden, unexpected death.

The exercise treadmill test, as previously noted, is a valuable method of noninvasive testing for coronary artery disease. However, most athletes who die suddenly have no reported symptoms prior to their death.[28] Therefore, exercise testing would have to be included as part of the preparticipation physical examination of the asymptomatic athlete to detect most cases of coronary artery anomaly or premature atherosclerotic coronary artery disease.

As already discussed, there are a large number of false-positive tests in this young population due to the low prevalence of the disease. Also, the cost of this type of examination for all college athletes would be prohibitive. The health history questionnaire should select symptomatic athletes who would require a treadmill test. All athletes with a history of syncope, unusual unexplained fatigue, palpitations, or exercise-induced chest pain require a maximal exercise treadmill exam.

Editor's Note: Since sudden death in athletes above the age of 30 is most commonly due to coronary artery disease, exercise testing should be used more frequently in this age group, since it is apparent that the older the athlete, the more useful exercise testing becomes. For example, a person, in his or her fifties, sixties, or seventies, performing more strenuous athletics would need electrocardiographic and exercise testing much more frequently than a man or woman of teen age or in their twenties. – WPH

Examination of the Athlete Preparticipation

Routine use of electrocardiographically monitored maximal exercise testing as a screening tool in athletes prior to participation in a sport *cannot be recommended*. The main reasons are the cost of the examination (which is unlikely to be supported by the school, university, or insurance policies), the low prevalence of disease that could be detected by treadmill testing in the high school and college-age population, and the time constraints involved in mass screening. If treadmill testing is used in an effort to detect coronary artery disease or anomalies, every effort should be made to improve the sensitivity, specificity, and predictive accuracy of the test.

Exercise Test Protocols

Treadmill Protocols

The most commonly used testing protocols in the United States involve the treadmill and are the Bruce, Balke, and Naughton protocols. Of these, the Bruce protocol is most suited for athletes because of the high level of mets (one met = 3.5 milliliters of oxygen per kilogram per minute) required for the later stages of exercise. The Ellestad protocol is also acceptable for athletes. Tall athletes, however, often have problems with running on high percent grades (>14%), which are required during the higher levels of the Ellestad and Bruce protocols. When these protocols are used in basketball players, for instance, it is not rare to have to abort the test because of an athlete's low back pain.

At treadmill grades >14%, it is difficult for the athlete to run comfortably without holding on or at least using the handrail for balance. Athletes prefer to run on a zero grade at a higher treadmill speed rather than on a lower treadmill speed and a higher percent grade. Except in the most elite runners, however, treadmill speeds above 10 miles an hour are difficult for the athlete to negotiate.

Bicycle Protocols

In Europe, bicycle ergometers are more frequently used than treadmills, both in the exercise laboratory and in clinical practice. Bicycle ergometers have the advantage of being smaller, less expensive and making less noise. With bicycle ergometers the athlete can be in multiple positions, which could help certain handicapped athletes. The ergometer may be used by the hands or the legs, which not only allows testing of different muscle groups, but training for the athlete using different muscle groups at times of injuries. Also, bicycle testing allows for a cleaner electrographic pattern, more accurate blood pressure recording at near-maximal exercise, and additional exercise echocardiographic and Doppler studies. The body weight of the athlete has a much smaller effect on bicycle ergometer performance than on the treadmill. Also, the danger of falling while running on a treadmill at maximum levels of exertion is greater than that of cycling.

Electronically-braked bicycles now can provide a constant workload despite changes in pedaling rate. The bicycle protocols in general involve continuous pedaling at incremental workloads of 25 watts (150 kilogram-meters per minute) for 1 to 3 minute stages. However, in well trained college athletes, incremental workloads of 50 watts may be more practical.

Arm Ergometry

Arm ergometry protocols involve arm cranking at incremental workloads of 10 to 200 watts (60 to 120 kilogram-meters per minute) for two to three minute stages. It is mandatory to place the ECG leads below the clavicles and to take special precaution with the wires. Blood pressures can only be obtained if the athlete takes one arm off the crank.

Summary

Exercise testing offers valuable information about athletes. It has potential value to prevent sudden death in athletes, although this has not been proven. Electrocardiographically-monitored exercise testing in athletes can help rule out coronary artery disease, due either to premature atherosclerosis or anomalous coronary artery anatomy. However, due to the low prevalence of these disease states in young athletes, the predictive accuracy of these tests is very low. The risk of obtaining a false-positive test exists, which may unnecessarily preclude an athlete's participation in a sport or, at the least, require unnecessary and expensive additional tests. Exercise testing as a preparticipation screening test offers many potential advantages. It is not a cost-effective procedure but is one that is valuable if appropriate funds, personnel, and equipment are available.

The personnel interpreting the exercise test must have adequate knowledge about exercise physiology and the reason the test is being performed. Frequently the test will not uncover the athlete's symptom or will have no direct relationship to the athlete's sport. The maximal exercise protocol should resemble the athlete's workload in his or her sport if detection of symptoms or prediction of performance is the goal.

Exercise testing in athletes has its greatest value in the following areas:

• Determining VO_2 max and anaerobic threshold, which allows an accurate exercise prescription to be written for endurance training.

• Evaluating an athlete's symptom that has occurred while participating in his or her sport or while exercising.

• Evaluating an athlete's capability and safety to participate in a sport.

• Comparing the athlete's performance with that of other athletes who have been successful in that sport.

References

1. Schlant RC, et al: A report of the American College of Cardiology/American Heart Association, task force on assessment of cardiovascular procedures (subcommittee on exercise testing). *J Am Coll Cardiol* 8:No 3, 725, 1986.
2. Maron BJ, et al: Sudden death in young athletes. *Circulation* 62:218, 1980.
3. Topaz O and Edwards JE: Pathologic features of sudden death in children, adolescents and young adults. *Chest* 4:476, 1987.
4. Maron BJ, Epstein SE, and Roberts WC: Causes of sudden death in competitive athletes. *J Am Coll Cardiol* 7:204, 1986.
5. Mitchell JH, Maron BJ, and Epstein SE: 16th Bethesda Conference: Cardiovascular abnormalities in the athlete: Recommendations regarding eligibility for competition. *J Am Coll Cardiol* 6:1189, 1985.
6. Saltin B and Astrand PO: Maximal oxygen uptake in athletes. *J Appl Physiol* 23:353, 1967.
7. Blair SN, et al: Guidelines for exercise testing and prescription. Lea and Febiger, Philadelphia, p 1.
8. Sheffield LT: Exercise stress testing. In Braunwald E (ed): Heart Disease, a Textbook of Cardiovascular Medicine. W.B. Saunders Co., Philadelphia, 1988, p 225.
9. Singh BN: A symposium: Detection quantification and clinical significance of silent myocardial ischemia in coronary artery disease. *Am J Cardiol* 58:1B, 1986.
10. Kurita A, Chaitman BR, and Bourassa MG: Significance of exercise-induced junctional ST depression in evaluation of coronary artery disease. *Am J Cardiol* 40:492, 1977.
11. Lozner EC and Morganroth J: New criteria for evaluation of positive exercise tests in asymptomatic patients. *Am J Cardiol* 39:288, 1977.
12. Huston TP, Puffer JC, and Rodney WM: The athletic heart syndrome. *N Engl J Med* 313:24, 1985.
13. Spirito P, et al: Prevalence and significance of an abnormal ST segment response to exercise in a young athletic population. *Am J Cardiol* 51:1663, 1983.
14. Zeppilli P, et al: Comparative electrovectorcardiographic: echocardiographic study in athletes with ST-T wave abnormalities (pseudoischemic patterns). In Lubich T and Venerando A (eds): Sports Cardiology. Aulo-gaggi, Bologna, 1980, p 415.
15. Nishimura T, et al: Noninvasive assessment of T-wave abnormalities in precordial electrocardiograms in middle-aged professional bicyclists. *J Electrocardiol* 14:357, 1981.
16. Morris SN, et al: Incidence and significance of decreases in systolic blood pressure during graded treadmill exercise testing. *Am J Cardiol* 41:221, 1978.
17. Weiner DA: The diagnostic and prognostic significance of an asymptomatic positive exercise test. *Circulation* 75:11-20, 1987.
18. Balady GJ, Cardigen JB, Ryan TJ: Electrocardiogram of the athlete: An analysis of 289 professional football players. *Am J Cardiol* 53:1339, 1984.
19. Zipes DP, et al: 16th Bethesda Conference: Task Force VI: Arrhythmias. *J Am Coll Cardiol* 6:1225, 1985.
20. Visser FC, et al: Arrhythmias in athletes: Comparison of stress test, 24-hour Holter and Holter monitoring during the game in squash players. *Eur Heart J* 8: Supplement D 29, 1987.
21. Pitano JA and Oriel RJ: Prevalence and nature of cardiac arrhythmias in apparently normal, well-trained runners. *Amer Heart J* 104:762, 1982.
22. McNamara EG, et al: Task Force I: Congenital heart disease. *J Am Coll Cardiol* 6:1200, 1985.
23. Cheitlin MD, et al: Task Force II: Acquired valvular heart disease. *J Am Coll Cardiol* 6:1209, 1985.
24. Savage EE, et al: Mitral valve prolapse in the general population. 1. Epidemiological features: the Framingham study. *Am Heart J* 106:571, 1983.
25. Rink LD, Garl T, Bomba B: Unpublished material, 1988.
26. Musante R, et al: Ergometric evaluation of physical fitness of athletes affected by mitral valve prolapse: Study of 80 cases. *Eur Heart J* 8:33, 1987.
27. Frolich EE, et al: Task Force IV: Systemic arterial hypertension. *J Am Coll Cardiol* 6:1218, 1985.
28. Epstein SE and Maron BJ: Sudden death and the competitive athlete: Perspectives of preparticipation screening studies. *J Am Coll Cardiol* 7:220, 1986.

CHAPTER 7

HOLTER RECORDING IN ATHLETES: PURPOSES AND APPLICATIONS

Gerald F. Fletcher, MD

Professor and Chairman
Department of Rehabilitation Medicine
Emory University School of Medicine
Atlanta, Georgia

Editor's Note: It is, of course, evident that Holter recording is not a routine screening test for athletes. However, it can be of great help in identifying and documenting arrhythmias that may occur in athletes.

As discussed in Chapter 3, you can simulate by hand motion various arrhythmias that a patient may describe. – WPH

The healthy, asymptomatic athlete has often alarmed his or her physician because of seemingly dangerous disturbances of heart rate, rhythm, and/or conduction. However, these disturbances in the highly trained athlete are often functional, resulting from increased vagal tone rather than definitive pathologic changes in the heart. [1-9] Certain arrhythmias are relatively common in athletes, such as sinus bradycardia, sinus arrhythmia, Wenckebach type of second-degree atrioventricular block, atrioventricular junctional rhythm, and wandering atrial pacemaker. [10-18]

Zeppili et al[19] reported 10 cases of spontaneous or induced Wenckebach second-degree atrioventricular block in trained athletes. In 9 of the 10 subjects, conduction disturbances were improved or abolished by reflex sympathetic maneuvers, autonomic (vagolytic) drug administration, or exercise.

Wenckebach atrioventricular block initially was thought to be rare in persons without heart disease. In one study, only one of 67,375 men had Wenckebach atrioventricular block on a standard resting 12-lead ECG. [20] Wenckebach findings, however, subsequently were found to be more common in highly trained persons. [10-13,17] A study of 126 top Israeli athletes found that 11 had first-degree block and three had Wenckebach atrioventricular block. [12]

In another study, Talan et al[21] obtained 24-hour continuous ECG recordings in 20 young (19- to 28-year-old) male long-distance runners (50 miles/week) during activities other than running. All 20 runners had premature atrial complexes, but only one had >100/24 hours. Fourteen runners (70%) had premature ventricular complexes, but only two (10%) had >50 in 24 hours and none had ventricular couplets or tachycardia.

In a study by Pantano and Oriel,[22] 60 high-level runners (24-177 km/week, median 48.5) had Holter recordings only during the period of exercise. Sixty percent had ventricular arrhythmias during the recorded run: bigeminy in 10%, couplets in 10%, and multiform premature ventricular contractions in 5%. Forty percent of the group had atrial arrhythmias during the recorded run. Occasional to frequent premature atrial complexes were the most common; however, seven subjects had atrial couplets or paroxysmal atrial tachycardia. This study is limited in scope, however, because of the brief time of Holter recording.

In our study[23] of 24-hour continuous electrocardiography both during running and other activity, there was no significant difference in the occurrence of rhythm and conduction disturbances in the different groups at varying levels of exercise intensity. The most common abnormalities were ventricular ectopic complexes, seen in 40 subjects, <50/min in 34 and >50/min in 6. The high-grade ventricular ectopic activity – five-beat run of ventricular tachycardia (immediately after exercise) and two instances of ventricular couplets during exercise – were of concern and subjects were referred for further medical evaluation. However, no data are available on the medical evaluation. Table 7-1 reflects data from the aforementioned studies.

Healthy, well-trained endurance runners com-

Table 7-1
Results of Three Long-Term Electrocardiographic Studies of Apparently Healthy Runners

Study and No. of Subjects	Total with ESCs		>100 ESCs/ 24 hr		Atrial Couplets or Tachycardia		Total with EVCs		>50 EVCs/ 24 hr		Paired Ventricular Extrasystoles		Ventricular Tachycardia		Mobitz 1 AV Block	
	n	%	n	%	n	%	n	%	n	%	n	%	n	%	n	%
Talan et al[21] 20 – FA only	20	100	1	5	2	10	14	70	2	10	0	0	0	0	8	40
Pantano et al[22] 60 – DR only	24	40	—	—	7	12	36	60	—	—	6	10	0	0	0	0
Pilcher et al[23] 80 – DR and FA																
Group I	7	35	0	0	0	0	9	45	0	0	0	0	0	0	0	0
Group II	10	53	0	0	0	0	13	68	1	5	1	5	0	0	0	0
Group III	7	33	1	5	0	0	6	29	1	5	1	5	1	5	0	0
Group IV	9	45	0	0	0	0	13	65	4	20	0	0	0	0	0	0

Abbreviations:
AV = atrioventricular; DR = during running; ESCs = ectopic supraventricular complexes (predominantly premature atrial);
EVCs = ectopic ventricular complexes; FA = during free activity; — = no information

monly have variations in heart rhythm that might be considered serious in a different clinical setting. Further, the frequency and grade of these arrhythmias are not predictable by the routine maximal exercise test nor can they be extrapolated to a level of exercise far beyond the capacity of most healthy persons. Caution also must be exercised in using the Lown grading system to describe arrhythmias found in normal subjects, as the categories were originally used in relation to patients with coronary artery disease. Assigning increasing severity of ventricular arrhythmia in normal subjects to increasing Lown grade is open to speculation.

Arrhythmias occur throughout all phases of human endeavor, from sedentary activities to exhaustive testing procedures. Numerous studies have documented various types of ventricular arrhythmias, including ventricular tachycardia, in healthy individuals during routine activities,[24-29] during supervised workouts[29,30] and during treadmill tests.[31-34] A study of the Indiana State Police Force indicated that ventricular arrhythmias during maximal exercise can be demonstrated in 30 to 32% of men in the 35 to 44-year-old age group and are generally confined to heart rates greater than 85% of predicted maximal.

Application to Athletic Evaluations

As the American public becomes more health conscious, there is considerable increase in awareness for symptoms such as palpitations, "skipped" heart beats, or speeding and slowing of the heart. Such symptoms are often described by athletes. It is often clinically difficult to ascertain the exact type of arrhythmia involved in such a setting, or the frequency with which it occurs. The Holter recording is a relatively inexpensive and convenient method to assess such symptoms. Optimal evaluation is obtained by 24-hour recording, including both leisure activity and exercise. Results are quite unpredictable: the aforementioned symptoms may be substantiated by the detection of premature atrial contractions, premature ventricular contractions, sinus arrhythmia, or sinus tachycardia; to the contrary there may be no changes whatsoever.

Another symptom complex reported in athletes is chest discomfort or chest pain. Such is often musculoskeletal in origin and in no way relates to the cardiovascular system. However, infrequently there are considerations of hypertrophic cardiomyopathy, mitral valve prolapse, or even a rare occurrence of occlusive coronary artery disease.

Holter recording may well be indicated in these groups if indeed there are symptoms of heart irregularity. In addition, in rare instances, chest discomfort associated with myocardial ischemia and ST segment displacement may be reliably detected by Holter recording.

Another concern in athletes is a "slow heart rate." This, of course, is often only the resulting bradycardia of the training effect, but in some settings there are escape cardiac beats (usually ventricular escape beats) and the subject may be quite aware of the post-extrasystolic pause followed by the post-extrasystolic accentuation of the next contraction. The latter is often a cause for alarm in otherwise healthy athletes. In accord with this, the role of the autonomic nervous system must be considered in a trained person. Often in youth, sinus arrhythmia is present and the fluctuations of heart rate are considerable. In athletes, the autonomic nervous system may have even more effect on cardiac rate, with periods of slowing and occasional bursts of sinus rhythm rate increases, which may indeed cause symptoms.

It is important to recognize that ectopic atrial and ventricular contractions, atrioventricular Wenckebach, ventricular escape beats, sinus arrhythmia, and periodic episodes of fast heart rate in athletes (and in other normal people) are normal variations of cardiac rhythm. Table 7-2 lists such types of "normal" rhythm, in athletes. These rhythms may "wax and wane" during the period of athleticism and oftentimes will resolve with increasing age. It is important not to exhibit excessive concern to the athlete about these aberrations because often the subject will become overly alarmed, as may coaches, family, and others involved in their career.

However, with some Holter recording abnormalities in athletes, clinical judgement may demand further tests. Prior to Holter recording, a medical history and physical examination should have been done, and usually a 12-lead resting electrocardiogram. While it is not the purpose of this chapter to address in detail the resting 12-lead electrocardiogram (discussed in Chapter 4), suffice it to say that slow sinus rhythm, early repolarization changes of the ST segment (more marked in black athletes), and left ventricular hypertrophy patterns are commonly seen.

If (for instance) frequent ectopic beats are seen during Holter recording, exercise testing may be in order to determine the behavior of such ectopy with an exercise stress under ECG monitoring. Bradycardia, atrioventricular escape rhythm, or atrioventricular Wenckebach conduction also can be further assessed by exercise testing.

In the presence of a prominent left ventricular impulse and/or systolic murmur on physical examination with a history of chest discomfort and abnormal findings on Holter recording, an echocardiogram can be quite effective in elucidating the dynamics of the ventricular septum with regard to possible hypertrophic cardiomyopathy and of the mitral valve with regard to possible prolapse or mitral regurgitation. In addition, structural changes of the left ventricle can be delineated, which may be important if there is ventricular enlargement.

More elaborate diagnostic studies such as nuclear exercise testing or radionuclide wall motion analysis and cardiac catheterization are usually reserved for athletes who have a significant history, physical findings, and electrocardiographic abnormalities, either at rest or with Holter recording, which (in the judgment of the physician in charge) dictate more specific testing and further evaluation. The need for catheterization obviously is quite rare in athletes, but may be dictated by certain clinical settings. Figure 7-1 depicts a

---

Table 7-2
Rhythm and Conduction Disturbances Frequently Seen in Normal Athletes

- Extreme Sinus Bradycardia (35-40 beats per minute)
- Sinus Pauses
- Sinus Arrhythmia
- First Degree Atrioventricular Block
- Atrioventricular Junctional Escape Rhythm
- Atrioventricular Wenckebach Conduction
- Ectopic Supraventricular Beats
- Ectopic Ventricular Beats

step-by-step approach to the cardiovascular evaluation of athletes.

The problem of sudden cardiac death in athletes, while quite rare, is of concern because of such occurrences in high school, college, and professional athletes. The etiology of sudden death in athletes, although less well substantiated than in others, is still most likely arrhythmogenic. Aortic dissection with thoracic aorta rupture, cardiomyopathy with compromise in cardiac output, and pulmonary emboli are all possible structural or specific etiological causes of sudden cardiac death. However, in any setting, the final event is usually ventricular arrhythmia with ventricular fibrillation.

Such terminal ventricular arrhythmias may have their prodromal changes elucidated through careful cardiac evaluation and Holter recording. In rare instances when, for example, frequent high-grade ventricular ectopy is discovered, certain drugs and/or changes in type or levels of physical exercise may be recommended. However, the efficacy of routine screening of athletes with Holter recordings has not been accepted as prudent, nor has it been thought to be cost effective in the long-term prevention or management

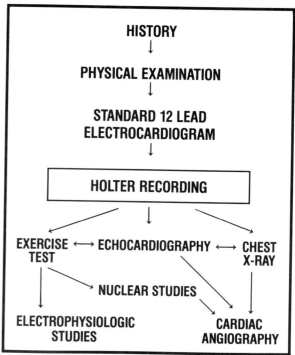

Figure 7-1: Step-by-step guide – to the cardiovascular evaluation of athletes. The arrows depict rational alternatives in evaluation based on variables of the clinical setting and the initial data base. Evaluation may be completed at any point or level, at which time treatment is prescribed or disposition is made.

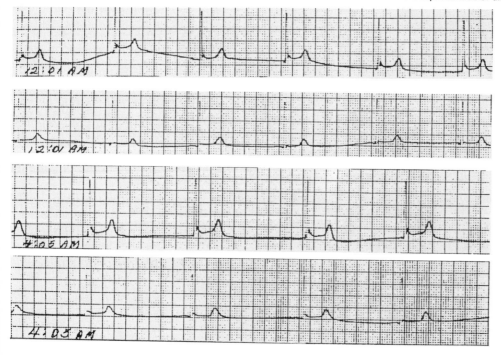

Figure 7-2: Bradycardia – A 23-year-old, well trained male athlete with no clinical evidence of cardiac disease was evaluated because of "slow heart beat." Extreme bradycardia (34-42 beats/minute), either sinus or low atrial, was recorded during sleep. No treatment was administered and the subject has remained healthy. (From Fletcher GF,[4] with permission.)

of such potential problems. It is generally accepted that routine Holter recording is not indicated in athletes who do not exhibit the aforementioned symptoms or signs. Perhaps in the future, such additional testing will be considered as more attempts are made to screen athletes for such possible problems.

Case Examples

The Holter recordings shown in Figures 7-2, 7-3, 7-4, and 7-5 display data from a broad spectrum of otherwise healthy athletes who continued playing their sports. Figure 7-6 is from an athlete with abnormal Holter results in whom further evaluation revealed significant myocardial dysfunction.

Summary

When considering Holter recording in an athlete, the following points must be emphasized:

1. The basic history and physical examination are the most important initial aspects of the cardiovascular evaluation.

2. The Holter recording should be utilized after this initial evaluation only if there are data to suggest a cardiac rate or rhythm disturbance.

3. Arrhythmias are common in athletes. These should be assessed in the clinical perspective of the "total subject" and not as isolated events.

4. The subject and his or her family should not be alarmed with regard to normal arrhythmias. If treatment is initiated in the otherwise normal athlete, it must be re-evaluated in the future, as often arrhythmias will spontaneously resolve, dictating cessation of treatment.

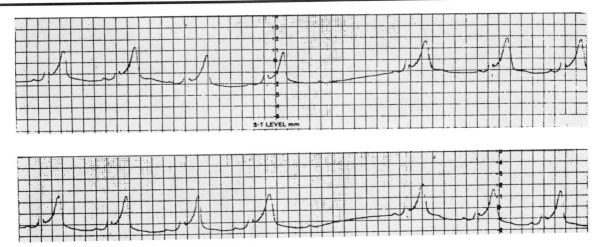

Figure 7-3: "Skipped Beats" – A 52-year-old subject who regularly ran 25 to 30 miles per week presented with "dropped beats." Holter recording revealed sinus bradycardia of 50 beats per minute with periods of atrioventricular block, probably Wenckebach (Type I). No therapy was initiated and the subject has continued to run regularly without any difficulty. (From Fletcher GF,[4] with permission.)

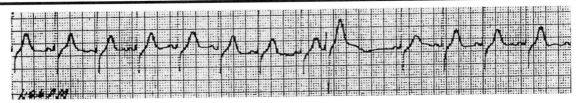

Figure 7-4: "Palpitations" – This 32-year-old physically active pathologist presented with "palpitations." Clinical data revealed no evidence of heart disease. Holter recording detected only occasional premature ventricular beats. No treatment was indicated and the subject has done well. (From Fletcher GF,[4] with permission.)

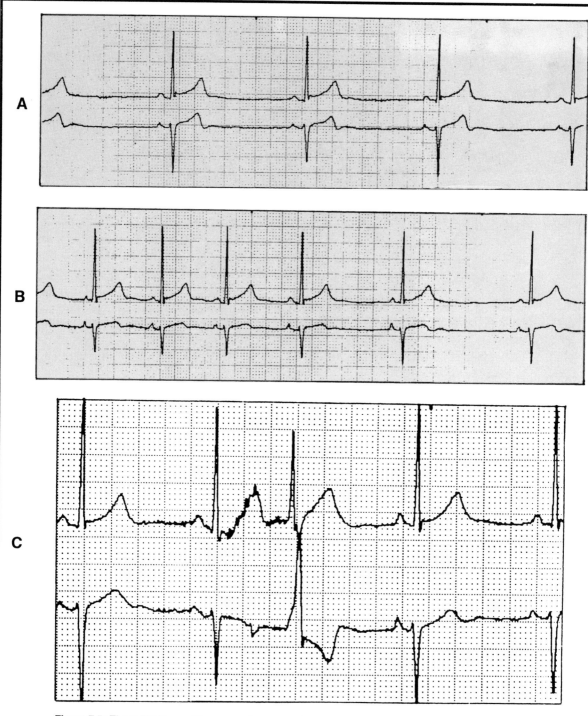

Figure 7-5: Three Findings – These recordings were taken from a 38-year-old high-level runner (20 to 60 miles per week) with no symptoms. They reveal (A) sinus bradycardia of 30 beats/minute at 4:30 a.m., (B) periods of sinus arrhythmia, and (C) infrequent single, ventricular ectopic beats.

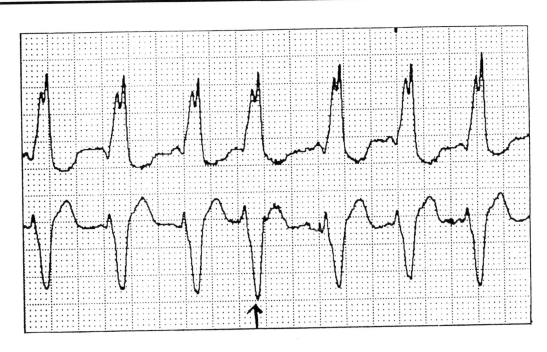

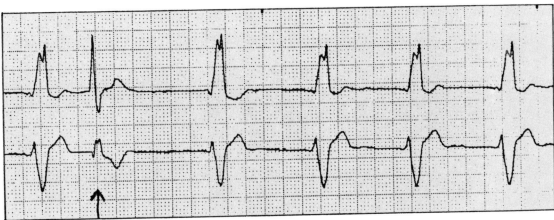

Figure 7-6: Probable Cardiomyopathy – A 17-year-old high school football player had brief periods of syncope. Clinical evaluation revealed a resting ECG consistent with preexcitation. (a) A 2-channel Holter recording of the preexcitation pattern (extremely short P-R interval) with rare supraventricular ectopic contractions (▲). (b) A rare ventricular ectopic beat (▲). Variable supraventricular tachycardias were documented by electrocardiography and electrophysiological studies. Further evaluation by echocardiography revealed global hypokinesis with a dilated left ventricle and paradoxical septal motion consistent with the preexcitation. Arrhythmias were treated with 1000 mg procainamide (long-acting) three times daily and physical activity was decreased. The patient was felt to have a cardiomyopathy, but has done well clinically with no recurrence of high-grade arrhythmias.

Editor's Note: As a personal opinion, athletes such as this young man, having syncopal episodes plus the other findings, would be advised not to continue to play football. – WPH.

References

1. Fletcher GF: Dynamic Electrocardiographic Recording. Futura Publishing, Mount Kisco, NY, 1979.

2. Salerno DM, Granrud G, Hodges M: Accuracy of commercial 24-hour electrocardiogram analyzers for quantitation of total and repetitive ventricular arrhythmias. *Am J Cardiol* 1987;60:1299-1305.

3. Fletcher GF: Dynamic Electrocardiographic Recording. Futura Publishing, Mount Kisco, NY, 1979, p 122, 127, 157.

4. Young D, Eisonberg R, Fish B, Fisher J: Wenckebach atrioventricular block (Mobitz Type 1) in children and adolescents. *Am J Cardiol* 40:393-398, 1977.

5. Hall V: The relation of heart rate to exercise fitness: an attempt at physiological interpretation of the bradycardia of training. *Pediatrics* (Suppl)II: 723-729, 1963.

6. Gambetta M, Denes P, Childers R: Vagally induced second degree block Mobitz Type I, and the hyporeactive SA node. *Chest* 62:152-154, 1972.

7. Lightfoot P, Sasse L, Mandel W, Kazakawa H: His bundle electrocardiograms in healthy adolescents with persistent second degree A-V block. *Chest* 63:358-362, 1973.

8. Dighton D: Sinus bradycardia: autonomic influences and clinical assessment. *Br Heart J* 36:791-797, 1974.

9. Rasmussen V: Vagotonia in rigorously trained athletes. *Primary Cardiol* 8:Jan:175-185, 1982.

10. Cullen K, Collin R: Daily running causing Wenckebach heart block. *Lancet* 2:729-730, 1964.

11. Sargin O, Alp C, Tansi C, Karaca L: Wenckebach phenomenon with nodal and ventricular escape in marathon runner. *Chest* 57:102-105, 1970.

12. Meytes I, Kaplinsky E, Yahini J, Hanne-Paparo N, Neufeld H: Wenckebach A-V block: A frequent feature following heavy physical training. *Am Heart J* 90:426-430, 1975.

13. Goldschlager N, Cohn K, Goldschlager A: Exercise-related ventricular arrhythmias. *Mod Concepts Cardiovasc Dis* 48:Dec:67-72, 1979.

14. Beckner G, Winsor T: Cardiovascular adaptations to prolonged physical effort. Circulation 9:835-846, 1954.

15. Hunt E: Electrocardiographic study of 10 champion swimmers before and after 110 yard sprint swimming competition. *Can Med Assoc J* 88:1251, 1963.

16. Smith W, Cullen K, Thorburn I: Runners in 1962 Commonwealth games. *Br Heart J* 26:469, 1964.

17. Lichtman J, O'Rourke R, Klein A, Karliner J: Electrocardiogram of the athlete. *Arch Intern Med* 132:763-770, 1973.

18. Hanne-Paparo N, Proory Y, Schoenfeld Y, Shapria Y, Kellerman J: Common ECG changes in athletes. *Cardiology* 61:267, 1976.

19. Zeppilli P, Fenici R, Sassrra M, Pirranis M, Caselli G: Wenckebach second degree A-V block in top-ranking athletes: an old problem revisited. *Am Heart J* 100:281-294, 1980.

20. Averill K, Lamb L: Electrocardiographic findings in 67,375 asymptomatic subjects. *Am J Cardiol* 6:76-83, 1960.

21. Talan DA, Bauernfeind RA, Ashley WW, Kanakis C, Rosen KN: Twenty-four-hour continuous ECG recordings in long-distance runners. *Chest* 82:19-24, 1982.

22. Pantano JA, Oriel FJ: Prevalence and nature of cardiac arrhythmias in apparently normal well-trained runners. *Am Heart J* 104:762-768, 1982.

23. Pilcher GF, Cook AJ, Johnston BL, Fletcher GF: Twenty-four-hour continuous electrocardiography during exercise and free activity in 80 apparently healthy runners. *Am J Cardiol* 52:859-861, 1983.

24. Hiss RG, Averill KH, Lamb LR: Electrocardiographic findings in 67,375 asymptomatic subjects. III. Ventricular rhythms. *Am. J. Cardiol;* 6:96, 1960.

25. Gaughan GL, Gorfinkel HJ: Physiologic and biologic variants of the electrocardiogram. *Cardiovas Clin* 3(3)7, 1977.

26. Clarke JM, Shelton JR, Hamer J, Venning GR: The rhythm of the normal human heart. *Lancet* 2:508, 1976.

27. Brodsky M, Wu D, Denes P, Kanakis C, Rosen KM: Arrhythmias documented by 24 hour continuous electrocardiographic monitoring in 50 male medical students without apparent heart disease. *Am J Cardiol* 39:390, 1977.

28. Kennedy HL, Underhill SL: Frequent or complex ventricular ectopy in apparently healthy subjects. *Am J Cardiol* 38:141, 1976.

29. Ekblom B, Hartley LH, Day WC: Occurrence and reproducibility of exercise-induced subjects ventricular ectopy in normal subjects. *Am J Cardiol* 43:35, 1979.

30. Shepard RJ: Sudden death: A significant hazard of exercise? *Br J Sports Med* 8:101, 1974.

31. Viitasalo MT, Kala R, Eisal A, Holonen PI: Ventricular arrhythmias during exercise testing, jogging and sedentary life. *Chest* 76 (1):21, 1979.

32. Blackburn H, Taylor HL, Hamrell B, Buskirk E, Nicholas WC, Thorsen RD: Premature ventricular complexes induced by stress testing: Their frequency and response to physical conditioning. *Am J Cardiol* 31:44, 1973.

33. Jelinik MV, Lown B: Exercise stress testing for exposure of cardiac arrhythmias. *Prog Cardiovasc Dis* 16:497, 1974.

34. McHenry PL, Fisch C, Jordan JW: Cardiac arrhythmias observed during maximal treadmill exercise testing in clinically normal men. *Am J Cardiol* 29:331, 1972.

CHAPTER 8

NONFATAL CORONARY, VALVULAR, AND MYOCARDIAL HEART DISEASE UNMASKED BY EXERCISE

Bruce F. Waller, MD
Clinical Professor of Pathology and Medicine
Indiana University School of Medicine;
Director, Cardiovascular Pathology Registry
St. Vincent Hospital, Indianapolis
Cardiologist, Nasser, Smith, Pinkerton Cardiology, Inc.
Indianapolis, Indiana

Editor's Note: This chapter is a very important one. It reminds us of the serious complications that can be caused or brought to light by exercise. The patients are unfortunate, because the exercise "unmasked" their heart disease. On the other hand, they are fortunate that the exercise did not result in sudden death, which we know too well can and does occur.

Worthy of emphasis is that careful screening can often "spot" the patient with heart disease. This person should not engage in strenuous or competitive athletics, thereby preventing serious problems. This entails the so-called "5 finger approach" of cardiovascular evaluation: a careful, detailed history, meticulous physical examination (auscultation), electrocardiogram, chest x-ray, and simple laboratory tests. – WPH

Exercise stress testing may bring out symptoms, abnormal cardiovascular physical findings, or electrocardiographic changes indicative of underlying cardiovascular disease which are not present at rest. Professional running, amateur jogging or other sport activity may serve as a self-performed exercise test and may similarly uncover an underlying cardiovascular abnormality, perhaps sooner than might have been apparent without exercise. This chapter describes six men in whom symptoms developing during running or swimming led to the diagnosis of previously unrecognized aortic-valve stenosis and coronary heart disease.

Three Patients With Valvular Heart Disease

While running, each of three men aged 35, 55 and 60 years (Table 8-1) developed symptoms of dyspnea, syncope, and/or chest pain which had not been present at rest. Patient 1 had been exercising for four to five years, with no symptoms. Then he began to feel fatigued, light-headed, and dyspneic during short distances of jogging. He experienced "near-syncope" while running one-half mile on a hot, humid day.

Cardiac evaluation disclosed left ventricular hypertrophy on electrocardiogram, precordial systolic ejection murmur (Grade 3/6) and diastolic blowing murmur (Grade 1/6), and 112 mmHg peak systolic gradient (psg) between left ventricle (LV) and aorta (Ao). Although a "nonspecific" precordial systolic murmur had been heard several years earlier, the patient had no previous cardiac symptoms. He underwent aortic valve (AV) replacement; the excised valve (Figure 8-1) was congenitally unicommissural with moderately heavy calcific deposits.

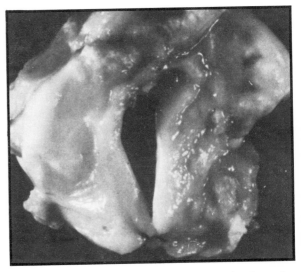

Figure 8-1: Patient 1 – Operatively-excised stenotic unicommissural (unicuspid) aortic valve.

Table 8-1
Six Cases of Nonfatal Heart Disease Unmasked by Exercise

	Valvular Heart Disease			Coronary Atherosclerotic Heart Disease		
	Patient #1	Patient #2	Patient #3	Patient #4	Patient #5	Patient #6
Age (years)	35	55	60	50	46	20
Sex	M	M	M	M	M	M
Type of Exercise	Running	Running	Running	Swimming	Running	Running
Exercise History:						
Miles	<1.5/day	<1/day	<.5/day	.5/day	3-4/day	5/day*
Duration	<5 years	<2 mos	<2 wks	>1 year	Several years	14 yrs
Symptoms during						
exercise	Dyspnea	Syncope	CP	CP	CP	CD
Family history heart disease?	0	0	0	+	+	+
Angina Pectoris	0	0	0	0	0	0
History of AMI	0	0	0	0	0	0
SAP (mmHg)	105/75	135/70	170/80	150/100**	120/80	SH
Total serum cholesterol (mg/dl)	160	–	–	259	171	–
Abnormal ECG:						
Resting	+	+	+	0	0	0
Exercise	–	–	–	0***	0	–
LV-Ao (mmHg)	112†	55††	70†††	0	0	0
Abnormal CA by angiography	0	0	0	+	+	+
Treatment	AVR	AVR	AVR	PTCA	PTCA	PTCA
Resumed Exercise	Yes	No	Yes	Noᵃ	Yes	Yes
Type of Cardiac Abnormality:						
Coronary artery	0	0	0	+	+	+
Valvular	+	+	+	0	0	0
Myocardial	0	0	0	0	0	0

Abbreviations:
AMI = Acute myocardial infarction
Ao = Aorta
AR = Aortic Regurgitation
AVR = Aortic valve replacement
CA = Coronary artery
CD = Chest discomfort
CP = Chest pain

LV = Left ventricle
PCW = Pulmonary capillary wedge pressure
PTCA = Percutaneous transluminal coronary angioplasty
SAP = Systemic arterial pressure
SH = Systemic hypertension

* Approximate daily average. Patient ran more several years earlier.
** Systemic hypertension for four years, treated with nadolol.
*** ST-segment changes only with reproduction of chest pain.
† Ao = 106/75; LV = 218/14; LV-PCW = 0; 1 + /4 + AR
†† Ao = 135/70; LV = 190/8; LV-PCW = 0; 1 + /4 + AR
††† Ao = 170/80; LV = 240/22; LV-PCW = 0; 2 + /4 + AR
a = Planning to resume daily swims.
+ = Present
0 = Absent
– = No information available

Editor's Note: This obviously was not an innocent "non-specific" murmur. This 35-year-old man's murmur is that of aortic stenosis.

An innocent murmur is early to mid-systolic in timing, generally short in duration, not harsh in quality (like the clearing of one's throat), has no ejection sound, and does not transmit into the neck; nor is it heard over the clavicles. The murmur of congenital stenosis, usually bicuspid in type, has an ejection sound heard at the apex as well as at the base, it is generally longer, more harsh in quality than the innocent and can usually be heard over the clavicles, suprasternal notch, and supraclavicular area; there would be approximately a 50% chance of an early blowing aortic diastolic murmur also being present (if carefully searched for). This was indeed present in the man and, in itself, mitigated against an innocent or "insignificant" murmur. An S4 was also likely present. Even when the murmur was first de-

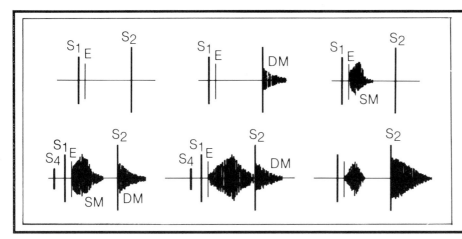

Figure 8-2: The spectrum of possible findings on auscultation of the congenital bicuspid aortic valve vary from only an ejection sound (E) *(no murmur)* to a systolic murmur (SM), or a diastolic murmur (DM), or combinations of both. The murmurs also are variable in intensity. An atrial sound (S_4) is likely to be present with more severe degrees of stenosis.

S_1 - First heart sound

S_2 - Second heart sound

tected, the ECG would probably have shown LVH. Once such a diagnosis is made, strenuous sports, including jogging, would not be advised.

The spectrum of possible auscultatory findings from a bicuspid aortic valve are shown in Figure 8-2. – WPH

Patients 2 and 3 had just started jogging to help reduce body weight. Patient 2 had run short distances for less than two months when he had syncope while jogging. Cardiac evaluation disclosed left ventricular hypertrophy on electrocardiogram, precordial systolic murmur (Grade 3/6), and 55 mmHg psg between LV and Ao at catheterization. He underwent aortic valve replacement; the excised valve was congenitally bicuspid (Figure 8-3).

Editor's Note: The typical clinical findings of aortic stenosis can be accurately diagnosed in the physician's office or at the bedside. At his age of 55, he ran a very high chance (probably 90%) of having a bicuspid valve, which are almost always calcific. He was overweight, otherwise his systolic murmur probably would have been louder and there would be about a 50% chance of an aortic diastolic murmur being heard.

Personally observed has been a boy, age 15, who died suddenly while playfully wrestling with a friend on the beach. He had been completely asymptomatic. He had a congenital bicuspid aortic valve with only a moderate degree of stenosis. – WPH

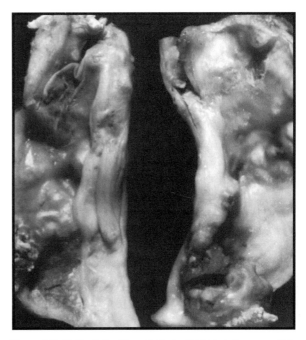

Figure 8-3: Patient 2 – Operatively-excised stenotic congenital bicuspid aortic valve.

Patient 3 was 60 years old. He had been running one to two times per week, gradually reaching distances of one-and-one-half miles, when he developed chest pain while running. Cardiac evaluation disclosed systemic hypertension, left ventricular hypertrophy on electrocardiogram, precordial systolic ejection murmur (Grade 3/6), diastolic blowing murmur (Grade 2/6), and 70 mmHG psg between LV and Ao. He underwent aortic valve replacement; the excised valve (Figure 8-4) was stenoid, non-rheumatic, and tricuspid. Two of the three men have resumed mild exercise.

Editor's Note: Patients aged 60 and above with aortic stenosis have a greater chance of having a tricuspid aortic valve, as was found in this patient.

"Two of the three men have resumed mild exercise" – Hopefully it was walking rather than more strenuous types.

I have a practical clinical guide to physical activity which I suggest to my patients with known heart disease: "Do only what you can do in comfort, avoiding extremes of exertion in extremes of weather." The extremes of weather are: the "bitter" cold (the worst cardiac-wise) and the hot humid. I call this my "old fashioned rule." Over the years it has proved satisfactory and it works! For these last two patients who were trying to lose weight, dieting rather than running is wiser and safer.

All three of these patients can be accurately screened in the physician's office and advised concerning physical activity. – WPH

Three Patients With Coronary Atherosclerotic Heart Disease

Each of three other men, aged 32, 42, and 44 years (Table 8-1), began to develop chest pain or discomfort while swimming or running. Previously they had felt no discomfort while exercising. Patient 4 had been swimming regularly for over one year when he developed substernal heaviness after swimming 100 to 200 yards of a half-mile swim. Subsequently, pain developed with brisk walking. Cardiac evaluation disclosed systemic arterial hypertension and hypercholesterolemia. Coronary angiography disclosed severe narrowing of the proximal right coronary artery (75% diameter reduction), with total occlusion of the distal right. It also revealed separate origin of the left anterior descending (LAD) and left circumflex arteries from the ascending aorta. Percutaneous transluminal coronary angioplasty (PTCA) successfully reopened the distal and dilated the proximal lesion.

Patient 5 had been running regularly for several years when he developed chest pain after running

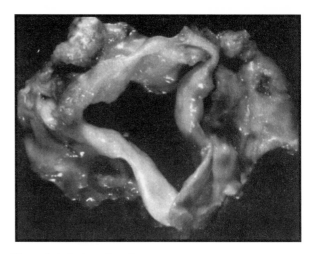

Figure 8-4: Patient 3 – Operatively-excised stenotic tricuspid (non-rheumatic) aortic valve.

3.5 miles. One month later, medical examination disclosed normal systemic pressure, normal total serum cholesterol, and normal resting electrocardiogram. An exercise treadmill test was negative for ischemia. He was advised to use trinitroglycerin prophylactically before running. Four months later he had recurrent chest pain. Coronary angiography disclosed severe narrowing (>75%) of the proximal LAD coronary artery. He had successful PTCA but angina recurred one month post-PTCA. A second dilation of the previous lesion was complicated by coronary dissection. He subsequently had aortocoronary bypass grafting to the LAD and has resumed running regularly.

Patient 6 had been running regularly for at least 14 years, and had completed several marathon races. He had a history of labile systemic hypertension since age 20, treated with diet restriction and exercise. During one run, he experienced chest discomfort and tightness after two or three miles. He stopped running and the discomfort disappeared, permitting resumption of running. Six weeks later, chest discomfort developed after one-quarter mile. Returning home, he experienced chest tightness at rest and sought medical attention. Cardiac evaluation disclosed systemic hypertension (185/115 mmHg) and a normal electrocardiogram. Subsequent coronary angiography disclosed severe narrowing of the proximal LAD, which was successfully dilated at PTCA (Figure 8-5).

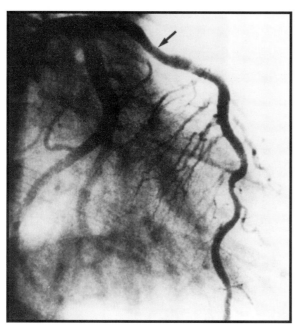

Figure 8-5: Patient 6 – Angiographic frames after percutaneous transluminal coronary angioplasty of the left anterior descending coronary artery (arrow).

Previous Reports of Heart Disease Unmasked in Athletes

The literature shows at least seven reports of nonfatal heart disease unmasked in athletes during vigorous exercise (Table 8-2).[1-6] Four of the seven athletes[1,2,4] were competitive, well conditioned long-distance runners. Five developed chest pain during exercise. One of these[1] experienced chest pain after running 2¼ miles. He later developed angina with 1 mm ST-segment depression on an exercise electrocardiogram. Angiography showed that the diameter of the LAD artery was reduced by 90%, and the LOM, 50%. He was able to resume exercise after PTCA.

In another runner[2], who had successfully completed seven marathons and a number of other races ranging from 6.2 to 52 miles, the LAD artery was found to be reduced by 99%. He also underwent PTCA.

Another marathoner[3], who had logged over 20,000 miles in training, suffered an acute myocardial infarction during exercise. Ten months later, angiography showed that the LAD artery was reduced in diameter by 50 to 75%, whereas the LM, LC, and R arteries were normal. A dilated left

ventricular cavity with anterior akinesis was also revealed.

A 50-year-old man[4] who had completed 18 marathons had a history of one episode of chest pain while running, five years earlier. He experienced the onset of angina pectoris during a marathon. Forty-eight hours after completing the race, he had an acute myocardial infarction. One month later, angiography demonstrated "significant" distal R narrowing, a normal left coronary system, and a dyskinetic apex on LV angiogram. He later resumed marathoning.

A 46-year-old athlete[4] who engaged in various forms of vigorous exercise experienced the onset of chest pain while running. An ECG five days later showed an acute myocardial infarction. Two years later, angiography found the PD reduced 70%, the LAD artery reduced by 80%, and mild but diffuse LC disease. A left ventricular angiogram disclosed an anterior akinetic area. He also resumed his previous activity.

A varsity swimmer[5] had competed frequently in the preceding six months and had achieved national-level performance times for the 200-meter butterfly event. He experienced the onset of severe chest pain while performing a routine nine-mile training session. The pain was unaffected by position or breathing movements and gradually resolved after one hour of rest. He remained asymptomatic until 3 A.M. the following morning, when he was awakened by similar pain that prompted medical attention.

Resting ECG showed ST-segment elevation in leads I, II, III, AVL, AVF, and V_2-V_6; ST-segment depression in AVR and V_1; and premature ventricular contractions. On day four, the ECG had evolved T inversion in I, II, III, AVF, and V_4-V_6, and upright T waves in AVR and V_1. Serum creatine kinase was markedly elevated, with 11% MB fraction. A technetium pyrophosphate scan showed localized uptake in the left anterolateral myocardial wall. Eight days after the onset of acute myocardial infarction, selective coronary artery angiograms disclosed normal coronary arteries with a 2 to 3 cm myocardial bridge in the middle left anterior descending coronary artery. A ventriculogram disclosed hypokinesis of the anterolateral wall. The swimmer was able to return to his previous level of activity, however.

A 20-year-old girl[6] suffered cardiac arrest dur-

Table 8-2
Literature Reports of Athletes with Nonfatal Cardiac Disease Unmasked by Exercise

	Asay[1] 1981	Handler[2] 1982	Cantwell[3] 1969	Noakes[4] 1977		Hanson[5] 1982	Fletcher[6] 1981
Age (years)	54	48	48	50	46	20	20
Sex	M	M	M	M	M	M	F
Type of Exercise	Running	Running	Running	Running	Run, Swim, 0	Swimming	Running
Exercise History:							
Miles	2-4/day*	50-70/wk	80-90/wk	40/wk	–	–	–
Duration	20 years	>8 years	10 years	10 years	14 years	Several yrs	–
Symptoms during exercise	CP	CP	AMI	CP	CP	CP	SD**
Family history of heart disease?	+	0	+	+	–	0	0
Angina Pectoris	+	+	0	+	+	0	0
History of AMI	0	0	0	0	0	0	0
SAP (mmHg)	130/78	–	130/90	110/80	130/90	135/95	–
Total serum cholesterol (mg/dl)	212	185	268	216	–	–	–
Abnormal ECG:							
Resting	0	0	+	+	+	+	–
Exercise	+	+***	–	–	+†	–	–
Abnormal CA by angiography	+	+	+	+	+	0	0
Treatment	PTCA	PTCA	0	0	0	0	Digoxin
Resumed Exercise	Yes	No	Yes†	Yes†	Yes†	Yes	Yes
Type of Cardiac Abnormality:							
Coronary artery	+	+	+	+	+	+	0
Valvular	0	0	0	0	0	0	0
Myocardial	0	0	0	0	0	0	+

Abbreviations:
0 = – =
AMI = Acute myocardial infarction
CA = Coronary artery
CP = Chest pain
ECG = Electrocardiogram
SAP = Systemic arterial pressure
SD = Sudden death

* 3 to 6 runs/week.
** Successfully resuscitated.
*** Developed angina with 1 mm ST-segment depression.
† Ventricular bigeminy.
†† Continues to run marathons.

ing jogging, but was successfully resuscitated from ventricular fibrillation. At cardiac catheterization, the LV end-diastolic pressure rose to 55 mmHg after exercise. The left ventricular dysfunction was interpreted as that of an idiopathic cardiomyopathy. She was treated with digoxin and resumed exercise.

Implications

In the first three patients reported here (Table 8-1), running produced symptoms of underlying valvular stenosis that may well have been clinically recognized had medical attention been sought for other reasons. This did not happen, but the running produced the symptoms for which they sought medical evaluation, and therefore led to the diagnosis of AV stenosis.

The other three patients shown on Table 8-1 , with coronary atherosclerotic heart disease, had been exercising for several years. Each, however, had at least one risk factor for coronary atherosclerosis: other family members with coronary atherosclerotic heart disease (all three patients), systemic hypertension (two patients), and hypercholesterolemia (one patient). Similar risk factors apply to several of the other athletes reported in the literature.[1-6]

Thus, running, swimming, and other forms of exercise may unmask valvular, coronary, or myocardial heart disease which previously had been clinically silent. The experience of the three patients with valve disease re-emphasizes the need for individuals to seek medical evaluation before commencing participation in amateur sports. Individuals with one or more risk factors for coronary atherosclerotic heart disease, in particular, should begin a gradual and graduated exercise program. New onset of any chest symptoms or arrhythmias during exercise should be an indication to seek prompt medical attention. It is interesting to speculate that running or other sports may unmask coronary atherosclerosis or cardiomyopathies at an early stage, when the disease, particularly coronary atherosclerosis, may be more amenable to therapy.

Editor's Note: One sees it all the time – patients such as these want to, and continue to, do their former physical activities. However, I am appalled; I would not do so myself and consequently would advise against it. Once is enough! Of course, many people perform certain physical activities knowing full well that risks and serious dangers are involved. It represents the erroneous way of thinking – "it won't happen to me, but to someone else" – like the teenager who smokes cigarettes but can't fathom that lung cancer could subsequently result in his or her case. – WPH

References

1. Asay RW, Vreweg WVR: Severe coronary atherosclerosis in a runner: an exception to the rule? *J Cardiac Rehab* 1:413-421, 1981.
2. Handler JB, Asay RW, Warren SE, Shea PM: Symptomatic coronary artery disease in a marathon runner. *J.A.M.A.* 248:717-719, 1982.
3. Cantwell JD, Fletcher GF: Cardiac complications while jogging. *J.A.M.A.* 210:13-131, 1969.
4. Noakes T, Opie L, Beck W, McKechnie J, Benchimol A, Desser K: Coronary heart disease in marathon runners. *Ann NY Acad Sci* 301:593-619, 1977.
5. Hanson PG, Vander CR, Besozzi MC, Rowe GG: Myocardial infarction in a national-class swimmer. *J.A.M.A.* 248:2313-2314, 1982.
6. Fletcher GF: The dangers of exercise. In "The Heart. Update V." (Hurst JW, ed.), pp. 161-174, New York: McGraw-Hill, 1981.
7. McManus BM, Waller BF, Grayboys TB, Mitchell JH, Siegel RJ, Miller HSJr, Froelicher VF, Roberts WC: Exercise and sudden death, part II, *Cur Prob in Cardiol* 6(10):33-50, 1982.

CHAPTER 9

MITRAL VALVE PROLAPSE: IMPLICATIONS FOR THE ATHLETE

Robert M. Jeresaty, M.D.

Professor of Medicine
University of Connecticut
School of Medicine
Chief, Section of Cardiology
Saint Francis Hospital and Medical Center
Hartford, Connecticut

Editor's Note: This chapter is an excellent presentation on mitral valve prolapse by one of our country's top experts on this subject – Dr. Robert M. Jeresaty.

Mitral valve prolapse is a very common heart lesion, affecting approximately 15 million Americans. The best way to make the diagnosis is with your stethoscope, despite the erroneous impression of many that the optimal diagnostic test is echocardiography. The possible auscultatory findings in mitral valve prolapse cover a wide spectrum, as shown in Figure 9-1 below. We must be aware of these various auscultatory possibilities and actively search for them.

Once the diagnosis is confirmed in an athlete, how should we proceed? Dr. Jeresaty describes his recommendations regarding participation in various sports. – WPH

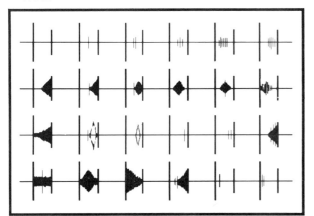

Figure 9-1: Spectrum of possible auscultatory findings in mitral valve prolapse.

Mitral valve prolapse (MVP) is defined as systolic protrusion of the mitral valve leaflets into the left atrium, as demonstrated by angiography, echocardiography, and pathological studies. On auscultation, it is often manifested by a midsystolic click with or without a late systolic murmur.

Mitral valve prolapse was first identified as an entity in the mid 1960's, when the midsystolic click and the late systolic murmur were recorded in the left atrium with intracardiac phonocardiography, and angiographic protrusion of the mitral leaflets into the left atrium and late systolic mitral regurgitation were demonstrated in patients with a click and murmur. A syndrome consisting of nonspecific symptoms, electrocardiographic abnormalities, and arrhythmias has been recognized by many investigators,[1,2] but serious doubt has recently been raised about its existence.[3-7]

Mitral valve prolapse continues to generate considerable interest in view of its prevalence, the controversy surrounding a distinct syndrome, and particularly its complications, which are rare but represent important aspects of modern cardiology.[8]

Careful studies of mitral valve prolapse in athletes are lacking.[9] Little information is available regarding eligibility of athletes with mitral valve prolapse for competitive activity and the relationship between this type of activity and some of the complications of prolapse, i.e., progression of mitral regurgitation, ruptured chordae tendineae, arrhythmias, and sudden death.

Mitral valve prolapse is probably the most common cardiac valve disorder and should be looked upon as a generally benign entity by the physician evaluating athletes.[9,10] The high prevalence of mitral valve prolapse, the symptoms that have been attributed to it, and its serious, yet uncommon complications would often bring the patient to the attention of the physician and would require assessment regarding work-up, participation in athletics, and disqualification.

This chapter will review the etiologic, pathologic, auscultatory, echocardiographic, and electrocardiographic features of mitral valve prolapse, and describe its complications, thus providing a background for evaluating athletes for mitral valve prolapse and for determining the advisability of participation in athletics by patients with documented prolapse.

Etiology, Classification, and Morphologic Abnormalities

In early studies of the etiology of mitral valve prolapse, two theories were proposed.[2] The myocardial theory, based on angiographic and hemodynamic findings, postulated a primary myocardial disorder. In view of the high prevalence of mitral valve prolapse and its generally benign outlook, however, a myocardial component appears highly unlikely. There is little evidence to warrant the diagnosis of myocardial disease in the young athlete with mitral valve prolapse. Thus, the myocardial theory is no longer advanced as a tenable hypothesis.

The second theory, the valvular theory, looks upon myxomatous transformation of the mitral valve as the underlying disorder, with thickened spongiosa encroaching on the fibrosa, causing a basic weakness of the supporting structure and leading to redundancy and prolapse. The valvular theory has been well documented in the advanced forms of mitral valve prolapse, the so-called "floppy mitral valve," in which voluminous, thickened mitral leaflets, mitral annular dilation, and myxomatous transformation are evident. Similar morphologic changes have been demonstrated in more than 50 patients with mild forms of mitral valve prolapse associated with a non-ejection click and late systolic murmur.[2] Very few cases of isolated clicks or "silent" mitral valve prolapse have come to autopsy and surgery. A centralized registry to collect these cases has been proposed.[6]

Among the proponents of the valvular theory, some investigators have postulated a primary inherited abnormality of the mitral collagen tissue manifested as myxomatous transformation leading to valvular distortion. Others have advanced the theory of response to injury secondary to variation of chordal and leaflet architecture inducing "wear and tear" on the valve structure. Recognition of mitral valve prolapse as a major manifestation of Marfan's syndrome, a connective tissue disorder, adds a major argument in favor of mitral

valve prolapse as a part of a generalized connective disorder.

Prolapse can be further classified as primary due to intrinsic structural abnormalities of the mitral valve and secondary due to a reduction of the left ventricular cavity caused by anorexia nervosa, secundum atrial septal defect, and other conditions, with intrinsically normal leaflets. Although the concept is controversial,[6] mitral valve prolapse associated with Marfan's syndrome and other systemic diseases of the connective tissue should be classified as primary, and "secondary prolapse" should be used only in describing echocardiographic or angiographic protrusion of the mitral valve secondary to reduction in the left ventricular cavity, with normal valve structure. In the secondary form, the prolapse is an incidental and insignificant finding, there is an element of reversibility associated with change in the volume of the left ventricular cavity, and the prognosis and complications are independent of the mitral valve involvement. It is possible that some cases of mild "echo only" mitral valve prolapse may represent a normal variant with no pathological abnormality of the mitral valve.[8]

Editor's Note: Mitral valve prolapse (floppy mitral valve) is a congenital valvular problem. The congenital aspect appears to be the increased leaflet area. The acquired component to the floppy valve syndrome is annular stretching or dilation. As the annulus dilates, progressive mitral regurgitation ensues. – BFW

Prevalence, Sex and Age Distribution

The prevalence of mitral valve prolapse is quite variable and depends on the population studied, the diagnostic tools used (auscultation, echocardiography or pathological findings) and the criteria used for diagnosis.[11] It is estimated that 4 to 5% of the population have mitral valve prolapse.[2] The prevalence increases with age, suggesting a "wear and tear" phenomenon superimposed on a congenital abnormality of the valve, or progression of an intrinsic structural abnormality of the mitral collagen tissue. Mitral valve prolapse has been reported in children and young adolescents with a prevalence of 1 to 1.5% in most reports.[12] A female preponderance has been reported, women constituting two-thirds of subjects. An autosomal form of inheritance with incomplete penetrance and reduced expressivity in the male and the young has been noted.

Symptomatology

In the setting of tertiary referral cardiology centers, atypical chest pain, dyspnea, fatigue, dizziness and palpitations, as well as arrhythmias and electrocardiographic changes, are commonly encountered in mitral valve prolapse, leading to the concept of a mitral valve prolapse syndrome.[1,2] Chest pain is usually sharp, left precordial, and can be either fleeting or last for several hours. In one group of 100 patients,[2] chest pain occurred in 61 (61%), being unrelated to physical activity in 83% of the 61, exertional in 8%, and both exertional and non-exertional in 9%. It is less related to a specific effort than to accumulation of fatigue. The absence of a physiologic explanation linking mitral valve prolapse to symptoms and electrocardiographic abnormalities has raised doubt about the existence of a true syndrome.

In epidemiological surveys, most patients diagnosed as having mitral valve prolapse have been asymptomatic,[13] and the nonspecific symptoms that have been attributed to mitral valve prolapse are common in the general population. Moreover, there is often a selection bias in the referral centers: The patients may be referred for unexplained symptoms associated with unrelated auscultatory abnormalities. Ascertainment bias also was postulated because the above-mentioned symptoms often prompt consideration and recognition of mitral valve prolapse.[6] Several studies were reviewed that examined the strength of association between components of the mitral valve prolapse syndrome by comparing echocardiographically documented prolapse and control subjects in the general population. The frequency of symptoms and echocardiographic findings were not significantly different in subjects with or without mitral valve prolapse in the general population.

The flaws of a major epidemiological survey documenting this lack of difference in symptoms and electrocardiographic findings were reviewed[8] and alluded to by one of the co-authors.[6] Another study[14] showed only association between mitral valve prolapse and thoracic bony abnormalities, low body weight, low systolic blood pressure, and palpitations. Further epidemiological studies will undoubtedly shed light on this controversy. It may well be that an etiological relationship will be found between mitral valve prolapse and at least two symptoms (i.e., chest pain and palpitations), but that the mitral valve prolapse syndrome will not be found to be as ubiquitous as originally thought.

Autonomic dysfunction with a predominantly hyperadrenergic state has been noted in symptomatic patients with mitral valve prolapse in comparison with controls, but many investigators have been unable to confirm this finding. It is probable that symptoms attributed to mitral valve prolapse are adrenergically mediated and reflect manifestations of anxiety rather than a direct correlation with the valve abnormality. Many of the studies reporting autonomic dysfunction have compared symptomatic patients with mitral valve prolapse to asymptomatic controls, thus introducing a definite selection bias.

Auscultatory Findings

On auscultation, non-ejection click remains the diagnostic hallmark of mitral valve prolapse.[8] The click moves earlier in systole with sitting and standing. Since few cardiac and extra-cardiac abnormalities are associated with this type of click, its mere presence is virtually diagnostic of mitral valve prolapse. Unfortunately, phonocardiography is no longer generally available for confirmation of the presence and mobility of the click and, on auscultation alone, a split first heart sound or a gallop rhythm have sometimes been misdiagnosed as a click. Thus, there is need for phonocardiographic confirmation of a click when equipment is available, and for echocardiographic confirmation of mitral valve prolapse in cases where there is doubt about the presence of a true click. The click in mitral valve prolapse may not always be evident in the supine position; to detect it, auscultation should be carried out in supine, left decubitus, sitting, standing, and squatting positions.

The late systolic murmur is another diagnostic hallmark of mitral valve prolapse in young individuals. In older individuals, it can be a sign of conditions such as papillary muscle dysfunction, hypertrophic cardiomyopathy, or calcification of the mitral valve annulus. Midsystolic murmurs are not infrequently misdiagnosed as late systolic murmur.[6] In general, echocardiographic confirmation of mitral valve prolapse would be advisable in the presence of isolated late systolic murmurs. The murmur in mitral valve prolapse may be pansystolic or may be heard as a precordial honk. Moreover, an auscultatory silent form has been described.[2] In these cases, echocardiographic studies are a prerequisite for the diagnosis of mitral valve prolapse.

The inability to demonstrate prolapse by echocardiography in some patients with typical nonejection clicks does not necessarily cast doubt on the diagnostic reliability of the click, but points to the shortcomings of echocardiography, which may fail to adequately visualize a complex structure such as the mitral valve.

Echocardiographic Features

Echocardiography has become accepted as a major diagnostic tool in mitral valve prolapse. Although two-dimensional echocardiography allows better visualization of the valve, M-mode echocardiography, when two-dimensionally guided, remains a helpful technique for the diagnosis of mitral valve prolapse. The typical findings on M-mode study are pansystolic hammocking and late systolic dipping. Unfortunately, hammocking is a very sensitive sign and requires, therefore, confirmation by 2D echocardiography. However, late systolic dipping, particularly when pronounced (3 mm) is virtually diagnostic of mitral valve prolapse.

On 2D echocardiography, mitral valve prolapse is recognized as billowing of the mitral leaflets across the plane of the mitral annulus. The diagnostic criteria are systolic arching of these leaflets in the parasternal long-axis view, posterior systolic bowing in the apical four-chamber view, and systolic coaptation of both leaflets at or behind the plane of the mitral valve annulus.[8] Minimal bowing of the anterior leaflet in the apical four-chamber view is a nonspecific finding and is probably due to the nonplanar "saddle" shape of the mitral annulus.[15]

Thickening and redundancy of mitral leaflets point to intrinsic involvement of the mitral valve. They may be seen on M-mode echocardiography but are best visualized on the 2D study.

Doppler echocardiography, preferably with color flow mapping, is helpful in the diagnosis and assessment of the severity of mitral insufficiency. This technique may be too sensitive when only minimal mitral regurgitation is noted, and its clinical significance awaits further studies.

Electrocardiographic Findings and Arrhythmias

Electrocardiographic abnormalities, noted primarily in the inferior limb leads, have been reported in mitral valve prolapse.[1,2] They consist of initially inverted or totally inverted T waves with or without S-T depression. The causal relationship between mitral valve prolapse and these nonspecific S-T and T changes has been questioned and awaits further study. Moreover, biphasic or negative T waves are not uncommon in the athlete and are not necessarily due to mitral valve prolapse.

S-T segment changes suggestive of ischemia have been reported on exercise tests in patients with mitral valve prolapse. Thallium 201 scintigraphy, when results are normal, is helpful in eliminating coronary artery disease as a cause of these changes.

A wide variety of arrhythmias have been reported in mitral valve prolapse, but premature ventricular complexes are the most prevalent rhythm disturbances.[16,17] Ventricular fibrillation is the probable mechanism of the rare cases of sudden death. Inappropriate sinus tachycardia is probably common in some patients with mitral valve prolapse.[8] There seems to be an association between mitral valve prolapse and pre-excitation, but the true prevalence of arrhythmias in mitral valve prolapse and their causal relationship to this entity remains controversial. Using ambulatory electrocardiographic monitoring, one group[16] observed premature ventricular complexes in 58%, supraventricular arrhythmia in 35%, and bradyarrhythmia in 29%, whereas another group[17] reported a 75% incidence of ventricular arrhythmias. In both investigations, ambulatory monitoring was more sensitive than stress testing in the detection of arrhythmias.

Unfortunately, many of these studies were carried out in symptomatic patients referred to tertiary centers and it has been shown that both atrial and ventricular arrhythmias are highly prevalent in normal subjects even in the absence of mitral valve prolapse. A low prevalence of arrhythmias has been reported in the pediatric age group.[18]

A statistically significant increase in supraventricular arrhythmias was demonstrated by one group,[19] with a modest trend to more complex or frequent premature ventricular beats. These authors have also stressed the importance of mitral insufficiency with or without mitral valve prolapse as a responsible factor for atrial and ventricular arrhythmias.[20] Unfortunately, they have compared a group with *severe* mitral regurgitation (with or without mitral valve prolapse), an entity that is known to be associated with a high prevalence of arrhythmias, to patients with mitral valve prolapse and *no* mitral regurgitation, and they have failed to evaluate the less severe forms of mitral insufficiency usually encountered in mitral valve prolapse. This study has been misinterpreted as indicating that mitral regurgitation alone was responsible for the increased arrhythmia in mitral valve prolapse.

It is worth noting that of 19 athletes with tachyarrhythmias reported in one study,[21] nine had mitral valve prolapse. Tachycardia in these 19 patients frequently occurred during exercise. The arrhythmia in the nine mitral valve prolapse patients was identified as paroxysmal atrial fibrillation in four, paroxysmal supraventricular tachycardia in one and ventricular tachycardia in four.

Angiographic Findings

Left ventriculography shows the mitral cusps to bulge toward the left atrium in systole.[2] The angiographic hallmark in the right anterior oblique view is systolic protrusion along the postero-inferior pole of the mitral valve, with associated convex deformity toward the left atrium. The left anterior oblique position is helpful in confirming the diagnosis of mitral valve prolapse and in identifying the involved leaflet. As an invasive procedure, however, left ventriculography is no longer used for the diagnosis of mitral valve prolapse except in those patients with severe mitral insufficiency who undergo cardiac catheterization with a view to surgery. In such patients, the diagnosis of mitral valve prolapse has already been made noninvasively and left ventriculography provides only confirmatory evidence.

Prognosis and Complications

The prognosis in mitral valve prolapse is generally favorable,[1, 2] particularly in children and in patients with an isolated click and those with the silent form. Its course may be infrequently complicated by the progression of mitral insufficiency, ruptured chordae tendineae, infective endocarditis, transient ischemic attacks, malignant arrhythmias, and sudden death. Considering the high prevalence of mitral valve prolapse and the relatively rare occurrence of complications, we must infer that this syndrome has a generally benign course. Patients with mitral valve prolapse and the murmur of mitral regurgitation (late systolic or holosystolic) and those with thickened, redundant mitral valve on echocardiography[22] are at a greater risk of developing these complications than those without these features.

It is now generally accepted that mitral valve prolapse is probably the most common cause of severe pure mitral insufficiency in developed countries,[23] which have witnessed, despite recent small outbreaks, an almost complete extinction of rheumatic fever. In ruptured chordae tendineae, mitral valve prolapse is the underlying pathological abnormality in the majority of patients.[24] Theoretically, patients with mitral valve prolapse and proven underlying structural abnormality of the mitral valve (regurgitant murmur, redundant leaflets by echocardiography) may be at a risk of developing ruptured chordae tendineae during strenuous activities, particularly those associated with isometric strain and body contact. However, except for two reported cases occurring during wood chopping[24] and a "particularly vigorous sprint"[25] respectively, evidence for this increased risk is lacking and, thus, no recommendation can be made at this time to restrict athletic activity in patients with mitral valve prolapse to prevent ruptured chordae tendineae.

Mitral valve prolapse is emerging as a major, if not *the* major, risk factor in endocarditis now that rheumatic heart disease has been decreasing in frequency. Endocarditis has been reported in mitral valve prolapse associated with a regurgitant murmur, but rarely in the silent form or in patients with isolated clicks. Male gender and the presence of a systolic murmur, particularly in persons above the age of 45, identify patients at increased risk of endocarditis.[26]

The risk of infective endocarditis warrants the use of antibiotic prophylaxis in patients with mitral valve prolapse when a regurgitant murmur is present and when thickened and redundant leaflets are identified on echocardiography. In the absence of a murmur, the clinical significance of mitral regurgitation demonstrated by Doppler echocardiography has not been elucidated.

Transient ischemic attacks and partial strokes are recognized as a complication of mitral valve prolapse and account for 40% of cases under the age of 45.[27] As an explanation for this complication, most investigators have postulated an embolic mechanism due to a clot or platelet aggregate originating from the rough surface of the prolapsed mitral valve or from the traumatized adjacent left atrial surface. Antiplatelet therapy is indicated following the occurrence of a cerebral ischemic episode.

Editor's Note: Some are presently advocating the use of daily aspirin for the prevention of accumulation of fibrin platelets in the acute angle formed by prolapsing leaflet tissue. – BFW

Sudden death is the most feared but, fortunately, the least common complication of mitral valve prolapse[2, 19, 28-31] (See Chapter 1). The author is aware of only 15 cases of sudden death associated with well-documented mitral valve prolapse, including four previously reported[2] who had no other diseases and were seen personally or whose clinical and pathological findings were reported to him. Approximately 100 other cases have been reported in the literature.

Although the rare occurrence of sudden death in this common entity has raised questions about the causal relationship between them, the absence of other accepted causes of sudden death in these patients makes it difficult to deny this relationship.

The age of the patients who died suddenly ranges from 9 to 79; only five were 20 years of age or younger (age 9, 14, 17, 19, and 20 respectively).[9] In 12 children, adolescents, and young adults with mitral valve prolapse who died suddenly, there was a family history of sudden death in three.[31] Death occurred during physical stress and

athletic activity in only six patients: The first, a 39-year-old man, died while mowing his lawn; the second, age 31, died after a game of tennis; the third, a 17-year-old boy, died during football scrimmage; the fourth and fifth, a woman age 29 and a man age 35, died during "athletic activity;" the sixth, age unreported, with known atrial fibrillation and pronounced left ventricular hypertrophy (the heart weighed 550 gm) died during a game of squash.[9, 31, 32]

Sudden death has been reported in only one patient with "silent mitral valve prolapse" and only a few patients with isolated clicks.[9] It would seem that patients with mitral valve prolapse and a regurgitant murmur and/or thickened valve on echocardiography are at a higher risk of dying suddenly and of developing ruptured chordae tendineae and infective endocarditis than patients with "silent mitral valve prolapse" or isolated clicks. The rare occurrence of sudden death in mitral valve prolapse should not be mentioned to the patient or their families for fear of causing undue anxiety or possibly inducing psychoneurosis.

Clinical Presentations, Diagnostic Criteria, and Work-up of the Athlete with Mitral Valve Prolapse

Mitral valve prolapse can present as an auscultatory abnormality characterized by a nonejection click with or without a late systolic murmur. Identification of a typical click is sufficient to diagnose this entity. The click and/or late systolic murmur are often evident on a routine physical examination of an athlete and are particularly sought in the presence of a symptom complex characterized by chest pain, fatigue, dyspnea, palpitations, dizziness, syncope, and arrhythmias. Despite doubt recently expressed about the existence of a true mitral valve prolapse syndrome, the occurrence of these symptoms in the athlete or the individual being evaluated for athletic activity would warrant a thorough auscultation. An echocardiographic work-up in this setting is probably not warranted.

In order to avoid over-diagnosis and the labeling of a normal variant as a disease, echocardiographic criteria for the diagnosis of mitral valve prolapse should be tightened. On two dimensional echocardiography, moderate to pronounced bowing of the mitral leaflets in the apical four-chamber view, visualization of the systolic coaptation point of the mitral leaflets at or behind the plane of the annulus, and preferably the demonstration of prolapse of the mitral leaflets on the parasternal long axis view should be required as diagnostic criteria. Thickening and redundancy of the mitral leaflets reinforce the diagnosis by pointing to intrinsic involvement of the mitral valve and by providing arguments against a normal variant.

Doppler echocardiography, preferably with color flow mapping, is helpful in the diagnosis and assessment of the severity of mitral regurgitation.

In the presence of asymptomatic mitral valve prolapse, there is controversy regarding the indications for ambulatory electrocardiographic monitoring or exercise testing. Such tests do not appear to be indicated in the asymptomatic athlete with mitral valve prolapse, or in individuals with mitral valve prolapse being evaluated regarding eligibility for competition in athletics. However, the Committee on Congenital Cardiac Defects of the Council on Cardiovascular Disease in the Young, American Heart Association, has recommended exercise testing prior to athletic competition in these individuals.[33]

In the presence of symptoms, particularly palpitations,[10] dizziness, near syncope or syncope, or in the presence of premature beats on auscultation or electrocardiography, both Holter monitoring and exercise testing are recommended for evaluation of the mechanism of symptoms and to help the physician formulate a recommendation. It is important to recognize that patients with mitral valve prolapse may have symptoms in the absence of arrhythmias, and that symptoms should be correlated with electrocardiographic changes as noted on Holter monitoring and exercise testing.[17] Electrophysiological studies[34] should be reserved for sustained ventricular tachycardia, syncope or near syncope (particularly when the relationship to arrhythmias has been demonstrated), episodes of cardiac arrest successfully resuscitated, and ventricular arrhythmias in patients with a family history of sudden death.

In evaluating the young athlete with mitral valve prolapse, Marfan's syndrome should be ruled out because the risk of aortic rupture and dissection in this syndrome represents a contraindication to competitive activities or contact sports, particularly if dilation of the ascending aorta is present. It should be noted that despite the high prevalence of mitral valve prolapse in Marfan's syndrome, an uncommon disease, there is a rare occurrence of Marfan's syndrome in mitral valve prolapse, a common disorder.

Criteria for Disqualification of Athletes with Mitral Valve Prolapse from Competition

The question of eligibility for athletic competition and criteria for disqualification of athletes with mitral valve prolapse from such competition have been discussed as a part of the 16th Bethesda Conference of the American College of Cardiology[10] and in the statement for physicians by the Committee on Congenital Cardiac Defects of the Council on Cardiovascular Disease in the Young, American Heart Association.[33] The 16th Bethesda Conference[35] has classified sports according to the type and intensity of exercise performed and to the danger of body collision. It has divided exercise into two general types: Static (isometric) and dynamic (isotonic), and has categorized the intensity of exercise into low, medium, or high. It also listed those sports that posed significant danger of body collision and those with further danger if syncope occurs.

The American Heart Association's special committee classified recreational activities into:
• Category 1: no restriction
• Category 2: moderate exercise (activities include regular physical education classes, tennis, baseball)
• Category 3: light exercise (activities include swimming, jogging, cycling, golf)
• Category 4: moderate limitation (no participation in physical education classes)
• Category 5: extreme limitation (homebound or wheelchair activities).

Some authors favor classifying jogging under category 2 rather than category 3.

Patients with mitral valve prolapse seen in tertiary centers, particularly those with symptoms, may not be athletically oriented. Such individuals should be encouraged to participate in exercise programs prescribed on the basis of Holter monitoring and exercise testing when they are indicated. It is likely, but yet unproven, that such programs may be associated with improvement of symptoms, particularly inappropriate sinus tachycardia, dyspnea, and fatigue.

Hard data on which to base a judgement for participation of individuals with mitral valve prolapse in athletic activities are not yet available. The dearth of documented serious complications, particularly in the young, and the lack of correlation between these complications and physical effort would warrant a permissive attitude toward participation in athletics. The prognosis of both ventricular and supraventricular arrhythmias detected with either exercise testing or ambulatory electrocardiography in these individuals is unknown.[36] The demonstration of no, infrequent, or benign premature ventricular or supraventricular complexes on Holter monitoring, and the lack of occurrence of complex ventricular arrhythmias on stress testing would provide the physician with objective evidence favoring a permissive attitude toward athletic participation. It is more difficult to arrive at a definite recommendation when apparently important arrhythmias are noted. Documentation of mitral insufficiency and demonstration of thickening of the mitral valve by echocardiography may warrant a more conservative approach in some patients.

The American Heart Association Committee[33] recommends no restriction on recreational activity in mild mitral valve prolapse associated with no symptoms and, after the performance of satisfactory exercise testing, no restriction in athletic competition (category 2). In the presence of premature ventricular contractions in the normal heart or mild mitral regurgitation without cardiac enlargement, no restrictions are recommended. Moderate exercise is allowed for patients with moderate mitral regurgitation (category 2). Moderate limitation (category 4) is recommended in the presence of severe mitral regurgitation with marked cardiomegaly and atrial fibrillation.

Recommendations from the Bethesda Conference

Recognizing the lack of definitive data at the present time, it would appear reasonable to consider disqualifying individuals with mitral valve prolapse from athletic competition or other equally strenuous activities except for participation in low-intensity competitive sports such as bowling, cricket, golf, rifling, etc.,[9, 10, 33, 35] if they fall into any of the following categories:

1. Patients with a history of syncope.[35] In mitral valve prolapse patients who died suddenly, a history of syncope was frequently elicited.[2, 29, 30] Since syncope may be due to arrhythmias, vasovagal reaction, orthostatic hypotension, etc., it is advisable to evaluate with Holter monitoring and exercise testing all patients with mitral valve prolapse and a history of syncope. The American Heart Association Committee[33] recognizes that "in certain recreational and occupational activities, the risk of even brief episodes of dizziness or syncope creates hazards much greater than might be implied by the degree of work itself."

2. Patients with a family history of sudden death due to mitral valve prolapse.

3. Patients with disabling chest pain, particularly if the pain is made worse by exercise. This combination is a rare occurrence in mitral valve prolapse and requires, under some circumstances, a work-up to rule out coronary artery disease, hypertrophic cardiomyopathy, or congenital anomalies of the coronary arteries.

4. Patients with complex ventricular arrhythmias (frequent, multifocal, repetitive). These arrhythmias are especially of concern if they are induced or made worse by exercise. When this is not the case, this recommendation is "soft."

5. Patients with significant mitral regurgitation associated with moderate to marked cardiomegaly on chest films and moderate to marked left ventricular enlargement by echocardiography. As mentioned above, no restriction is warranted in mild mitral regurgitation without cardiac enlargement.

6. Patients with Marfan's syndrome and associated mitral valve prolapse, because of the risk of aortic rupture and dissection.

Summary

Mitral valve prolapse is probably the most common valvular disorder, affecting approximately 5% of the population. Its diagnostic hallmark is a non-ejection click. In its absence, strict M mode and two dimensional echocardiographic criteria are required to reach the diagnosis. Minimal to moderate bowing of the mitral valve on two dimensional echocardiography probably represents a normal variant.

The prognosis of mitral valve prolapse is generally favorable. However, in a few patients, progression of mitral insufficiency with or without chordal rupture, infective endocarditis, transient ischemic attacks, and, rarely, sudden death do occur.

A permissive attitude toward participation in athletics is warranted by the available evidence. However, a restrictive approach is recommended in the presence of syncope, disabling chest pain, prolonged Q-T interval, complex arrhythmias, significant mitral regurgitation, Marfan's syndrome, or a family history of sudden death.

References

1. Barlow JB, Pocock WA: The mitral valve prolapse enigma – two decades later. *Mod Concepts Cardiovasc Dis* 53:13, 1984.
2. Jeresaty RM: Mitral Valve Prolapse. New York, Raven Press, 1979.
3. Retchin SM, et al: Mitral valve prolapse: Disease or illness? *Arch Intern Med* 145:1081, 1986.
4. Savage DD, Devereux RB, Garrison RJ, et al: Mitral valve prolapse in the general population II. Clinical features: The Framingham Study. *Am Heart J* 106:577, 1983.
5. Uretsky BF: Does mitral valve prolapse cause non-specific symptoms? *Int J Cardiol* 1:435, 1982.
6. Devereux RB, et al: Diagnosis and classification of severity of mitral valve prolapse: Methodologic, biologic, and prognostic considerations. *Am Heart J* 113:1255, 1987.
7. Arfken CK, Lachman AS, Schulman P, et al: Lack of association of cardiac symptoms with mitral valve prolapse in sixth grade schoolchildren. (Abstract) *J Am Coll Cardiol* (suppl A) 7:29a, 1986.
8. Jeresaty RM: Mitral valve prolapse – An update. *JAMA* 253:793, 1985.
9. Jeresaty RM: Mitral valve prolapse: Definition and implications in athletes. *J Am Coll Cardiol* 7:231, 1986.
10. Maron BJ, Gaffney FA, Jeresaty RM: Task Force III: Hypertrophic cardiomyopathy, other myopericardial disease and mitral valve prolapse. *J Am Coll Cardiol* 6:1215, 1985.
11. Levy D, Savage D: Prevalence and clinical features of mitral valve prolapse. *Am Heart J* 113:1281, 1987.
12. Sakamoto T: Phonocardiographic Assessment of the Prevalence of Mitral Valve Prolapse in the Prospective Survey of Heart Disease in Schoolchildren: A Seven Year Cumulative Study. *Acta Cardiologica* 38:261, 1983.
13. Procacci PM, Savran SV, Schreiter SL, et al: Prevalence of clinical mitral valve prolapse in 1,169 young women. *N Engl J Med* 294:1086, 1976.
14. Devereux RB, et al: Relation between clinical features of the mitral prolapse syndrome and echocardiographically documented mitral valve prolapse. *J Am Coll Cardiol* 8:763, 1986.
15. Levine RA, et al: The relationship of mitral annular shape to the diagnosis of mitral valve prolapse. *Circulation* 75:757, 1987.
16. DeMaria, et al: Arrhythmias in the mitral valve prolapse syndrome. *Ann Intern Med* 84:656, 1976.
17. Winkle RA, et al: Arrhythmias in patients with mitral valve prolapse. *Circulation* 52:73, 1975.
18. Bisset GS, et al: Clinical spectrum and long-term follow up of isolated mitral valve prolapse in 119 children. *Circulation* 62:423, 1980.
19. Kligfield P, et al: Arrhythmias and sudden death in mitral valve prolapse. *Am Heart J* 113:1298, 1987.
20. Kligfield P, et al: Complex arrhythmias in mitral valve prolapse: Contrast to arrhythmias in mitral valve prolapse without mitral regurgitation. *Am J Cardiol* 55:1545, 1985.
21. Coelho A, et al: Tachyarrhythmias in young Athletes. *J Am Coll Cardiol* 7:237, 1985.
22. Nishimura RA, et al: Echocardiographically documented mitral valve prolapse. *N Engl J Med* 313:1305, 1985.
23. Waller BF, Morrow AG, Maron BJ, et al: Etiology of clinically isolated, severe, chronic, pure mitral regurgitation. Analysis of 97 patients over 30 years of age having mitral valve replacement. *Am Heart J* 104:276, 1982.
24. Jeresaty RM, Edward JE, Chawla SK: Mitral valve prolapse and ruptured chordae tendineae. *Am J Cardiol* 55:138, 1985.
25. Zimmerman FH, Mogtader AH: Ruptured chordae tendineae and acute pulmonary edema induced by exercise. *JAMA* 258:812, 1987.
26. MacMahon SW, et al: Mitral valve prolapse and infective endocarditis. *Am Heart J* 113:1291, 1987.
27. Barnett HJM, et al: Further evidence relating mitral valve prolapse to cerebral ischemic events. *N Engl J Med* 302:139, 1980.
28. Chesler E, King RA, Edwards FE: The myxomatous mitral valve and sudden death. *Circulation* 67:632, 1983.
29. Kramer MR, Drori Y, Lev B: Sudden death in young soldiers – High incidence of syncope prior to death. *Chest* 93:343, 1988.
30. Pocock WA, et al: Sudden death in primary mitral valve prolapse. *Am Heart J* 107:378, 1984.
31. Topaz O, Edwards JE: Pathologic features of sudden death in children, adolescents, and young adults. *Chest* 87:476, 1985.
32. Northcote RJ, Flannigan C, Ballantyne D: Sudden death and vigorous exercise – A study of 60 deaths associated with squash. *Br Heart J* 55:198, 1986.
33. Gutgesell HP, Gessner IH, Vetter VL, Yabek SM, Norton JB: Recreational and Occupational Recommendations for Young Patients with Heart Disease – A Statement for Physicians by the Committee on Cardiovascular Disease in the Young, American Heart Association. *Circulation* 74:1195A, 1986.
34. Rosenthal ME, et al: The yield of programmed ventricular stimulation in mitral valve prolapse patients with ventricular arrhythmias. *Am Heart J* 110:970, 1985.
35. Mitchell JH, Blomqvist CG, Haskell WL: Classification of sports. *J Am Coll Cardiol* 6:1198, 1985.
36. Kennedy HL: Comparison of ambulatory electrocardiography and exercise testing. *Am J Cardiol* 47:1359, 1981.

CHAPTER 10

CARDIOVASCULAR EVALUATION FOR SPORT SCUBA DIVING

Jacqueline O'Donnell, MD

Associate Professor of Medicine
Department of Medicine/Division of Cardiology
Krannert Institute of Cardiology
Indiana University School of Medicine

Editor's Note: Most of us have had little or no experience with scuba diving and, in particular, with the health hazards associated with it. This chapter will, therefore, serve as a desk reference, to help us in advising our patients who participate in this sport. – WPH

Sport scuba diving is a popular recreational activity enjoyed by an estimated two to three million divers.[1,2] More than 200,000 persons enroll in scuba classes each year.[3] Certain geographical areas in the United States such as California and Florida (particularly the Florida Keys) have both the warm climate and water temperatures to support such activities. The Caribbean has also become a popular dive location, since it is very accessible; most Caribbean destinations are within a one to three hour flight from the United States.[4]

In addition, the manufacturing industry has promoted the popularity of sport scuba diving by developing new products with fashionable colors, using the latest design and materials in dive gear, and expanding product lines to include women and adolescents.

Although there are several scuba diving certifying agencies such as PADI,* NAUI, YMCA, etc., there are no regulations specifying the standards for sport scuba diving as there are in military and commercial diving. In most areas, a certification card from one of the above agencies is all that is necessary to dive; this is the extent of the regula-tions. Refresher courses are not mandatory and, in fact, are difficult to find. Therefore, it is up to each diver to maintain physical fitness, have equipment in working order, and be knowledge-able in diving skills.

Hazards of Scuba Diving

The underwater environment is unique and poses special problems for the diver.[5] Increased pressure effects, depth, visibility, temperature, and water currents are all factors that affect the scuba diver. Pressure changes that occur as the diver descends and ascends affect all air-filled spaces, particularly the sinuses, middle ear, and lungs. Inability to equalize pressure in the sinuses and middle ear can result in sinus squeeze or middle ear barotrauma. In the lungs, the change in pressure can result in pulmonary overpressure accidents, leading to arterial gas embolism or spontaneous tension pneumothorax (Boyle's Law in physics).

Another hazard is increased nitrogen uptake by various tissues, which can be manifested as nitrogen narcosis and decompression sickness. The increase in nitrogen uptake is explained by Henry's Law: The solubility of a gas in liquid solution at equilibrium is proportional to the partial pressure of that gas. Therefore, the dissolution of nitrogen in the blood and tissues increases as the pressure increases.

Loss of body heat[5] can occur even in tropical waters, and all divers must contend with some degree of hypothermia. It is of major importance in temperate or cold climates. The longer the immersion and the colder the temperature, the greater the risk for hypothermia. Wet suits, dry suits or dive skins are worn to protect against loss of body heat. A decrease in body temperature makes exercise much more difficult and exaggerates certain physiologic responses. Hypothermia

---

*PADI – Professional Association of Diving Instructors
NAUI – National Association of Underwater Instructors
YMCA – Young Mens' Christian Association.

also impairs fine motor movements, which are needed for making dive gear adjustments, abandoning gear in emergency situations, or manipulating a dive buddy's equipment for rescue procedures.

Control of buoyancy[5] is a critical factor with which the diver must contend. Many factors affect buoyancy, including the amount of muscle versus body fat, fresh versus salt water, and amount and weight of equipment. The diver must achieve neutral buoyancy so that he neither bobs to the surface nor sinks to the bottom, but swims weightlessly in the water.

Water currents can frequently pose problems, particularly for divers who are cold, fatigued, disoriented, or poor swimmers. If the current is not properly assessed, the diver can find himself a long distance from the shore or boat and may be required to swim at the end of a dive while very cold, fatigued and with the added resistance of his scuba gear.

Preparticipation Evaluation

Aside from being knowledgeable regarding the mechanisms and physics of diving plus being at ease in the water and assessing the environmental conditions, physical fitness to dive is a vital issue. Although diving itself does not require great physical prowess, the entire diving experience, including collecting, carrying, and loading equipment, entering and exiting the water with equipment in rough seas, and the occasional instance of needing to swim against the current to the boat or beach on the surface can demand a great deal of physical stamina and strength. Thus, sport scuba diving is an athletic endeavor and participants must have a high degree of physical and mental fitness. For example, an average diver in good condition should be able to swim a minimum of a quarter of a mile in eight minutes or less with fins and mask without stopping. A diving instructor should be able to swim a half mile in fifteen minutes.[6, 7]

Diving differs from other sports in that a temporary alteration in consciousness occurring under water at depth would most assuredly result in a fatal outcome. If the same alteration of consciousness occurred in a person skiing, playing tennis or football, the person would likely survive. Therefore, any condition that might result in

syncope, near-syncope or loss of consciousness is disqualifying.

History and Physical Examination

In the cardiac evaluation of a potential sport scuba diver, a comprehensive history and physical is mandatory. If any abnormality is found, further testing is required in order to exclude particular disease states that are felt by diving physicians to be a contraindication to scuba diving (Table 10-1). With respect to history taking, it is important that the following conditions be emphasized and fully evaluated:

1. Any history of chest pain
2. History of loss of consciousness, syncope or near syncope
3. History of palpitations, rapid heart rate, or any rhythm abnormality
4. History of rheumatic fever or heart murmur heard at birth, in infancy or adolescence
5. Hypertension
6. Diabetes mellitus
7. Lung problems, wheezing, asthma, recurrent bronchitis, or pneumonia.

The physical examination of the potential sport scuba diver should include the patient's actual height and weight and assessment of body habitus. Examination of the peripheral vascular system should be performed to exclude presence of arterial or venous insufficiency. During the cardiac examination, the physician should listen for any abnormal heart sounds such as clicks, ejection sounds, gallops, murmurs, or rubs. The lung sounds should be normal without rales, rhonchi, or reduced diaphragmatic excursion.

Cardiovascular Guidelines

If any aspect of the cardiovascular history or physical examination is abnormal, the minimal evaluation should include a resting and exercise electrocardiogram, chest x-ray, echocardiogram, 24-hour ambulatory monitoring, and repeat blood pressure determinations. Referral to a physician with diving experience is strongly recommended. The Divers' Alert Network (DAN) (919-684-2948) can provide the names and phone numbers of experienced diving physicians throughout the United States who are available for consultation.

Particular attention should be given to known risk factors for heart disease such as hyperten-

Table 10-1
Conditions For Which Disqualification From Scuba Diving is Recommended*

- Tympanic membrane perforation or aeration tubes
- Inability to autoinflate the middle ears
- External ear exostoses or osteomas adequate to prevent external ear canal pressure equilibration
- Meniere's Disease or other chronic vertiginous conditions; status post-surgery, such as subarachnoid endolymphatic shunt for Meniere's Disease
- Stapedectomy and middle ear prosthesis
- Chronic mastoiditis or mastoid fistula
- Any oral or maxillofacial deformity that interferes with retention of the mouthpiece
- Corrected near visual acuity not adequate to see tank pressure gauge, watch, decompression tables, and compass underwater. Uncorrected visual acuity not adequate to see the diving buddy or locate the boat in case corrective lenses are lost underwater
- Radial keratotomy or other recent ocular surgery
- Claustrophobia of a degree to predispose to panic
- Suicidal ideation
- Psychosis
- Significant anxiety states
- Severe depression
- Manic states
- Alcoholism
- Mood altering drug use
- Improper motivation for diving
- Episodic loss of consciousness
- History of seizure. History of seizures in early childhood must be evaluated individually
- Migraine
- History of cerebrovascular accident or transient ischemic attack
- History of spinal cord trauma with neurologic deficit – whether fully recovered or not
- Demyelinating process
- Brain tumor with or without surgery
- Intracranial aneurysm or other vascular malformation

- History of neurological decompression sickness with residual deficit
- Head injury with sequelae
- History of intracranial surgery
- Sickle cell disease
- Polycythemia or leukemia
- Unexplained anemia
- History of myocardial infarction
- Angina or other evidence of coronary artery disease
- Unrepaired cardiac septal defects
- Aortic stenosis or mitral stenosis
- Complete heart block
- Fixed second degree heart block
- Exercise-induced tachyarrhythmias
- Wolff-Parkinson-White Syndrome with paroxysmal atrial tachycardia or syncope
- Fixed rate pacemakers
- Any drugs that inhibit the normal cardiovascular response to exercise
- Peripheral vascular disease, arterial or venous, adequate to limit exercise tolerance
- Hypertension with end-organ finding – retinal, cardiac, renal, or vascular
- History of spontaneous pneumothorax
- Bronchial asthma. History of childhood asthma requires special studies
- Exercise or cold-air-induced asthma
- Chronic obstructive pulmonary disease
- X-ray evidence of pulmonary blebs, bullae, or cysts
- Insulin dependent diabetes mellitus. Diet or oral medication-controlled diabetes mellitus if there is a history of hypoglycemic episodes
- Any abdominal wall hernia with potential for gas trapping, until surgically corrected
- Paraesophageal or incarcerated sliding hiatal hernia
- Sliding hiatus hernia if symptomatic due to reflux esophagitis
- Pregnancy

*Consensus recommendations for sport scuba diving only, prepared by a group of multispecialty physicians who are scuba divers, and from consultation with physiologists and experts on diver training. (From Davis, [8] with permission).

sion, history of previous cardiac disease, hyperlipidemia, tobacco history, positive family history for heart disease, and history of diabetes mellitus.

Diving candidates over the age of 40, or poorly conditioned candidates under 40 should have an exercise tolerance test including an exercise ECG. These candidates must be able to achieve 14 METs of exercise with a normal ST segment response. (One MET, or metabolic equivalent, is the energy expended per kilogram of body weight per minute by an average person at rest and is calculated to be approximately 1.4 calories per minute or 3.5 ml 0_2 per minute.) The average energy requirement for scuba diving is 8 METs, varying from 2 METs (sitting quietly on the ocean bottom) to 18 METs (towing a buddy against a strong current). Therefore, it is felt that the minimum fitness level for all sport divers is 10 METs.[9]

• **A history of coronary artery disease** manifested by myocardial infarction or angina pectoris is an absolute contraindication. There are a few exceptional individuals who may dive following coronary artery bypass surgery, if they are able to demonstrate excellent physical conditioning and exercise tolerance and a normal cardiac evaluation.

Candidates who have undergone percutaneous transluminal coronary angioplasty in the treatment of coronary artery disease may be cleared for diving if they have no evidence of myocardial infarction, if the angioplasty was successful (<30% residual stenosis), and if a subsequent exercise test (combined with either echocardiography or thallium imaging) is normal to 14 METs.

• **Pacemakers** represent a relative contraindication. Unpublished data from the Medtronics (Versatrax, Mirel, and Spectrax) and Cordis companies report tests on pacemaker function at depths up to more than 165 feet of sea water (FSW). During compression, prolonged exposure, and decompression, no changes in structural integrity or electrical performance were found down to 6 atmospheres (165 FSW). The Versatrax ceased operation between 6 and 8 atmospheres. From these preliminary data, the primary concern appears to be the underlying cardiac pathology that required the pacemaker, not the pacemaker's performance, and the patient's ability to exercise adequately.

• **Cage ball or disc prosthetic heart valves** are disqualifying. Tissue heterograft valves generally are also disqualifying, but rare exceptions can be made after full cardiac evaluation.

Any drugs that significantly inhibit the normal cardiovascular response to exercise are generally contraindicated in diving. Each case must be individually evaluated by a cardiologist, however. Major consideration should be directed toward the underlying pathology that requires the drug.

Blood pressure is not significantly affected by hydrostatic pressure, but it may be raised by other factors such as cold water, panic, stress, or exertion. A hypertensive diving candidate whose blood pressure is well controlled by weight loss, physical conditioning, and/or diuretics may be cleared for sport diving after a complete cardiac evaluation with close medical supervision. As noted above, however, patients who require antihypertension drugs that produce significant blockade of the autonomic nervous system must be disqualified. Selection of indicated drugs for a given patient must not be tempered by the patient's desire to dive, but should be determined by the need for adequate control of moderate hypertension. In older patients and anyone with severe hypertension, a search for end-organ (for example, retinal, renal, or cardiac) involvement should be made. Such damage would obviously disqualify the diver.

The following additional cardiovascular defects also would disqualify a candidate from participation in sport scuba diving:
• Central arteriovenous communication (such as atrial septal defect, ventricular defect, patent ductus arteriosus), because of the risk of paradoxical venous to arterial gas embolism
• Aortic stenosis or mitral stenosis
• Coarctation of the aorta
• Cyanotic heart disease
• Peripheral vascular disease of either the arterial or venous system, of a degree to limit exercise tolerance, is a contraindication. Because of cold water exposure, Raynaud's phenomenon is disqualifying.
• Arrhythmias:
    Complete heart block
    Fixed types of second-degree heart block
    Exercise-induced tachyarrhythmias
    Wolff-Parkinson-White syndrome with parox-

ysmal atrial tachycardia, because of the unpredictable risk of atrial and ventricular tachycardia, which could lead to hypotension and drowning.

• **Mitral valve prolapse** without associated tachyarrhythmias or other hemodynamic problems need not disqualify the candidate. A very common disorder (see Chapter 9), it usually does not hamper exercise capacity or performance. Of course, diving would be contraindicated in individuals with significant mitral regurgitation,[10] which can cause an increase in myocardial work and may be associated with an inability to increase exercise capacity.

• **Paroxysmal atrial tachycardia** may occur in the normal individual with excess caffeine, cigarettes, alcohol, and stress. If cardiac evaluation reveals no underlying pathology and the episodes are fully controlled by lifestyle modification, diving can be allowed.

• **Type I or Wenckebach-type heart block** usually suggests variable refractoriness of the A-V node. This can be due to a variety of causes, from myocardial ischemia to increased vagal activity caused by drugs such as digitalis. Rarely, a changing P-R interval with an occasional non-conducted P wave ("dropped beat") that occurs with respiration may be seen in well-trained individuals. If the conduction abnormality disappears with exercise, the heart rate response to exercise is appropriate, and no other underlying disease is found, the person may be cleared for diving.

• **Mild valvular regurgitation** with normal ventricular response to exercise and no ventricular enlargement need not disqualify a candidate from diving. If clinical examination, echocardiogram, or ECG indicate ventricular enlargement, however, diving is contraindicated. Murmurs must be evaluated for exact hemodynamic significance. An obstruction to forward flow, such as aortic or mitral stenosis, is disqualifying because of the inability to increase the cardiac output to provide needed flow during exercise, leading to a risk of syncope and drowning.

Editor's Note: I recall a 60-year-old man who had significant aortic stenosis, but had no symptoms referable to his heart; he was referred to me for advice concerning his continuing participation in scuba diving. He loved this sport and had been diving for many years. He had never experienced any difficulty. He had no history of chest discomfort, palpitation, unusual fatigue, dizziness, nor syncope during his diving episodes.

I would have liked for him to follow the advice as given in the above discussion; however, he stated even if it was advised that, to be on the safe side, he discontinue scuba diving, he would continue to dive. He was a very intelligent man, fully cognizant of the possible danger. He said scuba diving represented one of the greatest pleasures in his life, and he did not want to give it up. I understood…and I wonder if I might not have made the same decision if I were in his place. An interesting "cardiac pearl" is that a patient with a "tight mitral stenosis" may become short of breath by merely getting into water up to his neck – as might occur at the seashore or in a swimming pool. By submerging in the water, an increase in venous return to the right side of the heart can occur. This can cause significant dyspnea, even though there has been no physical effort.

I learned this pearl from the late Professor George Burch of Tulane. Since looking for this, I have seen the same thing in some of my patients. – WPH

---

*Author's Note: I must disagree with Dr. Harvey's view regarding the 60-year-old man with aortic stenosis. Patients with significant aortic stenosis must be advised **against** diving – even those who are asymptomatic. The patient would not only endanger his own life but that of his "buddy" and other potential rescuers. – JO'D*

Pulmonary Guidelines

The most dramatic and life-threatening medical emergencies in compressed air diving are pulmonary overpressure accidents, which result from lung overinflation during breathholding, or pathological air trapping in part of the lung during ascent from depths as shallow as four feet of water. Under high pressure, gas bubbles can enter the pulmonary circulation, then cross the pulmonary capillary bed, enter the left side of the heart and potentially embolize the coronary or cerebral circulation (air embolism) and result in immediate life-threatening situations. Pulmonary interstitial emphysema and mediastinal and subcutaneous emphysema are also seen.

The history and examination of the lungs must be directed toward prevention of these serious complications. Diving instruction and psychological assessment of the diving candidate are the best preventive measures against panic and breathholding on ascent. The physician's responsibility is to minimize the risk of local air trapping by advising candidates at increased risk not to dive.

A baseline chest x-ray is desirable for all divers, to rule out blebs (remembering that small blebs may not be detectable), bullae, or other air-containing cavities. Certainly, a chest x-ray must be part of the examination of cigarette smokers and those with any history suspicious of pulmonary disease. Pulmonary function testing and referral to a pulmonary medicine specialist is indicated for questionable cases.

• **Bronchial Asthma** – Whether to allow patients with bronchial asthma to dive is sharply debated among physicians. The diagnosis is usually made by a history of episodic wheezing, dyspnea, cough, and pulmonary function studies that demonstrate reversible airflow obstruction. Such patients are at increased risk of bronchospasm, which may be triggered by cold water, panic, or heavy exertion underwater, with resultant pulmonary overpressure during ascent.[11] These individuals **must** be excluded from diving.

Questions may arise, however, concerning more subtle cases, such as patients with only cough or dyspnea as initial symptoms. Indeed, some have few symptoms to suggest bronchial hyperactivity, so that bronchial inhalation challenge testing may be needed to arrive at a rational decision.

Most diving medicine specialists recommend that patients with currently active bronchial asthma be strictly forbidden to dive. The physician should not be swayed by arguments that the air of scuba is free of pollens or that other asthma patients dive successfully. The stresses of diving and the life-threatening consequences of an underwater bronchospastic episode are too dangerous. Although some asthma patients dive without

incident (just as some drunk drivers avoid wrecks), it is a matter of odds; few would deny that the risk is increased.

Any patient with a history of significant childhood asthma, symptoms suggestive of asthma during past years, exercise-induced wheezing, or wheezing on inhalation of cold air should be referred to a pulmonary medicine specialist for examination, including challenge testing, before diving recommendations can be made.

• **The Dangers of Shallow Diving** – It must be emphasized that the greatest volume changes in the lungs of a diver with air trapping occur at shallow depths. **Never** clear such a diver for "shallow diving only" – shallow depth is the most dangerous.

• **Other Disqualifying Conditions** – A history of spontaneous pneumothorax is considered disqualifying because there exists a high risk of recurrence at ground level, even without the pressure changes encountered in diving. A pneumothorax occurring underwater becomes a potentially fatal tension pneumothorax as pleural cavity gas volume expands during ascent.

Opinions are divided regarding diving after resection of pulmonary blebs. Some specialists believe the risk of local air trapping during decompression (ascent) still exists, while others hold that the risk has been removed by surgery. To be safe, these patients should not dive.

Whether a history of healed and fully resolved thoracotomy should preclude diving is also the subject of differing opinion. The conservative approach is to be concerned about possible scarring and local air trapping. Each case should be evaluated on an individual basis, taking into account the reason for the thoracotomy (trauma, lobectomy, or underlying pulmonary disease), and a pulmonary medicine specialist should be consulted. Most diving medicine specialists are concerned that differing lung stiffness due to old scars can cause tears with the great pressure imbalances that exist even at shallow depths.[12]

Chronic obstructive pulmonary disease generally represents a contraindication, but in borderline cases a complete pulmonary medicine evaluation should be undertaken.

Other conditions considered disqualifying include any active infection, pneumonitis, bronchitis, bronchiectasis, emphysema, pulmonary fibrosis, or pulmonary tuberculosis in active form. All studies in patients with a history of pulmonary tuberculosis must indicate that the disease is fully arrested without evidence of cavitation or extensive fibrosis before diving can be allowed. Mycotic disease with cavitation and residual scars or calcifications deserves individual consideration, with pulmonary medicine consultation. Overall, however, these conditions also are considered to be disqualifying.

Summary

Danger from trapped gases on the decompression of ascent, along with the physical exertion that may be required in scuba diving and the threat to life that may result from underwater episodes that would be much less hazardous on land require that screening for scuba diving be rigorous. Diving should not be permitted if any disorders are found that put the candidate in jeopardy of air-trapping or of syncope or near-syncope. Even diving at shallow depths requires strict adherence to medical recommendations, since that is when the greatest pressure changes occur. Consultation with an appropriate specialist for additional testing is indicated if there is any doubt about the candidate's suitability for diving.

References

1. Bove Alfred A: Diving Medicine. *Skin Diver* 34(12):14, 1985.
2. Davis JC: Decompression Sickness in Sport Scuba Diving. *The Physician and Sports Medicine* 16 (Feb):108-21, 1988.
3. Tzimonlis Paul J: (Editorial) Scuba: Safety Comes First. *Skin Diver* 35(3):8, 1986.
4. Tzimonlis Paul J: (Editorial) Scuba: Sand in Their Shoes. *Skin Diver* 36(4):10, 1987.
5. Richardson Drew: (ed): *PADI Open Water Diver Manual.* PADI, Santa Ana, CA, 1988.
6. Tzimonlis Paul J: (Editorial) Spring Body Tune-up. *Skin Diver* 34(5):4, 1985.
7. Tzimonlis Paul J: (Editorial) Winter Work-outs Maintain Dive Fitness. *Skin Diver* 35(1):6, 1986.
8. Davis JC: (ed): *Medical Examination of Sport Scuba Divers.* Medical Seminars, Inc., San Antonio, 1983.
9. Bove Alfred A: Diving Medicine: Improving Diver Fitness. *Skin Diver* 36(4):30, 1987.
10. Bove Alfred A: Diving Medicine: Mitral Valve Prolapse. *Skin Diver* 35(8):16, 1986.
11. Bove Alfred A: Diving Medicine: Asthma. *Skin Diver* 35(6):60, 1986.
12. Bove Alfred A: Diving Medicine. *Skin Diver* 36(8):24, 1987.

CHAPTER 11

CONSIDERATIONS IN THE CARDIOVASCULAR ASSESSMENT OF ULTRAENDURANCE ATHLETES

Mary L. O'Toole, PhD

University of Tennessee-Campbell Clinic
Department of Orthopaedic Surgery
Memphis

Pamela S. Douglas, MD

Harvard Medical School
Beth Israel Hospital Cardiovascular Section
Boston

Editor's Note: This chapter provides us with an excellent, authoritative discussion of a very specialized subject – evaluation of ultraendurance athletes. This is a topic with which most of us are unfamiliar; therefore this discussion is welcome and appropriate. – WPH

Ultraendurance exercise can be defined as exercise lasting longer than two hours. In recent years, ultraendurance racing events have become commonplace in sports such as running, bicycling, swimming, and triathlon. These events require continuous, vigorous physical activity of several hours duration, as well as the training necessary to compete in them. Although the millions of participants can collectively be called ultraendurance athletes, the demands on the cardiovascular system may be quite varied.

For example, much of the physiologic information currently available is based on studies of marathon runners. This leads the reader to believe that ultraendurance training consists almost entirely of aerobic exercise when, in fact, most ultraendurance athletes also engage in substantial amounts of high-intensity exercise that has a significant anaerobic or resistive component. For example, training records from participants in the Hawaii Ironman Triathlon (2.4 mile swim, 112 mile bike ride, 26.2 mile run) indicate that, on average, 46% of swim training is "interval" or high-intensity exercise. In this same group, interval training constitutes 21% of bike training and 19% of run training. Additionally, 27% of bike training and 24% of run training includes hill climbing.[1,2]

Thus, the cardiovascular adaptations in the ultraendurance athlete reflect both aerobic and anaerobic training, over a wide variety of intensities and durations. This diversity makes it difficult to identify a uniform set of characteristics that categorize the cardiovascular adaptation to ultraendurance exercise.

Conversely, one clear difference between ultraendurance exercise and other exercise is, by definition, the duration of the competitive event. As such, all types of ultraendurance exercise place demands on the cardiovascular system not seen during shorter exercise; performance of all ultraendurance exercise is limited in large part by the functional capacity of the cardiovascular system. Physiologic stressors on the cardiovascular system not seen in shorter exercise include the cumulative effects of dehydration, heat stress, and the increased use of fat as a substrate.

Cardiovascular adaptations, both central and peripheral, that occur with much less endurance training also are seen in the ultraendurance athlete. In this chapter, results of studies using ultraendurance athletes as subjects are presented with clinical and diagnostic implications discussed. Clinical exercise tests are discussed in terms of usefulness in evaluating ultraendurance athletes. A short discussion of ultraendurance exercise in the presence of heart disease is included.

Physiologic Considerations

• **Dehydration** – Dehydration is the most common medical problem encountered in ultraendurance racing.[3] Studies of both marathoners and triathletes[4-8] have consistently demonstrated that athletes become dehydrated during prolonged exercise even when adequate replacement fluid is available to them. During actual marathon races, runners in one study were shown to lose approximately 2.8 liters of sweat per hour[5] and in another to lose 1.6% of body weight per hour during the 3 hours, 15 minutes taken to finish the marathon.[7]

Studies of triathletes, during races of varying distances that lasted between 2 and 17 hours, have shown dehydration to be between 0.3 to 0.6% of body weight loss per hour.[8] Laboratory studies of runners[5] and triathletes[4] have shown mean decreases in body weight to be between 0.5 and 2.4% per hour. Claremont and associates[9] demonstrated the detrimental effects of dehydration by showing that, in long distance running, pace must be slowed by 2% for each 1% of body weight loss from dehydration.

Although cardiovascular parameters can be expected to reach a steady-state within five minutes after the initiation of continuous, rhythmical exercise, a "cardiovascular drift" occurs if exercise is prolonged.[10] This can, in part, be explained by dehydration, which causes a decrease in plasma volume that in turn reduces cardiac filling pressure, central blood volume, and stroke volume. Therefore, in order to maintain a cardiac output appropriate for the energy output, heart rate must be increased.[4, 11-16] Studies have shown a 10 to 15% decrease in plasma volume within the first 10 to 20 minutes of exercise,[12, 13, 17] even without dehydration. A further depletion of blood volume is likely after 30 minutes of exercise.[18]

• **Heat Stress** – Exercise by itself imposes a heat load on the exercising individual, since there may be a 10-fold increase in metabolic heat production resulting from skeletal muscle contraction during endurance exercise. Exercise in a hot environment adds to this load and imposes a more severe stress on the cardiovascular system.[12, 16] Since one of the main functions of the circulatory system is to transport heat from the muscles to the surface of the body, skin vasculature is dilated and competes with the active musculature for high perfusion rates. Since skin blood flow rises along with core temperature, the decrease in plasma volume seen with exercise is accentuated with exercise in the heat.[12, 16]

Although early thermoregulatory studies stated that women could not tolerate stress caused by exercise in the heat as well as men, more recent evidence shows these conclusions to have been artifactually based, since, in most cases, the women were less well-trained and worked at a higher percent VO_2 max.[19] Highly conditioned female ultraendurance athletes can be expected to tolerate combined exercise and heat stress as well as men.[20] However, women athletes have two potential disadvantages compared to men under these conditions, and one potential advantage:

First, women tend to have higher heart rates under all conditions.

Second, they have a lower blood volume per unit surface area (approximately 12%) so that cutaneous vasodilation produces a relatively greater peripheral shift of the available blood volume.[20] Both of these conditions would create a greater strain on the cardiovascular system.

To their advantage, women do not lose as large a volume of sweat as do men, thereby gaining an advantage by better maintaining blood volume.

• **Substrate Utilization** – The energy expenditure necessary for running a marathon (regardless of pace) has been calculated to be between 95-100 KCal per mile or approximately 2500 KCal,[14, 21, 22] and can be used to approximate the energy cost of longer events. During endurance exercise, the human body uses a combination of carbohydrate, fat, and protein as substrate. Proportions of the macronutrients vary among individuals and among exercise intensities. However, since the human body is capable of only storing approximately 1000 KCal of potential energy as muscle glycogen and another 300-600 KCal as glycogen in the liver, fat is, of necessity, a major substrate during ultraendurance events.[23]

Laboratory studies of prolonged exercise, lasting from two to eight hours, have consistently shown that the proportion of fat used as fuel increases as exercise is extended.[4, 14, 24] In a case study in which an athlete walked, ran, and rested for 70 hours, Costill reported that over the final hours of exercise, the athlete was deriving 90 to 100% of his energy from fat.[14] Since fat metabolism requires approximately 5 to 10% more oxygen to produce the same external work, the cardiovascular system must be able to deliver additional oxygen to the working muscles as work progresses.[25]

Clinical Evaluation
of the Ultraendurance Athlete

Clinically, cardiovascular evaluations can be made of the ultraendurance athlete at rest (without previous exercise), at rest following an extended exercise session, such as an actual competitive event, or during standard exercise tests in a laboratory.

Resting Evaluations
(No Previous Exercise)

Information about resting cardiac structure and function in ultraendurance athletes has been obtained through electrocardiography, echocardiography, and Doppler ultrasound measurements. Many studies have described changes in the electrocardiogram as a consequence of exercise training.[26, 29] (Also see Chapter 4).

Bradycardia is an almost universal finding in ultraendurance athletes, as it is in less well-trained athletes. This has been attributed to several interdependent factors, including changes in autonomic tone, cardiac dimensions, and intrinsic myocardial function.[30] There has long been general agreement that parasympathetic tone is increased at rest following dynamic exercise training; data regarding circulating catecholamines suggest that beta-receptor density decreases as a consequence of exercise training.[31] In athletes, it is also not uncommon to see QRS voltage increases, more prominent right ventricular forces, and repolarization abnormalities[32] (Table 11-1).

Table 11-1
ECG Abnormalities Found in Triathletes

Sinus bradycardia	93%
Early repolarization	22%
Inferior Q waves	11%
Premature depolarization	5%
Incomplete right bundle branch block	5%
Left bundle branch block	2%
Anterior Q waves	2%
Juvenile T waves	2%

(Adapted from Douglas[32])

• **Using echocardiography,** both cross-sectional and longitudinal studies have shown that myocardial hypertrophy with maintenance of the usual ratio of wall thickness to internal diameter occurs with endurance training.[33, 34] The hypertrophy may occur in as little as eight weeks and is reversible. However, if the hypertrophy is induced at an early age, it may be long-lasting.[34]

Although the increase in left ventricular (LV) size occurring with exercise training has been confirmed by several subsequent studies,[35-37] the lack of change in wall thickness and the suggested relationship of LV geometry to the sport pursued has not been borne out. Examining those pursuing a wide range of activities, most investigators find modest increases in both cavity size and wall thicknesses, with a normal or slightly increased relative wall thickness[38-44] and little correlation between exercise type and pattern of hypertrophy.

The finding of increased left ventricular volume in endurance athletes, however, is not universal. Douglas and colleagues,[39] among others, found normal left ventricular systolic and diastolic cavity dimensions, but increased wall thickness, increased relative wall thickness, and increased left ventricular mass in a group of ultraendurance triathletes compared to normal controls.

The effects of ultraendurance exercise training on intrinsic myocardial function remain uncertain. Most echocardiographic data provide no direct evidence for any significant training effects on contractile performance. In longitudinal studies,[36, 37] training (though not ultraendurance) was found to have no effect on ejection fraction at rest, during submaximal exercise, or during maximal exercise. In a cross-sectional study,[39] no differences were found in fractional shortening, end-systolic stress, or in diastolic function between ultraendurance athletes and sedentary controls. Blomqvist and Saltin[35] speculate that there is little to be gained (at least during maximal exercise) by increasing the myocardial contractile state, since the ejection fraction is already high and the end-systolic volume low even in normal, relatively untrained subjects.

In general, the clinical cardiovascular evaluation of the ultraendurance athlete is not known to be different from that in persons pursuing more moderate amounts of, but still vigorous, aerobic exercise. It appears that adaptations to exercise, such as bradycardia and physiologic hypertrophy, occur with relative ease, and that little further measurable change occurs despite continued training.

Although one reasonably expects to observe physiologic differences in the more highly trained ultraendurance athlete, these are difficult to identify at rest, using population studies. Thus, once the initial adaptive process has occurred, increases in the amount of exercise performed seem not to cause further cardiovascular remodeling. However, it is highly likely that some changes do take place, perhaps on a cellular or biochemical level, that are not well reflected in clinical evaluations. Indeed, some additional adaptation must occur as a consequence of more prolonged training: This is what makes the performance of ultraendurance race events possible.

As with the clinical examination, cardiovascular diagnostic testing is not known to be different in the ultraendurance athlete from that in other aerobically trained individuals (in part, perhaps, because few studies have undertaken such a comparison). One study[38] compared sprinters and endurance runners, finding a greater amount of left ventricular hypertrophy in the latter. This was manifested on the electrocardiogram by higher QRS voltage (Sokolow-Lyon criteria: sum of S wave in V1 + R wave in V5), and a longer P wave duration, and on the chest x-ray by a greater cardiothoracic ratio.

Echocardiographic studies showed the endurance runners to have a larger aortic root, larger left atrium, smaller systolic left ventricular dimension, and greater left ventricular posterior wall and septal thickness than sprinters.

Although it is not surprising that endurance runners may have a greater degree of physiologic left ventricular hypertrophy than those pursuing less prolonged exercise, the increased prominence of a concentric pattern of hypertrophy in endurance as opposed to sprinting events merits comment. These results are opposite from what would be expected from some analyses of the differences in the pattern of left ventricular structural adaptation to moderate intensity/long duration vs high intensity/short duration exercise, since some authors have stated that aerobic endurance exercise produces a thin-walled, dilated, or eccentrically hypertrophied heart, while

shorter duration, resistive exercise results in a more concentrically hypertrophied, pressure overloaded ventricle.[33] However, careful review of the existing literature on ultraendurance athletes reveals that the adaptation to exercise is similar to that noted above in athletes pursuing less prolonged training. The left ventricle of the ultraendurance athlete is usually characterized by top normal values of both wall thickness and cavity dimensions, an increased ratio of wall thickness to cavity radius (h/R ratio) and elevated mass, thus displaying a concentric rather than dilated pattern of hypertrophy.[38-44] (Table 11-2).

Table 11-2
Left Ventricular Echocardiographic Measures in Ultraendurance Athletes

	LVIDd (cm)	PWTd (cm)	RWT	FS (%)	Mass (gm)
*Colan et al[14]	5.2	.99	38**	30%	230
†Douglas et al[13]	5.4	1.0	37**	39%	255
†Douglas et al[12]	5.0	1.0	41	35%	226
*Ikaheimo et al[11]	5.3	1.2	45**	37%	219
*Niemela et al[17]	5.4	1.0**	37	38%	NA
*Paulsen et al[16]	5.6	1.0	36	NA	316
*Perrault et al[15]	4.9	.90	37	35%**	NA

* Subjects included endurance or marathon runners training
   >60 miles/week
† Subjects included athletes completing the Hawaii Ironman Triathlon
** Calculated from data given

LVIDd = LV internal dimension at end of diastole
PWTd = Posterior wall thickness at end of diastole
RWT = Relative wall thickness at end of diastole (2PWT/LVID × 100)
FS = Systolic fractional shortening
NA = Not available

Since it is physiologically unlikely that, in response to exercise training, the left ventricular cavity enlarges and then reduces in size if the intensity and duration of training increase, it is possible that the discrepancies found between various studies simply represent chance differences in the populations examined.

While the etiologic factors resulting in cardiac hypertrophy are unknown, because of the supposed structural differences in the hearts of athletes pursuing different sports, it has been postulated that the volume overload of the sustained increase in cardiac output that accompanies endurance exercise provides the stimulus for development of a dilated ventricle. Given the concentric pattern of hypertrophy seen in most ultraendurance athletes, as just discussed, this is unlikely to be the sole cause. However, the suggestion that some aspect of the acute stress imposed by exercise could be responsible for the hypertrophic reaction is quite plausible.

To further examine possible etiologic stimuli for the production of physiologic left ventricular hypertrophy, our group measured a series of cardiovascular parameters in 14 triathletes during an eight-hour exercise test.[39] Left ventricular mass was weakly related to both average cardiac output and stroke volume during exercise (r = .64 and .70, respectively), but was most closely related to average exercise systolic blood pressure (r = .88). While other factors such as circulating catecholamines cannot be excluded, this suggests, as does the finding of a concentric pattern of left ventricular hypertrophy, that the intermittent pressure overload of exercise is an important etiologic factor and supercedes the influence of the imposed volume load.

While left ventricular hypertrophy is considered to be characteristic, it is by no means found in *all* ultraendurance athletes. An echocardiographic study of participants in the Hawaii Ironman Triathlon found that 41% of men and 47% of women actually had normal left ventricular masses.[45] While these data cannot exclude substantial hypertrophy that was insufficient to cause mass to exceed the normal range, they suggest that hypertrophy is not a universal response, even when an athlete pursues extreme amounts of exercise training. They also suggest that physiologic hypertrophy or structural cardiac change is not a necessary component for the successful completion of an ultraendurance race event.

Resting Evaluations (Following Prolonged Exercise)

Historically, it has been held that the heart sustains no ill effects from exercise, and this does seem to be the case for relatively short exercise events. However, more recent studies of marathons and triathlons suggest that cardiac performance may be transiently impaired after such ultraendurance events. Investigators have documented a decrease in left ventricular systolic fractional shortening, an altered diastolic filling pattern, and reduced contractility in athletes studied immediately after crossing the finish line.[40, 42, 44, 46-48] In all cases, left ventricular function returned to normal following a recovery period of one to two days, and no study has been able to identify any evidence of cardiac damage.

The rapid resolution of abnormalities, the lack of electrocardiographic evidence of injury, and the lack of elevation in cardiac enzyme subfractions all suggest the presence of cardiac fatigue. In searching for what components of exercise might influence the development of fatigue, several investigations have noted that the extent of dysfunction was related to the intensity of exercise (the faster the race, the greater the decrement in performance).[40, 48] In another study, dysfunction did not appear until late in a 24-hour race, which suggests that the duration of exercise is important as well.[44]

• **Clinical Implications** – These findings have several substantial clinical implications and raise a number of unanswered questions. Since these studies were performed in athletes without heart disease, during a single race, it is unclear what the effects might be in those with abnormal hearts, in the elderly, or after many years of competition or repeated "insults." In addition, the possible contributions of other factors such as electrolyte disturbances, dehydration, or extreme environmental conditions are unknown. However, if anything, these would be expected to increase the likelihood of developing fatigue or to increase the severity of the functional impairment.

In addition, while it is unknown if athletes with pre-existing heart disease are at greater risk of developing fatigue, certainly they might reasonably be expected to be more likely to manifest clinical difficulties as a result of impaired cardiac performance. Therefore, it is probably sensible for the physician to advise athletes with myocardial dysfunction, from whatever cause, or with severe valvular disease to participate in ultraendurance events only with great caution, and with special attention to minimizing other stresses such as fluid or electrolyte imbalance.

An additional clinical implication of the development of fatigue is that cardiac dysfunction may play a role in those otherwise healthy athletes who are unable to complete ultraendurance race events. Whether this is true, or the extent to which it is important, is unknown. Certainly though, in light of increasing evidence for the existence and importance of fatigue, the race physician must keep this possibility in mind when caring for athletes in the medical tent, whether or not they have finished the race.

Exercise Evaluations

The cardiovascular system of ultraendurance athletes can also be evaluated during exercise. A short graded exercise test to maximal effort, or a prolonged submaximal exercise test, both with gas exchange and blood lactate measurements, will yield useful information, as will heart rate monitoring during either training or racing.

• **Maximal Exercise Tests** – The most commonly used exercise tests for ultraendurance athletes make use of a treadmill, a cycle ergometer and/or either tethered swimming or an arm crank ergometer.[14, 23, 49, 50] During a graded exercise test, each increase in workload will cause a proportionate increase in oxygen uptake (VO_2). Tests for ultraendurance athletes can be started at workloads requiring a VO_2 of 30 ml•kg^{-1}•min^{-1} or greater, with increments of 3 to 7 ml•kg^{-1}•min^{-1}. When maximal oxygen uptake (VO_2 max) has been reached, a further increase in workload will not be accompanied by an increase in VO_2.[51, 52]

• **Submaximal Exercise Tests** – Another method of evaluating ultraendurance athletes involves prolonged submaximal exercise tests. During these tests, the athlete may either be asked to continue until pace can no longer be maintained or may continue for a finite period of time at a specific exercise intensity. Physiologic variables of interest can be monitored at set intervals. During submaximal exercise tests lasting between 2 and 8 hours, the exercise workload has commonly been set between 50 and 70% of VO_2 max. Variables such as heart rate, cardiac output, minute ventilation, and blood lactate are usually measured each half hour. Ultraendurance athletes would be expected to maintain these values within narrow limits for long periods of time.

Similar short submaximal tests can be devised

to evaluate athletes during any other exercise mode (e.g., swimming or cycling). The importance of movement efficiency is of obvious benefit during ultraendurance exercise, where energy expenditure for an entire event is tremendously high.

Heart Rate Monitoring

To gain information more specific to a particular ultraendurance event, heart rate monitoring can be done during either training or racing. Monitors are now available that consist of a small transmitter held in place by a chest strap and a receiver worn like a wrist watch. The use of these heart rate monitors, in combination with information derived from more elaborate laboratory measurements, can lead to accurate monitoring of aerobic workloads during actual race conditions.

Ultraendurance Exercise and Heart Disease

In spite of the possible development of cardiac fatigue, the presence of significant heart disease has not prevented some individuals from successfully completing ultraendurance racing events. Athletes with severe atherosclerosis, coronary disease (including those with a history of myocardial infarction), hypertrophic cardiomyopathy, anomalous coronary anatomy, myopericarditis, and floppy mitral valve have all successfully completed marathons.[53-56] Indeed, rehabilitation programs specifically designed to train post-infarction patients for marathon runs have proven successful.[55] Douglas and colleagues[57] studied several athletes with severe aortic regurgitation and one heterotopic heart transplant recipient who competed regularly in international-distance triathlons (1.5 k swim, 40 k bike, 10 k run), and two athletes who had a history of both myocardial infarction and coronary artery bypass grafting and who successfully completed the Hawaii Ironman Triathlon. Not only were these athletes able to achieve the requisite degree of cardiopulmonary training, but the races themselves produced no measurable ill effects.[57]

A separate, important issue is the development of heart disease in the ultraendurance trained athlete. The extent to which such training may delay or partially prevent the development of heart disease is unknown, as is the amount of exercise necessary to achieve such effects. Preliminary data do suggest, however, that cardiovascular risk factors such as lipid profiles may be increasingly favorably affected by increasing amounts of exercise.[58]

Summary

The cardiovascular system of the ultraendurance athlete, stimulated by repeated bouts of prolonged exercise, has adapted to allow routine performance of ultraendurance exercise at relatively high workloads. The heart of the ultraendurance athlete generally shows the same pattern of physiologic LV hypertrophy as does that of other athletes: Modest increases in cavity size and wall thickness combined to increase LV mass. Although the stimuli producing such adaptations are ill defined, the increase in blood pressure during exercise is an important factor.

During the performance of ultraendurance events, these highly trained athletes have the advantage of performing at a given intensity with lower heart rates, larger stroke volumes, and a better distribution of cardiac output. Factors that affect performance in ultraendurance events, such as dehydration, heat stress, and substrate utilization, are all positively affected by training. Ultraendurance racing may have detrimental effects on both systolic and diastolic left ventricular performance, even in the healthy athlete. Since the effects of prolonged exercise in the presence of heart disease are unknown, such training and competition, while clearly not necessarily harmful, should be pursued with caution.

Editor's Note: To my way of thinking, it would seem prudent, in the presence of heart disease, to advise against this type of exercise. – WPH

Author's Note: Please see ref. 57. There are some individuals who have participated in endurance exercise either before heart disease was diagnosed or as a part of a rehabilitation program and wish to continue. While initiation of this type of exercise may well be inadvisable, we believe that each case should be considered individually. – MLO

References

1. O'Toole ML, WDB Hiller, F Massimino, RH Laird: Medical considerations in triathletes. A preliminary report from the Hawaii Ironman, 1984. New Zealand *J Sports Med* 13(2): 35, 1985.
2. O'Toole ML: Training for ultraendurance triathlons. *Med Sci Sports Exerc* 21(5) Suppl: S209, 1989.
3. Hiller WDB, ML O'Toole, EE Frotess, RH Laird, PC Imbert, TD Sisk: Medical and physiological considerations in triathlons. *Am J Sports Med* 15(2): 164, 1987.
4. O'Toole ML, WDB Hiller, PS Douglas, JB Pisarello, JL Mullen: Cardiovascular responses to prolonged cycling and running. *Ann Sports Med* 3(2): 124, 1987.
5. Costill DL, WF Kammer, A Fisher: Fluid ingestion during distance running. *Arch Environ Health* 21: 520, 1970.
6. Costill DL, JM Miller: Nutrition for endurance sport: Carbohydrate and fluid balance. *Int J Sports Med* 1: 2, 1980.
7. Pugh LGCE, JL Corbett, RH Johnson: Rectal temperatures, weight losses, and sweat rates in marathon running. *J Appl Physiol* 23(3): 347, 1967.
8. O'Toole ML: Prevention and treatment of electrolyte abnormalities. Medical Coverage of Endurance Athletic Events. Ross Laboratories Symposium: Columbus, OH, p93, 1988.
9. Claremont A, D Costill, W Fink, P van Handel: Heat tolerance following diuretic induced dehydration. *Med Sci Sports* 8: 239, 1976.
10. Saltin B, J Stenberg: Circulatory response to prolonged severe exercise. *J Appl Physiol* 19:833, 1964.
11. Stenberg J, P-O Astrand, B Ekblom et al: Hemodynamic response to work with different muscle groups. *J Appl Physiol* 22(1): 61, 1967.
12. Rowell LB: Human cardiovascular adjustments to exercise and thermal stress. *Physiol Rev* 54: 75, 1974.
13. Smith EE, AC Guyton, RD Manning et al: Integrated mechanisms of cardiovascular response and control during exercise in the normal human. *Prog Cardiovasc Dis* 18(6): 421, 1976.
14. Costill DL: Inside Running: Basics of Sports Physiology. Benchmark Press, Inc.: Indianapolis, p43, 1986.
15. Astrand P-O, K Rodahl: Textbook of Work Physiology. Physiological Bases of Exercise, ed. 3. McGraw-Hill, New York, 1986.
16. Brenglemann GL: Circulatory adjustments to exercise and heat stress. *Ann Rev Physiol* 45: 191, 1983.
17. Costill DL, WJ Fink: Plasma volume changes following exercise and thermal dehydration. *J Appl Physiol* 37: 521, 1974.
18. Wells CL, AC Schrader, JA Stern, GA Krahenbuhl: Physiological responses to a 20 mile run using three different fluid replacements. *Med Sci Sports Exerc* 17(3): 364, 1985.
19. Drinkwater BL: Women and exercise: physiological aspects. *Exercise and Sports Science Reviews*, 12:21, 1984.
20. Nunneley SA: Physiological responses of women to thermal stress: a review. *Med Sci Sports* 10(4): 250, 1978.
21. Locksley R: Fuel utilization in marathons: implications for performance. *West J Med* 133: 493, 1980.
22. Mahler DA, J Loke: The physiology of endurance exercise. The marathon. *Clinics in Chest Medicine* 5(1): 63, 1984.

23. Nadel ER: Physiological adaptations to aerobic training. *Am Scientist* 73: 334, 1985.

24. Costill DL: Metabolic responses during distance running. *J Appl Physiol* 28: 251, 1970.

25. Gollnick P: Metabolism during exercise and as modified by training. *Fed Proc* 44(2): 353, 1985.

26. Huston TP, JC Puffer, WM Rodney: The athletic heart syndrome. *N Eng J Med* 313:24, 1985.

27. Oakley DG, CM Oakley: Significance of abnormal electrocardiograms in highly trained athletes. *Am J Cardiol* 50:985, 1982.

28. Parker BM, BR Londeree, GV Cupp, JP Dubiel: The noninvasive cardiac evaluation of long-distance runners. *Chest* 73:376, 1978.

29. Roeske RW, RA O'Rourke, A Klein, G Leopold, JS Karliner: Noninvasive evaluation of ventricular hypertrophy in professional athletes. *Circ* 53:286, 1976.

30. Hammond HK, VF Froelicher: The physiologic sequelae of chronic dynamic exercise. Symposium on medical aspects of exercise. *Med Clinics North Am* 69(1):21, 1985.

31. Butler J et al: Relationship of B-adrenoreceptor density to fitness in athletes. *Nature* 298:60, 1982.

32. Douglas PS: Cardiac considerations in the triathlete. *Med Sci Sports Exerc* 21(5) Suppl: S214, 1989.

33. Morganroth J et al: Comparative left ventricular dimensions in trained athletes. *Ann Intern Med* 82: 521, 1975.

34. Saltin B, G Grimby: Physiological analysis of middle aged and old former athletes: Comparison with still active athletes of the same ages. *Circ* 38: 1104, 1968.

35. Blomqvist CG, B Saltin: Cardiovascular adaptations to physical training. *Ann Rev Physiol* 45: 169, 1983.

36. Peronnet R et al: Echocardiography and the athlete's heart. *Phys Sportsmed* 9:102, 1981.

37. Rerych SK et al: Effects of exercise training on left ventricular function in normal subjects. A longitudinal study by radionuclide angiography. *Am J Cardiol* 45: 244, 1980.

38. Ikaheimo MJ, IJ Palatsi, JT Takkunen: Noninvasive evaluation of the athletic heart: sprinters versus endurance runners. *Am J Cardiol* 44:24, 1979.

39. Douglas PS, ML O'Toole, WDB Hiller, N Reichek: Left ventricular structure and function by echocardiography in ultraendurance athletes. *Am J Cardiol* 58:805, 1986.

40. Douglas PS, ML O'Toole, WDB Hiller, K Hackney, N Reichek: Cardiac fatigue after prolonged exercise. *Circ* 76: 1206, 1987.

41. Colan SD, SP Sanders, KM Borow: Physiologic hypertrophy: effects on left ventricular systolic mechanics in athletes. *J Am Coll Cardiol* 9:776, 1987.

42. Perrault H et al: Echocardiographic assessment of left ventricular performance before and after marathon running. *Am Heart J* 112:1026, 1986.

43. Paulsen W et al: Left ventricular function in marathon runners: echocardiographic assessment. *J Appl Physiol* 51:881, 1981.

44. Niemela KO et al: Evidence of impaired left ventricular performance after an uninterrupted competitive 24 hour run. *Circ* 70:350, 1984.

45. Douglas PS, ML O'Toole, WDB Hiller, K Hackney: Electrocardiographic diagnosis of exercise induced left ventricular hypertrophy. *Am Heart J* 116:784, 1988.

46. Seals DR et al: Impaired left ventricular contractile function following exhaustive submaximal exercise in man. *Fed Proc* 44: 817, 1985.

47. Boynton M et al: Are echocardiographic estimates of left ventricular function altered by running a marathon? Abstract. *Med Sci Sports Exerc* 19: S84, 1987.

48. Chan K, A Pipe, M Barrie: Acute effect of marathon running on left ventricular function. Abstract. 19:S83, 1987.

49. O'Toole ML, WDB Hiller, LO Crosby, PS Douglas: The ultraendurance triathlete: a physiological profile. *Med Sci Sports Exerc* 19(1): 45, 1987.

50. Kohrt WM, DW Morgan, B Bates, JS Skinner: Physiological responses of triathletes maximal swimming, cycling and running. *Med Sci Sports Exerc* 19(1): 51, 1987.

51. Lamb DR: Physiology of Exercise: Responses and Adaptations, ed 2. MacMillan, New York, 1984.

52. McArdle WD, FI Katch, VL Katch: Exercise Physiology: Energy, Nutrition and Human Performance. Lea and Febiger, Philadelphia, 1986.

53. Noakes TD: Heart disease in marathon runners: a review. *Med Sci Sports Exerc* 19:187, 1987.

54. Maron BJ, YE Wesley, J Arce: Hypertrophic cardiomyopathy compatible with successful completion of the marathon. *Am J Med* 53:1470, 1984.

55. Kavanagh T, RH Shephard, V Pandit: Marathon running after myocardial infarction. *JAMA* 229: 1602, 1974.

56. Handler JB et al: Symptomatic coronary artery disease in a marathon runner. *JAMA* 248:717, 1982.

57. Douglas PS, A Sigler, ML O'Toole, WDB Hiller: Endurance exercise in the presence of heart disease. *Chest* 95:697, 1989.

58. Fortess EE, WDB Hiller, ML O'Toole, PS Douglas, RH Laird: Ultraendurance exercise and ischemic heart disease risk. Abstract. *Med Sci Sports Exerc Suppl* 19(2):S91, 1987.

CHAPTER 12

BLOOD DOPING, ERYTHROPOIETIN, AND DRUG TESTING IN ATHLETES

Brian Hainline, MD

Director, Clinical Neurology Service
and Sports Neurology
Hospital for Joint Diseases
New York, NY
Assistant Professor of Neurology
New York University School of Medicine

The use, misuse, and abuse of drugs have shaken the foundations of amateur and professional sports in recent years, but history indicates that long ago athletes sought a competitive advantage by using various substances to gain a competitive edge. Greek athletes ingested mushrooms in the third century B.C. in an effort to improve performance,[1] and gladiators used stimulants to overcome fatigue and injury in the famed Circus Maximus.[2] The first recorded fatality from a performance-enhancing drug occurred in 1886, when an English cyclist died from an overdose of "trimethyl."[3]

The problem of drug abuse in sports came under especially close scrutiny in the 1980's. In 1983, seven weightlifters were cited for using anabolic-androgenic steroids in the IX Pan American Games,[4] and in 1986, 21 college football players were banned from bowl games as a result of tests indicating anabolic-androgenic steroid use.[5] 1986 also saw the deaths of collegiate basketball superstar Len Bias and professional football player Don Rogers, both from an overdose of cocaine.[6] In 1988, worldwide attention was again directed to anabolic-androgenic steroid abuse in sports, when Ben Johnson was stripped of his gold medal at the XXIV Olympiad in Seoul for using this banned drug.[7]

Human growth hormone and recombinant human erythropoietin are two drugs that can now be produced in potentially unlimited quantities through genetic engineering, and they are of invaluable help for patients with endogenous deficiencies. It has not taken long for athletes to discover their potential use as ergogenic aids, and many believe that the potential widespread abuse of these drugs by athletes is a serious concern.[8-11, 41, 42]

Blood Doping

The term "drug abuse" in sports is not limited to the oral or parenteral intake of manufactured chemical substances, but also includes the intravenous infusion of blood. Blood is not commonly thought of as a drug, but blood transfusions are carefully regulated by the Food and Drug Administration, and facilities for blood collection and transfusion are registered, licensed, and inspected for compliance. Blood transfusions, like other drugs, are meant to be given only for medical indications.[12]

Blood doping refers to the practice of intravenously infusing blood into an individual in order to induce erythrocythemia. The procedure may be autologous (one's own blood) or homologous (donated blood). Reports of blood doping in a controlled scientific setting first appeared in 1947.[13] In 1966, Ekblom[14] began a series of studies addressing the question of improved aerobic capacity following blood doping. In the 1976 Olympic Games, reports began to circulate suggesting that the procedure was used by athletes as an ergogenic aid.[15] Several American cyclists admitted to blood doping for the 1984 Summer Olympics,[16] and common knowledge suggests that blood doping by athletes is often done for endurance events.[17]

Physiology of Blood Doping

Blood doping is used by athletes engaged in aerobic athletic activities, such as long distance running, cross-country skiing, and cycling. The expressed purpose is to increase the total aerobic power by increasing the transport of oxygen to the contracting muscle.

For example, raising the hemoglobin concentration to 16 gm per 100 ml produces 21.44 ml oxygen per 100 ml blood (1.34 x 16 = 21.44). Stated differently, it has been estimated that 500 ml of whole blood, or 275 ml of packed red blood cells, can add about 100 ml of oxygen to the total oxygen-carrying capacity of the blood. Because an athlete's total blood volume circulates five to six times each minute in maximal exercise, the potential extra oxygen available to the tissues from red cell reinfusion is about 0.5 liters per minute.[18, 19]

The notion of blood doping as an ergogenic aid stems from observations that blood loss and a concomitant fall in hemoglobin significantly reduces maximal oxygen uptake (VO_2 max) and working capacity.[20-22] Since aerobic performance is adversely affected following blood loss, it was postulated that improved oxygen delivery via an increase in hemoglobin could yield more energy-rich ATP, which could then enhance aerobically-dependent endurance activities.

Normally, blood doping is followed by certain compensatory physiologic adjustments that preserve the sought-after beneficial aerobic effect. Most notably, immediately following a blood transfusion, there is a shift of plasma from the intravascular space to the extravascular space, thereby restoring the blood volume to normal.[23, 24] This fluid shift occurs since blood volume is held relatively constant at the expense of plasma volume. The increased cardiac output which occurs immediately following a blood transfusion lasts only a few minutes, since the increased pressure at the capillary level leads to a transudation of fluid into the tissues, thereby returning blood volume to normal. Therefore, hematocrit levels increase with little change in total blood volume.

Even with an increase in hematocrit and oxygen-carrying capacity to the tissues, induced erythrocythemia would not improve aerobic capacity if oxygen delivery were impaired at the tissue level. Studies have shown that the affinity of the red blood cell for oxygen, as measured by 2, 3 diphosphoglycerate and P50, is unaffected by blood doping, indicating that there is no change in the ability of the red blood cell under conditions of induced erythrocythemia to release oxygen.[25-27]

Debate has often centered on whether the limiting factor in endurance exercise is oxygen delivery or the inherent oxidative capacity of the muscle.[12, 28] Ekblom and associates[29] have demonstrated that the oxygen uptake and the oxidative capacity of the muscle are not adversely affected with induced erythrocythemia. Others[30] have shown that both the volume of oxygen delivered by the left ventricle and the volume of oxygen actually used during maximal exercise are significantly increased following induced erythrocythemia.

Another theoretical benefit from induced erythrocythemia is an improved acid-base buffer system. Hemoglobin is a known excellent acid-base buffer, and lactic acidosis is a causative factor in producing physiologic fatigue.[31] A decrease in lactic acidosis following exercise at near maximal capacity has been demonstrated[32] following blood doping.

A major factor in determining whether induced erythrocythemia may lead to improved aerobic performance is the procedure used for blood doping. Homologous blood doping is rarely used by athletes today because of the high risk of developing transfusion-related complications. Autologous blood doping must be done under specified conditions if an increase in hematocrit is to be achieved. Studies have shown that following the removal of one to two units of blood, at least four weeks are required before prephlebotomy hemoglobin levels are achieved.[33] The reinfusion of one's own blood prior to this, i.e., while still anemic, would not result in induced erythrocythemia.

How It's Done

The general procedure for autologous blood doping is as follows:[14, 25, 34, 35]

1. About six to ten weeks prior to the athletic event for which blood doping is desired, two units of blood are removed from the individual.

2. The red blood cells are separated from the plasma, then preserved via glycerol freezing, allowing preservation for an indefinite period of time. If the red blood cells are refrigerated, the maximal storage time is decreased to only three weeks. Since prephlebotomy hemoglobin levels are not achieved in just three weeks, the full bene-

fit of reinfused red blood cells is not realized. Therefore, this latter method has fallen out of favor.

3. The individual retrains to full aerobic capacity during the six to ten weeks postphlebotomy.

4. At the time of reinfusion, the frozen red blood cells are thawed and reconstituted with a physiologic saline solution, then infused intravenously over one to two hours. Reinfusion is usually done one to seven days prior to the desired athletic event.

Erythropoietin

Erythropoietin is a naturally occurring glycoprotein growth factor synthesized by cells adjacent to the proximal renal tubules in the kidneys. Erythropoietin binds to and activates receptors on the erythroid progenitor cells in the bone marrow, thereby allowing the progenitor cells to develop into mature erythrocytes.[36] In 1987, Eschbach and associates[37] demonstrated the usefulness of recombinant human erythropoietin in the correction of the anemia of end-stage renal disease. Others have since successfully used recombinant human erythropoietin to treat patients with anemia from other causes.[38, 39, 40] Recombinant human erythropoietin makes it possible for autologous blood donors to donate more blood and to maintain a high baseline hematocrit.[36]

Use in Sports

No data exist regarding the incidence of blood doping or recombinant human erythropoietin use among endurance athletes, although anecdotal stories abound. It is not unusual for a runner or cyclist who performs unexpectedly well to be accused of blood doping.[43, 44] In 1984, Ireland's John Treacy stated that he saw an entire national team injecting themselves with a blood-colored liquid prior to the world cross-country championship. Also in 1984, the United States cycling team admitted to blood doping following their impressive showing at the Olympics.[43] Dr. Robert Voy, former director of science for the United States Olympic Committee, says that blood doping among athletes has gotten "completely out of control."[17] Dr. Voy further suggests that when a country comes out of nowhere to world prominence in an endurance event, the international athletic community nods knowingly and thinks "blood doping."[17]

Earlier studies did not support the contention that blood doping led to improved endurance performance,[45-48] but these studies can be criticized because of a flaw in blood doping technique that is now known to be a critical factor if blood doping is to be ergogenic.

The critical technical factors are total volume of red cells withdrawn and reinfused, the time interval between withdrawing and reinfusing blood, and the method used to store the blood. Specifically, about 900 ml of whole blood should be withdrawn and then frozen for storage. Reinfusion should be done about six to ten weeks later, in order to allow baseline hemoglobin levels to be achieved before reinfusion.[49]

Newer studies show that proper blood doping improves endurance performances.[26-28, 50, 51] The improvements have a clear-cut practical meaning: Statistically significant differences are noted in race times, using the athlete as his/her own control. Endurance capacity may improve up to 25% following blood doping.

Some modifying factors exist. For example, the magnitude of increase in maximal oxygen uptake is related to the individual's initial aerobic fitness.[51] Individuals in moderately good physical condition experience twice the increase in maximal oxygen uptake as individuals of greater or lesser fitness. The total amount of blood needed to be removed and reinfused to achieve a maximal effect has not been clearly established, but one group[50] found that the aerobic power of working muscles was not surpassed following three units of autologous blood transfusions in four highly trained endurance runners.

Recombinant human erythropoietin use by athletes has been reported by several authors[8-11, 52] and eighteen mysterious deaths among cyclists have been attributed to possible erythropoietin use,[53] although causative proof is lacking. Sport scientists have expressed a concern that mistakes will be made by athletes in dosing erythropoietin, thereby leading to a dangerously high hematocrit.[10]

Blood doping and erythropoietin use are banned by the International Olympic Committee (IOC) and the National Collegiate Athletic Association (NCAA).[54, 55] The American College of Sports Medicine views blood doping for ergogenic purpose as unethical and unjustifiable,[56] and strongly discourages the use of erythropoietin by athletes.[11] The Council on Scientific Affairs of the American Medical Association strongly recommends against the use of erythropoietin to enhance athletic performance.[10]

Evidence confirming blood doping or erythropoietin use leads to punitive actions according to IOC and NCAA guidelines, but no urine or blood test reliably detects their use. A combination of an increase in serum hemoglobin, bilirubin, and iron, coupled with a decrease in the serum erythropoietin level, is supportive evidence of blood doping, and a second comparison serum sample may give further supportive evidence. However, this testing procedure is invasive, and at present can detect only 50 to 75% of blood-doped individuals.[57, 58]

Adverse Effects

Homologous blood transfusions are now rarely given for blood doping, and the risk is clearly substantial. Three percent of such transfusions are complicated by immune side effects such as fever, urticaria, and more rarely, severe hemolytic reactions and anaphylactic shock. Viral infections are well known to occur and include hepatitis and the acquired immunodeficiency syndrome (AIDS).

Autogolous blood transfusions appear safe when performed by trained personnel, using approved techniques, and with storage and labeling in a registered blood bank.[12] Any flaw in technique may lead to complications ranging from bacterial infections to fatal reactions due to blood mislabeling. Induced erythrocythemia from blood doping carries with it the potential medical complications that have been well described with polycythemia, including hypertension, congestive heart failure, and stroke.

Hypertension develops in 30% of chronic renal failure patients treated with recombinant human erythropoietin and 5% of these patients will develop seizures.[36] Hypertension and other side effects have not been reported in nonrenal anemic patients treated with recombinant human erythropoietin.[36] Several authors[8-11] have expressed a deep concern about induced erythrocythemia from erythropoietin. With autologous blood doping, an athlete is limited by the amount of blood drawn off, making it difficult to increase the he-

matocrit above 60%. Miscalculating the dose of erythropoietin can, in theory, drive the hematocrit up to 80%.[8] Risk of recombinant human erythropoietin use and high hematocrit include encephalopathy, seizures, vascular distension, tissue hypoxia secondary to impairment of blood flow, and rapid clotting leading to phlebothrombosis, pulmonary embolism, myocardial infarction, and stroke.[10]

Drug Testing

In the 1960's, the concept of drug testing arose as a way of ensuring compliance with drug treatment programs for narcotic addicts. Drug testing in the athletic community was prompted by the amphetamine-related deaths of the Danish cyclist, Kurt Enemar Knud Jensen during the 1960 Olympiads[1] and the English cyclist Tommy Simpson during the 1967 Tour de France.[59] In 1965, Beckett and associates[60] used gas chromatographic testing techniques to control drug abuse at the Tour of Britain Cycle Races, and in 1967, the Medical Commission of the International Olympic Committee published a list of banned drugs for the 1968 Winter Olympics.[59] The 1972 Munich Olympic Games was the first international athletic event in which comprehensive drug testing was undertaken.[61] Since then, drug testing protocols have been introduced into most major amateur and professional sports.

The original intent of drug testing in sports was to eliminate any competitive advantage that might result from ergogenic aids. However, as "recreational" drug abuse in the sports community has become increasingly apparent, the intent of drug testing in sports has been expanded to include casefinding of individuals with a drug problem, screening teams or groups of athletes for evidence of drug abuse, protecting other athletes from injury caused by the drug-abusing athlete, enhancing the role-model perceptions of athletes, deterring drug abuse by athletes, and minimizing criminality.

Methodology

Regardless of the intent of drug testing, the application of testing results is limited by the sensitivity and specificity of a given drug-testing methodology. Most drug-testing protocols use urine as the body fluid to be analyzed. Urine analysis has several limitations:[62]

1. Unless the individual being tested is observed to urinate, the collection of the urine specimen is suspect since ingenious techniques of urine specimen tampering have been developed. However, some argue that providing an observed urine specimen is a violation of basic ethical and legal rights.

2. The presence of a drug in the urine does not necessarily correlate with any degree of purported performance enhancement. For most drugs, dose-response and time-action curves vis-a-vis drug ergogenicity are unavailable.

3. Urine analysis cannot detect the use of exogenous human growth hormone, recombinant human erythropoietin, or blood doping.

The use of blood or plasma to measure the concentration of a drug may permit better correlations with the effects of that drug or its active metabolites on athletic performance, but blood drawing is invasive and requires a technical proficiency which might not be available on a wide scale. Furthermore, the analyses of blood specimens are generally more expensive and more complex.

Human hair and saliva are also body specimens that can be used, but their application to clinical situations has only just begun to be validated.[62]

After the specimen for analysis is secured, the next major limiting factor is the laboratory technique. There are two general methodologic categories for evaluating urine for drug use: immunologic assays and chromatographic assays. The former includes radioimmunoassays (RIA) and enzyme immunoassays (EIA). The latter includes thin-layer chromatography (TLC), gas-liquid chromatography (GLC), high-pressure liquid chromatography (HPLC), and combined gas chromatography-mass spectrometry (GC/MS). Following is a brief discussion of each.

• **Immunoassay** – RIA and EIA are immunologic techniques based on the principles of antigen-antibody interaction.[63, 66] Both are useful for screening large numbers of specimens rapidly and inexpensively.[61] Neither procedure uses monoclonal antibodies, and therefore they are not absolutely specific for a given drug. The RIA technique utilizes known amounts of I-125 tagged antigen, and the EIA technique utilizes the enzyme glucose-6-phosphate dehydrogenase as the ac-

tive tag. Both procedures are generally used for screening urine specimens, and both are more sensitive and specific than TLC.

• **Thin-Layer Chromatography** – Chromatography is a technique used to separate a mixture of substances by taking advantage of the specific physicochemical characteristics of each of the components in the mixture.[67] The separation of the substances is achieved by virtue of differences in each substance's migration rate on or through a porous supporting medium called an absorbent.[68] TLC is an inexpensive, relatively crude chromatographic technique that primarily has been used in the emergency room setting to qualitatively detect high-dose drug abuse or toxic level of drugs in the comatose patient.[69] In the context of screening for banned drugs or drugs of abuse, TLC is inadequate and obsolete.[70]

• **Gas-Liquid Chromatography** – GLC is a process by which a mixture of compounds in a volatilized form is separated into its component parts by moving a mobile (gas) phase over a stationary (absorbent or liquid) phase.[64, 67, 71, 72] Therefore, this technique requires that the substance of interest be put into a gaseous (volatile) state. In routine gas-liquid chromatography, compounds are identified by their rate of speed traveling through the chromatographic column. This rate is referred to as the retention time and is unique and reproducible for each drug in a given type of chromatographic column. GLC is primarily used as a screening technique in drug testing.

• **High-Performance Liquid Chromatography** – HPLC is similar to gas chromatography, but does not require the preparation of a gaseous or volatile derivative of the substance being studied.[67] HPLC is primarily used as a screening technique, but it has been utilized to quantitate urinary caffeine levels at designated sporting events.[73]

• **Gas Chromatography-Mass Spectrometry** – The most precise way of accomplishing drug identification is to combine the chemical separating power of gas chromatography with the molecular identifying power of mass spectrometry, a procedure referred to commonly as GC/MS.[74] As each separated compound leaves the chromatographic column, it is introduced, one compound at a time, into a mass spectrometer. The mass spectrometer, under high vacuum, then bombards the separated compound with high-energy electrons. Because not all bonds in a drug molecule are of equal strength, the bombardment of the molecule by the high-energy electrons is more likely to break the weaker bonds than the stronger ones, thereby producing ionized fragments or breakage products. The fragmentation ions or patterns – the "molecular fingerprints" that are produced by this procedure – are unique for each compound. Like fingerprints, these fragmentation patterns are matched against known patterns in a computer library, thereby permitting precise identification.

GC/MS, which in most cases is about 100 to 1000 times more sensitive than TLC, is the most sensitive and accurate technique currently available in the field of drug testing, but it is also the most expensive.[59, 66, 68, 69, 75] GC/MS is regularly used to confirm presumptively positive urines as determined by the aforementioned screening techniques. In fact, the IOC and essentially all of the international sports federations have required GC/MS identification of the drugs or their metabolites for all positive screening tests.[61]

Application to Sports

Table 12-1 outlines the differences in detection limits and detection windows for various drugs utilizing the drug-testing methodologies discussed here. The successful implementation of a drug-testing program must take into consideration such differences. However, not only must the methodology be appropriate, but the intent of testing must be well-defined.

For example, cocaine is listed as one of the banned stimulants in both the IOC and the NCAA drug testing protocols.[54, 55] If an athlete uses cocaine, even in moderate amounts, on a Wednesday, and his or her urine is screened by TLC on Sunday, it will most likely test negative. If, on the other hand, his or her urine is tested by GC/MS, it may well test positive, depending on the detection windows that are used. Although there are sociologic and medical implications to Wednesday's cocaine use, there will undoubtedly be no performance enhancement from that drug usage.[76] If any performance enhancement is to occur

---

Table 12-1
Drug Testing Methodology and Drug Detectability

	Detection Limits (ng/ml)			Detection Windows (days)		
	TLC	EIA	GC/MS	TLC	EIA	GC/MS
Amphetamines	1000-2000	300	100	1	2	2-4
Barbiturates	1000-2000	300	100	1	2-3 +	7 [a]
Benzodiazepines	1000-2000	300	100	18 hr	3	7 [a]
Cocaine[b]	1000-2000	300	50	12 hr	2	5-6
Opiates	1000	300	100	1-2	2-3	5-6
Marijuana (cannabinoids)	—	20	10	—	10 [c]	10 [c]
Anabolic steroids [d]			10			
Alcohol[e]						

[a] As long as 2 to 3 weeks with long-acting sedatives
[b] Measured as benzoylecgonine
[c] As long as 30 days in chronic users
[d] A 6:1 testosterone/epitestosterone ratio is considered as evidence of exogenous testosterone usage. Exogenous steroids can be detected from 2 to 3 weeks (all) to as long as 12 months (parenteral).
[e] Sensitivity is 10 mg/dl in blood, 20 mg/dl in urine; blood level decrement is 15 mg/dl/hour; urine/blood ratio is approximately 1:3.

TLC = Thin-layer chromatography
EIA = Enzyme Immunoassay
GC/MS = Gas chromatography/mass spectrometry

following cocaine use, it probably happens at a very narrow range of blood concentration which has yet to be defined.[76]

If the intent of a drug-testing protocol is to eliminate the use of ergogenic drugs, then the quantification of a given drug in the urine becomes important. Such an approach is used by both the USOC and the NCAA with caffeine.[54, 55] Both institutions define a minimum concentration of caffeine that must be present in the urine before an athlete can be disqualified for caffeine abuse. Implicit in such an approach is the notion that a given concentration of a substance in the urine correlates with a quantifiable effect of that substance on performance. Unfortunately, data regarding drug concentration and athletic performance are sparse. Investigators do not even agree on which drugs are ergogenic under a variety of circumstances.

Some may argue that the mere presence of a drug such as an anabolic-androgenic steroid in the urine is sufficient evidence to disqualify an athlete if the governing body of the sporting event states that all ergogenic drugs are to be banned. However, for drugs such as ephedrine and phenylpropanolamine – two commonly used decongestants that are banned by both the USOC and the NCAA because of the possibility that they

may produce effects similar to amphetamines – correlating drug concentration with any possible performance-enhancing effect is essential if the protocol is to be fair and equitable. Otherwise, an athlete may be disqualified from competition for using a commonly prescribed drug for the symptomatic relief of a common ailment in accordance with the standards of good medical practice. Of note, one study[77] has demonstrated that a therapeutic dose of ephedrine is associated with no performance enhancement in several variables of relevance to the athlete.

Drug testing, therefore, should be viewed not only in a punitive context, but also as a vehicle for educating athletes, physicians, sports administrators, and all in the athletic community. The methodology and application of drug testing protocols should be constantly re-evaluated and modified in order to best achieve the intent of the specific drug-testing program.

Editor's Note: This excellent discussion by Dr. Brian Hainline is opportune as well as instructive. It is a logical companion for the next chapter by Dr. Bruce Waller on Cocaine and the Heart. – WPH

References

1. Puffer J: The use of drugs in swimming. *Clin Sports Med* 5:77, 1986.
2. Meer J: Drugs and Sports. In Snyder, SH (ed): *The Encyclopedia of Psychoactive Drugs*. Chelsea House, New York, 1987, p 19.
3. Dyment PG: Drugs and the adolescent athlete. *Ped Ann* 13:602, 1984.
4. Jeansonne J: Seven lifters named as drug users. *Newsday*, August 23, 1983.
5. Wilbon M: Number of banned players reaches 21. *Washington Post*, December 28, 1986.
6. Cantwell JD and Rose FD: Cocaine and cardiovascular events. *Phys Sportsmed* 14:77, 1986.
7. Johnson WO and Moore K: The loser. *Sports Illustrated*, October 3, 1988, p 20.
8. Cowart VS: Erythropoietin: A dangerous new form of blood doping? *Phys Sportsmed* 17:115, 1989.
9. Jereski L: It gives athletes a boost – maybe too much. *Business Week*, December 11, 1989, p 123.
10. Scott WC: The abuse of erythropoietin to enhance athletic performance. *JAMA* 264:1660, 1990.
11. Gall SC: Deterring EPO use in athletes. *Physician Sportsmed* 19:17, 1991.

12. Klein HG: Blood transfusions and athletics. Games people play. *N Engl J Med* 312:854, 1985.
13. Pace N, et al: The increase in hypoxia tolerance of normal men accompanying the polycythemia induced by transfusion of erythrocytes. *Am J Physiol* 148:152, 1947.
14. Ekblom B: Blood doping, oxygen breathing, and altitude training. In Strauss, RH (ed): *Drugs & Performance in Sports*. WB Saunders, Philadelphia, 1987, p 53.
15. Gledhill N, et al: Blood doping and related issues: A brief review. *Med Sci Sports Exerc* 14:193, 1982.
16. Jeansonne J: The controversy surrounding blood doping. *Newsday*, April 15, 1988.
17. Blood doping: The coming issue. *New Haven Journal Courier*, Jan 4, 1988.
18. Fox EL: *Sports Physiology, ed 2*. Saunders College Publishing, New York, 1984, p 9.
19. McCardle WD, Katch FI and Katch VL: *Exercise Psysiology – Energy, Nutrition, and Human Performance*. Lea and Febiger, Philadelphia, 1981, p 305.
20. Karpovich P and Millman N: Athletes as blood donors. *Res Quart* 13:166, 1942.
21. Balke B, et al: Work capacity after blood donation: *J Appl Physiol* 7:231, 1954.
22. Howell M and Coupe K: Effect of blood loss on performance in the Balke-Ware Treadmill Test. *Res Quart* 35:156, 1964.

23. Williams MH: Blood Doping. In Williams (ed): Ergogenic Aids in Sport. *Human Kinetics Publishers*, Champaign, 1983, p 202.

24. Williams MH et al: Effect of blood reinjection upon endurance capacity and heart rate. *Med Sci Sports* 5:181, 1973.

25. Brien AJ and Simon TL: The effects of red blood cell infusion on 10-km race time. *JAMA* 257:2761, 1987.

26. Buick FJ et al: Effect of induced erythtocythemia on aerobic work capacity. *J Appl Physiol* 48:636, 1980.

27. Williams MH et al: The effect of induced erythrocythemia upon 5-mile treadmill run time. *Med Sci Sports Exerc* 13:169, 1981.

28. Gollnick PD et al: Enzyme activity and fiber composition in skeletal muscle of untrained and trained men. *J Appl Physiol* 33:312, 1972.

29. Ekblom G, Golbard A and Gullbring B: Response to exercise after blood loss and reinfusion. *J Appl Physiol* 33:175, 1972.

30. Robertson RJ et al: Hemoglobin concentration and aerobic workout capacity in women following induced erythrocythemia. *J Appl Physiol* 57:568, 1984.

31. Hermansen L and Medbo JI: The relative significance of aerobic and anaerobic processes during maximal exercise of short duration. *Med Sport Sci* 17:56, 1984.

32. Gledhill N et al: Acid-base status with induced erythrocythemia and its influence on arterial oxygenation during heavy exercise. *Med Sci Sports Exerc* 12:122, 1980.

33. Wadler GI and Hainline B: *Drugs and the Athlete*. F.A. Davis, Philadelphia, 1989, p 172.

34. Eichner ER: Blood Doping: Implications of recent research. *Sports Med Digest* 9(3):4, 1987.

35. Wilmore JH: Blood doping. *Sports Med Digest* 9(11):6, 1987.

36. Erslev AJ: Erythropoietin. *N Engl J Med* 324:1339, 1991.

37. Eschbach JW et al: Correction of the anemia of end-stage renal disease with recombinant human erythropoietin. Results of a combined phase I and II clinical trial. *N Engl J Med* 316:73, 1987.

38. Erythropoietin for anemia. *The Medical Letter.* 31:85, 1989.

39. Fischl M et al: Recombinant human erythropoietin for patients with AIDS treated with Zidovudine. *N Engl J Med* 322:1488, 1990.

40. Ludwig H: Erythropoietin treatment of anemia associated with multiple myeloma. *N Engl J Med* 322:1693, 1990.

41. Erslev A: Erythropoietin coming of age. *N Engl J Med* 316:101, 1987.

42. Walker R and Brown A: Test drug surpassed doping. *Calgary Herald*, Feb 17, 1988.

43. Higden H: Blood doping among endurance athletes: rationalizations, results, and ramifications. *Am Med News*, Sept 27, 1985, p 37.

44. O'Brien R., Schlesinger D and Hirsch GA: Special report: Foreign intrigue. *Runners World*, June 1988, p 62.

45. Williams MH et al: Effect of blood reinjection upon endurance capacity and heart rate. *Med Sci Sports* 5a:181, 1973.

46. Videman T and Rytomaa T: Effect of blood removal and autotransfusion on heartrate response to a submaximal workload. *J Sports Med Phys Fitness* 17:387, 1977.

47. Pate R et al: Effects of blood reinfusion on endurance performance in female distance runners. *Med Sci Sports* 11:97, 1979.

48. Frye A and Ruhling R: RBC infusion, exercise, hemoconcentration and VO$_2$ *Med Sci Sports* 9:69, 1977.

49. Gledhill N: Blood doping and related issues: A brief review. *Med Sci Sports Exerc* 14(3):183, 1982.

50. Spriet LL et al: Effect of graded erythrocythemia on cardiovascular and metabolic responses to exercise. *J Appl Physiol* 61:1942, 1986.

51. Sawka MN et al: Erythrocyte reinfusion and maximal aerobic power: An examination of modifying factors. *JAMA* 257:1496, 1987.

52. Abuse of erythropoietin to enhance athletic performance. *Sports Medicine Digest* 13:6, 1991.

53. Fisher LM: Stamina-building drug linked to athletes' deaths. *The New York Times*, May 19, 1991, p 22.

54. U.S. Olympic Committee, Division of Sports Medicine and Science: Drug Education & Control Policy, 1988.

55. The 1988-89 NCAA Drug Testing Program. Mission, Kansas, NCAA Publishing, 1988.

56. American College of Sports Medicine Position Stand: Blood Doping as an Ergogenic Aid, Indianapolis, 1987.

57. Berglund B, Hemmingsson P and Birgegard G: Detection of autologous blood transfusions in cross-country skiers. *Int J Sports Med* 8:66, 1987.

58. Berglund B: Effects of blood transfusions on some hematologic variables in endurance athletes. *Med Sci Sports Exerc* 21:637, 1989.

59. Hanley DF: Drug and sex testing: Regulations for international competition. *Clin Sports Med* 2:13, 1986.

60. Beckett AH and Cowan DA: Misuse of drugs in sport. *Br J Sports Med* 12:185, 1979.

61. Catlin DH: Detection of drug use by athletes. In Strauss, RH (ed): *Drugs & Performance in Sports*. WB Saunders, Philadelphia, 1987, p 103.

62. Wadler GI and Hainline B: *Drugs and the Athlete*, F.A. Davis, Philadelphia, 1989, p 195.

63. Moyer TP et al: Marijuana testing – How good is it? *Mayo Clin Proc* 62:413, 1987.

64. Sandler KR: The role of the clinical laboratory in diagnosing and treating substance abuse. In: Biopsychiatric Insights on Substance Abuse (A Symposium). Psychiatric Diagnostic Laboratories, Inc., Princeton, 1986, p 68.

65. Gold MS and Dackis CA: Role of the laboratory in the evaluation of suspected drug abuse. *J Clin Psychiat* 47:17, 1986.

66. Erlich NEP: The athletic trainer's role in drug testing. *Athletic Training* 21:225, 1986.

67. Evenson MA: Principles of instrumentation. In Henry, JB (ed): *Todd-Sanford-Davidson Clinical Diagnosis and Management by Laboratory Methods, ed 17.* WB Saunders, Philadelphia, 1984, p 24.

68. Spitzer RH: Chromatography. In Teitz, NW (ed): *Fundamentals of Clinical Chemistry.* WB Saunders, Philadelphia, 1976, p 157.

69. Gold MS, Vereby K and Dackis CA: Diagnosis of drug abuse, drug intoxication and withdrawal states. *Fair Oaks Hospital Psychiatric Letter* 3:23, 1985.

70. Finkle BS: Drug-analysis technology: Overview and state of the art. *Clin Chem* 33/11(B):13B, 1987.

71. Chattoraj SC: Gas chromatography. In Teitz, NW (ed): *Fundamentals of Clinical Chemistry.* WB Saunders, Philadelphia, 1976, p 167.

72. Bauer JD: *Clinical Laboratory Methods, ed 9.* The CV Mosby Company, St. Louis, 1982, p 441.

73. Catlin D et al: Analytic chemistry at the games of the XXIIIrd Olympiad in Los Angeles, 1984. *Clin Chem* 33:319, 1987.

74. Council on Scientific Affairs, The American Medical Association: Scientific issues in drug testing. *JAMA* 257:1310, 1985.

75. Imwinkelried EJ: False positive – shoddy drug testing is jeopardizing the jobs of millions. *The Sciences,* September/October, 1987, p 23.

76. Wadler GI and Hainline B: *Drugs and the Athlete*, F.A. Davis, Philadelphia, 1989, p 87.

77. Sidney KH and Lefcoe WM: The effects of ephedrine on the physiological and psychological responses to submaximal and maximal exercises in man. *Med Sci Sports* 9:95, 1977.

CHAPTER 13

COCAINE AND THE CARDIOVASCULAR SYSTEM: RELEVANCE TO THE ATHLETE

Bruce F. Waller, M.D.

Clinical Professor of Pathology and Medicine
Indiana University School of Medicine;
Director, Cardiovascular Pathology Registry
St. Vincent Hospital, Indianapolis
Cardiologist, Nasser, Smith, Pinkerton Cardiology, Inc.
Indianapolis, Indiana

Editor's Note: This next chapter is sad, but true. The evidence is now in concerning the direct causal relationship between drugs such as cocaine and serious heart disease, including sudden death. The incredible use of cocaine is not just a national problem, but a worldwide one – including use by athletes. Of course, prevention by "saying no" to drugs is of prime importance, but this has been easier said than done.

A careful history on preparticipation screening must include diligent probing for any suggestion of drug use, and all involved in an athletic program – family, physicians, coaches, and administrative personnel – need to maintain a watchful eye throughout each season. Educational efforts to point out the serious consequences that can, and do, occur when athletes get involved with drugs should be a part of any athletic program. – WPH

Cocaine was implicated in the deaths of basketball star Len Bias and pro football player Don Rogers. The deaths of these prominent athletes have focused public attention on the potentially fatal effects of cocaine. Numerous coaching associations, professional and amateur athletic organizations, medical and non-medical athletic societies and associations, legal groups and doping control laboratories are addressing the issues of mandatory screening of athletes for the detection of cocaine and other illicit substances. Recently, a number of professional baseball, basketball, and football players have been suspended for detection of illicit substances in their urine samples.

This chapter will summarize the current effects and complications of cocaine usage, especially as it involves athletes.

The number of people in the United States who use cocaine has increased exponentially over the last 15 years. The increasing abuse of cocaine is related in part to cheaper forms ("crack") and the misbelief that cocaine is a benign and nonaddicting aphrodisiac.[1] Complicating the issue was the 1973 report of the Strategy Council on Drug Abuse, which stated that morbidity associated with cocaine abuse did not appear to be great, and that there were virtually no confirmed deaths attributed solely to cocaine overdose.[2]

Survey statistics indicate that in 1972 about 9% of young adults (ages 18 to 25 years) had tried cocaine. Between 1974 and 1985 the life-time prevalence of cocaine use drastically rose from 5.4 million to 22.2 million.[2,3] Current estimates indicate that about 25 million Americans have used or continue to use cocaine; that about 4 to 5 million people use cocaine on a regular basis, and about 1 million Americans are addicted to the drug.[3-5] There has been a sharp increase in cocaine treatment programs, emergency room treatment and admissions, and cocaine associated mortality.[3]

An alkyloid prepared from the erythroxylon coca plant, primarily located in South America, cocaine was first used as a local anesthetic in the late 19th century. Cocaine can be inhaled, smoked, or injected (intravenously, intramuscularly, or subcutaneously).

Ten years ago, little information was available about the cardiovascular effects and complications associated with cocaine. In more recent years, a number of reports have connected various cardiovascular events to the use of cocaine[3,6-31] (Figure 13-1): Myocardial ischemia,[10,27] over 50 clinical or necropsy-proven cases of acute myocardial infarction,[10-23,25-29] cardiomyopathy,[27,31] myocarditis,[3,21,23] malignant ventricular arrhythmias with or without fatal or nonfatal sudden cardiac arrest,[3,4,8,9,27] coronary spasm,[5,6,8,9,12,15,23] and rupture of the aorta.[19]

Pathogenesis of Cocaine-Related Cardiovascular Injury

Several mechanisms have been proposed to explain the pathogenesis of these injuries.[27]

Sympathomimetic Actions

Cocaine is a sympathomimetic agent and sensitizes tissues to catecholamines, in part through the inhibition of catecholamine reuptake at nerve terminals.[32] Tazelaar and associates[24] reported a 93% frequency of contraction-band necrosis in the myocardium of victims of cocaine-associated deaths, in comparison to a frequency of 45% in control subjects dying from sedative-hypnotic overdoses. The authors attributed the presence of contraction bands to cocaine-induced catecholamine myocardial injury. It is well known that catecholamines may induce myocardial injury in humans, in particular in those patients with pheochromocytoma.[33-35] In the study by Virmani and associates,[3] the frequency of contraction-band necrosis was much less (56%) than the frequency in Tazelaar's study and only slightly higher than control deaths (41%). Virmani et al[3] suggested that the marked difference in the frequency of contraction bands might be related to differences in populations studied, cocaine preparations, contaminants and adjuvants, route of delivery and chronicity of cocaine abuse.

As a sympathomimetic agent, cocaine can induce various tachycardias and produce severe systemic hypotension.[36] Myocardial ischemia and/or infarction may result from an increased myocardial oxygen demand.[13,14,23,27,29]

Vasoconstriction

Cocaine is a potent vasoconstrictor.[27] Several instances of coronary artery thrombosis and spasm have been reported in patients who abuse cocaine, including acute coronary thrombosis in association with angina, acute myocardial infarction, and sudden death.[13,23,28,29] In some instances, there is underlying atherosclerotic plaque; in others, the coronary arteries are normal. Coronary thrombosis occurring in coronary arteries free of atherosclerotic plaque suggests the role of cocaine-induced spasm or possible primary thrombogenicity of cocaine or its metabolites.[27]

Coronary spasm has been associated with cocaine usage and has been postulated as a mechanism of myocardial infarction in those users with clean coronary arteries.[5,6,8,9,12,15,23] Simpson and Edwards[21] reported coronary artery narrowing in a young patient without underlying atherosclerotic plaque. The coronary artery was severely narrowed by fibrointimal proliferation, which was attributed to underlying coronary artery spasm that caused focal vessel endothelial injury, platelet adherence, and aggregation. Platelets liberate platelet-derived growth factor (PDGF), which induces intimal proliferative lesions. In patients with underlying coronary plaque, cocaine-induced spasm also may produce endothelial disruption at the surface of the plaque and promote platelet aggregation and further vasoconstriction from the release of platelet prostaglandins.[3]

Myocarditis

Cocaine abuse has been associated with myocarditis.[3, 21, 23] The Virmani study[3] showed a 20% incidence of myocarditis in 40 necropsy patients who died from cocaine overdose or homicide. This represented a significantly greater number of cases compared to a control group of people who died from trauma (4%). The foci of myocarditis were small and sparse and were composed of lymphocytes only (7 of 9 cases) or lymphocytes and eosinophils (2 of 9 cases). The foci of myocarditis had cell necrosis and may have been the site origin of ventricular arrhythmias and sudden death.[37]

The etiology of cocaine-related myocarditis is unknown. Infectious agents (virus, bacterial, fungal) are possible, but reports to date have not proven this connection. As discussed previously, catecholamines induce necrosis, inflammation, and coronary vasoconstriction. Chronic administration of cocaine in the rat model has shown an increase in the concentration of left ventricular norepinephrine.[38] Norepinephrine is known to induce myocyte necrosis with an associated inflammatory component.[34,35] Cocaine may also have a direct effect on lymphocyte activity.[3] Intravenous cocaine usage can increase natural killer cell activity in the blood of humans,[3,39] and natural killer cells may be cytotoxic to cardiac myocytes.

It has been suggested[3, 27] that inflammatory infiltrates also may be an immunological response to other substances associated with adulterated cocaine. The presence of an eosinophilic infiltrate (as in the case of a 25-year-old chronic cocaine abuser who showed eosinophilic myocarditis)[17] suggests a hypersensitivity etiology to the cocaine-induced myocarditis. Such myocarditis may result from cocaine, its metabolites, or any contaminant substance.

Cardiac Arrest

A cocaine-induced cardiac arrest has been reported in association with underlying coronary atherosclerosis,[40] clean coronary arteries, and presumed coronary spasm and/or induction of ventricular arrhythmias. In the study by Virmani and colleagues,[3] 24 of 31 "natural cocaine-associated deaths" were sudden (18 unwitnessed, 6 witnessed). Others[40] reported 24 cases of sudden death associated with cocaine abuse, 15 of whom had severe underlying coronary atherosclerosis. As discussed earlier, cocaine-induced sudden death in these individuals may result from increased myocardial oxygen demands (ischemia), sympathomimetic action (vasospasm), and/or acute occlusion of diseased coronary arteries by platelet-fibrin thrombi (endothelial disruption, spasm).

Dilated Cardiomyopathy

Dilated cardiomyopathy has been reported in four patients.[27, 31] At least one, and possibly two, of these patients had myocardial infarcts that may have been related to coronary atherosclerosis (coronary dilated cardiomyopathy), but the remaining two patients had no other associated factor except chronic cocaine abuse (idiopathic dilated cardiomyopathy). The association suggests a possible myocardial toxic effect of cocaine.

Hypertensive Crisis

Rupture of the ascending aorta during cocaine intoxication was recently reported[19] in a 45-year-old man. The patient had chronic systemic hypertension, and his aorta probably ruptured in response to a cocaine-induced hypertensive crisis.

Cerebrovascular accidents also have been reported to occur within minutes of cocaine use. At least five cases of cerebrovascular accidents have been reported: three with underlying cerebrovascular aneurysms, one with an arteriovenous malformation and one with thrombotic occlusion.[41-44]

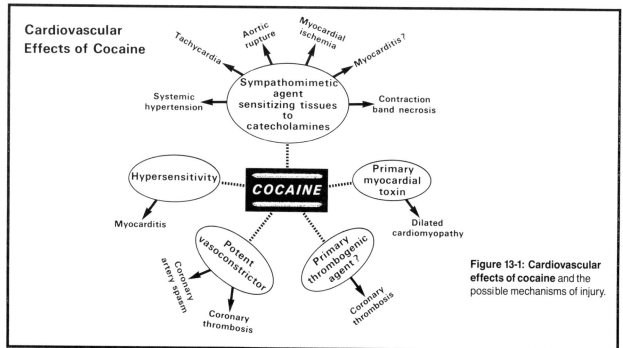

Figure 13-1: Cardiovascular effects of cocaine and the possible mechanisms of injury.

References

1. Cregler LL, Mark H: Medical complications of cocaine abuse. *N Engl J Med* 315:1495, 1986.
2. Kozel NJ, Adams EH: Epidemiology of drug abuse: An overview. *Science* 234:970, 1986.
3. Virmani R, Robinowitz M, Smialek JE, Smyth DF: Cardiovascular effects of cocaine: an autopsy study of 40 patients. *Am Heart J* 115:1068, 1988.
4. National Institute on Drug Abuse monograph series 1985; No. 85-1414.
5. Miller GW Jr: The cocaine habit. *Am Fam Physician* 31:173, 1985.
6. Weitli CV, Wright RK: Death caused by recreational cocaine use. *JAMA* 241:2519, 1979.
7. Mittleman RE, Wetli CV: Death caused by recreational cocaine use: an update. *JAMA* 252:1889, 1984.
8. Benchimol A, Bartall H, Desser KB: Acceleration of ventricular rhythm and cocaine abuse. *Ann Intern Med* 88:519, 1978.
9. Nanji AA, Filipenko JD: Asystole and ventricular fibrillation associated with cocaine intoxication. *Chest* 85:132, 1984.
10. Coleman DL, Ross TF, Naughton JL: Myocardial ischemia and infarction related to recreational cocaine use. *West J Med* 136:444, 1982.
11. Johnson S, O'Meara M, Young JB: Acute cocaine poisoning: Importance of treating seizures and acidosis. *Am J Med* 75:1061, 1983.
12. Schachne JS, Roberts BH, Thompson PD: Coronary artery spasm and myocardial infarction associated with cocaine use. *N Engl J Med* 310:1665, 1984.
13. Kossowsky WA, Lyon AF: Cocaine and myocardial infarction: A probable connection. *Chest* 86:729, 1984.
14. Pasternack PF, Colvin SB, Baumann FG: Cocaine-induced angina pectoris and acute myocardial infarction in patients younger than 40 years. *Am J Cardiol* 55:847, 1985.
15. Howard RE, Hueter DC, Davis GJ: Acute myocardial infarction following cocaine abuse in a young woman with normal coronary arteries. *JAMA* 254:95, 1985.
16. Cregler LL, Mark H: Relation of acute myocardial infarction to cocaine abuse. *Am J Cardiol* 56:794, 1985.
17. Gould L, Gopalswarny C, Patel C, Betza R: Cocaine-induced myocardial infarction. *NY State J Med* 95:660, 1985.
18. Wilkins CE, Mathor VS, Ty RC, Hall RJ: Myocardial infarction associated with cocaine abuse. *Texas Heart Inst J* 12:385, 1985.
19. Barth CW III, Bray M, Roberts WC: Rupture of the ascending aorta during cocaine intoxication. *Am J Cardiol* 57:496, 1986.
20. Weiss RJ: Recurrent myocardial infarction caused by cocaine abuse. *Am Heart J* 111:793, 1986.
21. Simpson RW, Edwards WD: Pathogenesis of cocaine-induced ischemic heart disease. Autopsy finding in a 21-year-old man. *Arch Pathol Lab Med* 110:479, 1986.
22. Rollinger IM, Belzberg AS, McDonald IL: Cocaine-induced myocardial infarction. *Can Med Assoc J* 135:45, 1986.
23. Isner JM, Estes M, Thompson PD et al: Acute cardiac events temporally related to cocaine abuse. *N Engl J Med* 315:1438, 1986.
24. Tazelaar HD, Karck SB, Stephens BG, Billinghan ME: Cocaine and the heart. *Hum Pathol* 18:195, 1987.
25. Zimmerman FH, Gustafson GM, Kemp HG: Recurrent myocardial infarction associated with cocaine abuse in a young man with normal coronary arteries: Evidence for coronary artery spasm culminating in thrombus. *J Am Coll Cardiol* 9:964, 1987.
26. Cantwell JD, Rose FD: Cocaine and cardiovascular events. *Phys Sports Med* 14:77, 1986.
27. Lam D, Goldschlager N: Myocardial injury associated with polysubstance abuse. *Am Heart J* 115:675, 1988.
28. Rod JL, Zucker RD: Acute myocardial infarction shortly after cocaine inhalation. *Am J Cardiol* 59:161, 1987.
29. Smith HWB III, Lieberman A, Brody S et al: Acute myocardial infarction temporally related to cocaine use. *Ann Intern Med* 107:13, 1987.
30. Altieri PI, Toro JM, Banch H, Carrion EH: Coronary artery spasm on patients with induced myocardial infarctions. *J Am Coll Cardiol* (Suppl A):172A, 1987.
31. Wiener RS, Lockhart JT, Scwartz RG: Dilated cardiomyopathy and cocaine abuse. Report of two cases. *Am J Med* 81:699-701, 1986.
32. Smith RB: Cocaine and catecholamine interaction. *Arch Otolaryngol* 98:139, 1973.
33. Tarizzo V, Ribio MC: Effect of cocaine on several adrenergic system parameters. *Gen Pharmacol* 16:71, 1985.
34. Karch SB, Billingham ME: Myocardial contraction bands revisited. *Hum Pathol* 17:9, 1986.
35. Reichenbach DD, Benditt EP: Catecholamines and cardiomyopathy: the pathogenesis and potential importance of myofibrillar degeneration. *Hum Pathol* 1:125, 1970.
36. Fischman MW, Schuster CR, Resnekov L et al: Cardiovascular and subjective effects of intravenous cocaine administration in humans. *Arch Gen Psychiatry* 33:983, 1976.
37. Vignola PA, Aonuma K, Swaye PS et al: Lymphocytic myocarditis presenting as unexplained ventricular arrhythmias: Diagnosis with endocardial biopsy and response to immunosuppression. *J. Am Coll Cardiol* 4:812, 1984.
38. Tarizzo V, Rubio MC: Effect of cocaine on several adrenergic system parameters. *Gen Pharmacol* 16:71, 1985.
39. Dyke CV, Stesis A, Jones R, Chuntharapai A, Seaman W: Cocaine increases natural killer cell activity. *J Clin Invest* 77:1387, 1986.
40. Mittleman RE, Weitli CV: Cocaine and sudden "natural" death. *J Forensic Sci* 32:11, 1987.
41. Brust JC, Richter RW: Stroke associated with cocaine abuse. *NY State J Med* 77:1473, 1977.
42. Caplan LR, Hier DB, Banks G: Current concepts of cerebrovascular disease-stroke: Stroke and drug abuse. *Stroke* 13:869, 1982.
43. Lichtenfeld PJ, Rubin DB, Feldman RS: Subarachnoid hemorrhage precipitated by cocaine snorting. *Arch Neurol* 41:223, 1984.
44. Schwartz KA, Cohen JA: Subarachnoid hemorrhage precipitated by cocaine snorting. (Letter). *Arch Neurol* 41:705, 1984.
45. Zalis EG, Lundberg GD, Knutson RA: The pathophysiology of acute amphetamine poisoning with pathologic correlation. *J Pharmacol Exp Ther* 158:115, 1967.

46. Bowen JS, Davis GB, Kearney TE: Diffuse vascular spasm associated with 4-bromo-2 5-dimethoxyamphetamine ingestion. *JAMA* 249:1477, 1983.

47. Smith HJ, Roche AHG, Jagusch MF, Herdson PB: Cardiomyopathy associated with amphetamine administration. *Am Heart J* 91:792, 1976.

48. Schwarzfarb L, Singh G, Marcus D: Heroin-associated rhabdomyolysis with cardiac involvement. *Arch Intern Med* 137:1255, 1977.

49. Scherrer P, Delaloye-Bishof A, Turnini G et al: Participation myocardique a la rhabdomyose non traumatique apres surdosage aux opiaces. *Schweiz Med Wochenschr* 115:1166, 1985.

50. Paranthaman SK, Khan F: Acute cardiomyopathy with recurrent pulmonary edema and hypotension following heroin overdosage. *Chest* 69:117, 1976.

CHAPTER 14

LEGAL ASPECTS OF CARDIOVASCULAR EVALUATION OF ATHLETES

David S. Starr, MD, JD

Georgetown, Texas

Editor's Note: There are a large number of physicians who are responsible for the medical screening and clearance of athletes who participate in an athletic program, whether at the grammar or high school level, or for college or professional sports.

Looming like a black cloud of a storm or a bad dream is the specter of a lawsuit against the physician in case some unforeseen medical problem (including even sudden death) occurs in an athlete that he has examined.

What are some of the medicolegal problems? How can we prevent them, or best deal with them if they do occur?

This chapter provides much needed practical information and wise advice for the physician as well as other medical personnel, coaches, and administrators who may have to face these problems. – WPH

The physician who conducts physical examinations of athletes prior to their participation in strenuous athletics often carries in the back of his mind the specter of some hidden cardiovascular disease, which, at a moment of peak effort, will cause the young athlete to fall dramatically, finally, and accusingly dead, in full view of hundreds, possibly millions of spectators. Boxing, marathon running, and most recently basketball have provided dramatic examples of this statistically rare, but memorable event. This chapter aims to give some practical guidance to the physician who performs such exams, whether as part of his or her regular practice, or as a part-time volunteer. Both of these groups run a definite but small statistical risk of such an untoward event

happening to an athlete whom they had previously cleared, potentially leading to the inevitable accusations and a lawsuit by disgruntled family members. However, before we look at practical steps we can take to minimize this risk, some general comments about the legal process are in order.

Standard of Care

The "standard of care" is the yardstick against which every defendant physician in a professional liability ("malpractice") suit is theoretically judged. However, the workday reality is that jury decisions are so variable that, for any given situation, there is no constant standard or "safety zone" that ensures immunity from lawsuits. Thus, similar cases within the same area of the country, or even in the same county, may have grossly dissimilar outcomes. The reason for this is that the standard of care in any individual case is set by the testifying experts, and the "quality" and believability of these experts are the centerpoint and determining factor in most lawsuits. Thus, the legal concept of a fixed "standard of care" is not, in fact, of much help in the battleground of the courtroom. Of more practical importance is a consideration of the factors that actually do determine the outcome in the minority (10%) of cases that go to the jury, thus determining the settlement value of the other 90% of cases.

Factors that Determine Outcome

Most physicians are surprised to learn that the medical facts are of secondary importance in determining the outcome of jury cases. The more important factors, in approximate order, are:

• The venue (location) of the case (which determines the makeup of the jury)
• The quality of the witnesses (including the defendant physician)
• The relative skill of the lawyers
• And last, the medical facts of the case.

In this context, the "quality" of the witnesses refers to jury appeal, consistency, clarity, and believability, since expert testimony from the two sides is usually directly contradictory and therefore confusing to the jury. Defendant physicians have an intrinsic advantage in most areas, winning over 70% of cases nationwide. However, jury awards are greater than for corresponding patient injuries from, say, auto accidents.

Precipitating Factors

Factors that precipitate lawsuits are just as counter intuitive as those that determine the outcome. Empiric studies consistently show that severity of injury, especially in a young person, large hospital bills, hostility towards the physician (whether groundless or not), and familiarity with the legal system are common precursors of a lawsuit. On the other hand, a large recent study indicates that most cases of negligence do not lead to lawsuits, nor are most lawsuits grounded in negligence (as judged by a retrospective review of hospital records). Thus, patients who have a hostile, negative attitude toward the physician, or who are connected with the legal system, are statistically "high risk" patients in that they are more likely than the average patient to initiate a lawsuit if problems develop. In my opinion, these patients should have special "defensive" notations on their charts, and be referred more often for specialty consultation. In this way, the cost of their litigious preference is not borne by the physician, but by themselves.

Medical Notes

In the face of conflicting testimony, juries place significant, and perhaps undue emphasis on medical records and patient information sheets made out at the time of the examination. Appropriate notations have been the basis of many successful defenses, while lack of them has led to many unduly generous settlements. While notes should be appropriate, they do not need to be in exhaustive narrative form: A history and physical checklist is very suited to the usual athletic examination, but just as important is the information sheet that the athlete receives. If the athlete is unable to testify as to what the doctor told him, whether through brain injury or death, or just fading memory, then a patient information sheet that explains the purposes and limitations of the athletic screening examination is a solid defense exhibit. In the case of a minor, the sheet should be addressed to the parents as well. If the physician recommends special investigations, then the record and information sheet should reflect this, since many athletes do not follow their physician's recommendations, or even tell their parents about the recommendations.

Protocols

A well designed and generally accepted protocol can be the defense lawyer's best friend. Although many physicians draw up their own individual protocols, one designed by a group of consultants or a professional body such as the American College of Cardiology has greater credibility with a lay jury. A protocol typically consists of a special "sports history and physical" form on which the physician can check the items as they are completed, combined with a set of recommended steps for positive findings (somewhat along the lines of an ACLS manual). In the case of positive findings, special investigations (eg, an EKG for a history of chest pain on exercise to detect hypertrophic cardiomyopathy) are indicated by the protocol steps.

Although some physicians find such cook-book medicine offensive, generally this system provides the physician with an excellent defense in the case of mishap. In the case of a protocol drawn up by an official body or from an accepted text, the protocol takes on the aura and prestige of its authors, and becomes the functional standard of care for the defending physician, usually to his advantage.

Risk Management

The term "risk management," borrowed from the insurance industry, refers to systematic behavior which attempts to reduce the statistical risk of injury and subsequent financial loss through lawsuits. In the context of the examining physician, this involves making several, usually minor changes to the practice format. Typical strategies include:

1. Communication – Information sheets should make the athlete (or parents) aware of the limitations of the preathletic examination. Any recommendations for further consultation or tests should be entered on an appropriate space on this form, as well as in the patient's record.

2. Records – Although records should be appropriate, they do not need to be exhaustive. Standardized forms and protocols streamline the record and ensure completeness. A clinical information sheet filled out by the athlete themselves provides an indisputable record of the athletes symptoms, thus avoiding later ambiguity. Test results should be reviewed by the physician and initialled upon communication to the athlete, thus ensuring a "paper trail" without creating undue inefficiency.

Editor's Note: The foregoing discussions of communication and records make wise good sense. Other lawyers also advise us to keep good records in writing. – WPH

---

3. Restrictions – Athletes are understandably annoyed and impatient with physician restrictions. In one bizarre case, the consulting specialist was sued for advising a professional athlete with hypertrophic cardiomyopathy against playing at all, thus "causing" substantial loss of income. The case was resolved by the subsequent death of the athlete during exertion, thus essentially proving the physician correct.

Editor's Note: I remember reading about this incredible case and thinking it almost unbelievable that such a good physician, who obviously made the correct diagnosis and gave the correct advice, could be sued. I also recall that this physician is reported to have said, in effect, that the athlete's death was not a good way to prove he was right. – WPH

The guiding principle legally (known as "patient autonomy") is that the physician's role is to inform, to present alternatives, to make a recommendation, and to explain the consequences of the various alternatives. The current legal model rejects the notion that a physician can make decisions for or "place restrictions" on a patient (despite the obvious reality to the contrary), and places the physician merely in the role of advisor. Thus, the progress notes should make clear what the physician recommended, and what the patient decides. Since many athletes disregard physician advice, such caution is appropriate.

4. Drug Testing – In accordance with the current consumerist model of medicine, a physician cannot force a patient to undergo drug (or other) testing. This said, the physician can perform any tests requested by the patient, even if the athlete feels "forced" to have them by contractual obligations or association rules. Whether the player will undergo testing is strictly a legal matter between the player and the coach or association, but the tests should only be ordered at the player's request.

5. Accreditation – Physicians with some special training or experience in the area in which they are practicing receive generally favorable treatment with juries. It makes sense that a physician doing a significant number of athlete examinations should attend courses and receive whatever certification seems appropriate and available.

6. Consultation – Appropriate consultation, whether by telephone or by referral, significantly reduces the likelihood of a successful malpractice suit. Several factors account for this: First, it seems like the sort of thing a prudent physician would do when unsure. Second, the second physician can often provide genuine new insight into the clinical problem. Third (and this from a defense lawyer's perspective), it creates an immediate interested expert witness for the defense! Consultation, even if for an opinion only, is underutilized as a risk management technique.

Some Case Examples

The Teenage Athlete – Alton was a 17-year-old high school football player; in fact, the star of the team. He was in excellent physical condition and seemingly healthy. He underwent physical examination at the beginning of the season, but died suddenly after walking away from a huddle halfway through a game, complaining of chest pain. There was no autopsy. His family, distraught at the loss of a second son (the first had died in a motor vehicle accident), sued the physician, the coaches, and the school. The local judge, a conservative rural veteran, dismissed the case, since the boy and his parents had signed a release and had been given a patient information sheet that explained the limitations of the preseason physical. It stated that injury, even death, was a recognized possibility from playing sports.

The Professional Athlete – JL was a basketball player for a minor league team, who had injured his knee in a pre-season game. After arthroscopy and repair of a partial tear to the medial meniscus, he was advised, according to his physician, to be non-weight bearing for two weeks, at least. After this time, without checking with his physician, he assumed it would be OK to return to "a little warmup game," but unfortunately he again twisted his knee, this time putting him out for the season. He sued the doctor for loss of income and failure to prevent recurrent injury. An examination of the physician's notes indicated quite clearly that the patient had been instructed to be non-weight bearing until he was cleared by the physician. The case was settled for a modest amount.

The Older Athlete – Mr. K, a 51-year-old male, underwent yearly physicals with his family practitioner. He had no risk factors except a strong family history of coronary artery disease. One afternoon, while competing in a league basketball tournament, he stated, "I don't feel too good," sat down and collapsed several minutes later. Although cardiopulmonary resuscitation was started immediately, he was unable to be resuscitated. His widow sued the family doctor. The physician could find no written record of his discussions with the patient regarding exercise restriction or recommendation that he have a treadmill stress test, although the physician remembered telling the patient that, with his family history, if he was going to play basketball, he should really have an exercise treadmill test. The case was settled for a moderate amount.

Editor's Note: This chapter also serves to reemphasize the need for careful initial screening, particularly by history and physical examination. It should be performed by a physician trained to detect any signs or symptoms of cardiovascular disease. With any question of a cardiac problem, additional diagnostic tests, plus additional consultations should be obtained. – WPH

The Inhibitory Effects of Litigation

The rising tide of litigation has affected all areas of American life, including participatory sports.

School boards, coaches, equipment manufacturers, and team physicians are all at risk for lawsuits that often follow severe athletic injuries or death in young people, and all have been held liable for player injuries. Although surveys indicate that fear of lawsuits has inhibited physician participation, it is difficult to estimate how many teams have been adversely effected. However, it is known that the risk of litigation, reflected in high insurance premiums or unavailability of insurance, has closed a number of play areas, and made athletic equipment (especially football helmets) more expensive. It seems reasonable to assume that the same factors limit physician availability. However, it is equally apparent that overall, many physicians are willing to shoulder the risk of litigation in order to take part in the rewarding and often exciting role of team physician. Often the physician was previously athletic himself, or has close links with the team he is serving. However, these important and positive reasons for participation should not blind the physician to the statistical risk he is running, or prevent him from adhering to the preventive programs noted earlier in this chapter.

The Future of Law and Sports Medicine

The pervasive effects of litigation on American life noted previously are effectively concealed by the predominant use of insurance, which has the effect of spreading the relatively large payments over a wide base. Since all the participants, including plaintiffs, insurance companies, lawyers both for the plaintiff and the defense, and even the judges, have a vested interest in this multibillion dollar industry, the legal system is unlikely to change until voter outrage forces reform at the ballot box. However, surveys indicate that, at present, most people are ambivalent about revision of the litigation system.

Despite this, professional liability ("malpractice") litigation is a likely candidate for early reform. Studies indicate that the present litigation process is wasteful, inefficient, and consistently fails to achieve its theoretical twin goals: compensation of injured patients and deterrence of substandard medical care. These data, combined with a need to reduce the practice of "defensive medicine" for cost reasons, may well lead to significant malpractice reform by Congress as the "inducement" part of a broader National Health package. Of the multiple bills before Congress at the time of this writing, one already proposes that such disputes should be heard by a medically qualified hearing officer, rather than a lay jury. Although such a system has drawbacks, the advantage of having technically trained people pass judgment on technical matters seems clear. The prestigious American Law Institute has also recently suggested several patient compensation schemes that bypass or minimize the judicial process. Which of these suggestions, if any, will survive the political process is uncertain. If these or similar changes are implemented, physicians participating in sports medicine will be among those to benefit.

Editor's Note: Dr. Starr has put his finger on a very important aspect of medical practice and patient care. Something has to be done about the national disgrace of the plethora of unjustified malpractice suits against physicians, medical institutions, and other medical personnel.

Dr. Starr advocates a "medically qualified hearing officer, rather than a lay jury." This would be advantageous, but I believe that if a panel, composed of unquestionably well trained and qualified members, screened and evaluated these suits, that most of them could be eliminated, or settled fairly out of court. If on this panel there were several physicians, several attorneys, several religious leaders, plus two or three other selected individuals, that prompt and efficient justice could be better administered. By its strength in numbers, such a large authoritative panel would carry more weight and be better than the opinion of one or two persons.

Also, it is likely that a marked reduction in the numbers of legal suits would occur if attorney contingency fees (such as one third of the award) were banned. I also favor, as some have suggested, that if the suit is determined to be unjustified, that the cost incurred by the defendant physician or other party being sued, be paid by the person (or persons) initiating the law suit. – WPH

CHAPTER 15

LEGAL CONSEQUENCES OF STANDARD SETTING FOR COMPETITIVE ATHLETES WITH CARDIOVASCULAR ABNORMALITIES*

John C. Weistart, JD, LLD

Professor of Law
Duke University School of Law

Summary

This chapter addresses the issue of whether establishing consensus standards for the treatment of particular medical conditions increases a physician's exposure to legal liability. The conclusion reached is that the legal effects of standard setting, rather than representing a significant threat of liability, should be seen as beneficial to the medical profession. A fundamental point is that the legal test for liability is entirely dependent on the medical profession's definition of what constitutes adequate care. The law incorporates the standard of care defined by the medical profession and does not impose an external norm. In the absence of formally stated standards, the process of defining relevant medical criteria will involve a great deal of uncertainty. Outcomes of legal contests will be affected by such extraneous factors as the relative experience of the lawyers involved, their access to knowledgeable expert witnesses, and their strategic decisions made with respect to tactics and procedures. Establishment of formal standards has the salutory effect of limiting the influence of these factors and thus reducing the randomness of the results reached. Formal standards also have the advantage of being easily replicated in unrelated proceedings and thereby contribute to the development of a consistent, evenly applied rule of liability. Finally, even if formal standards are either more, or less, progressive than the actual state of medical practice, there is relatively little risk that they will produce untoward results.

Organizations, conferences, papers and textbooks help set qualitative standards for cardiovascular evaluation of athletes and undoubtedly give rise to questions about the potential liability consequences for practicing physicians. Some readers of this book may be concerned that formal standards will produce automatic liability for practitioners who fail to satisfy the suggested criteria. Others may feel that even if liability is not automatic, its threat will be greatly increased because certain practices will now more obviously fail to measure up against an announced norm. In any event, it will frequently be assumed that the physician's exposure to the costs and turmoil of litigation will be enhanced.

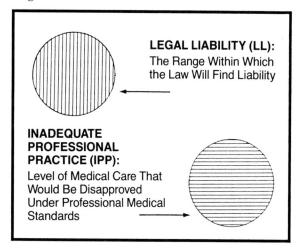

Figure 15-1: Legal Liability and Professional Practice – Symbols used to illustrate the relation between the scope of legal liability (LL) and inadequate professional practice (IPP), that is, the internal assessment of the medical profession, regarding whether a particular course of treatment is adequate. The symbol on the left depicts the range within which the law will find liability. The symbol on the right represents the sphere of medical care that would be disapproved under professional medical standards.

Reproduced with permission from Journal of the American College of Cardiology, Volume 6: 1191-1197, 1985.

If this were true, there would be rather ominous public policy implications. In effect, the medical profession would be discouraged from pursuing the improvement of patient care. Equally troubling would be the fact that it was the law and legal concerns that operated to deter better medical practice. The jurisprudential justification for a legal regime that had such an effect would be far from obvious. At least since the 13th century, it has been assumed that a regime of law should operate to improve the human condition.

This chapter attempts to provide reassurance that the law is not antagonistic to professional standard setting. Indeed, the essential message is even more positive: not only are liability implications not ominous, but the ultimate legal result may be quite favorable for the medical profession itself. If carefully devised and properly disseminated, standard setting should have the effect of reducing, rather than increasing, the instances of inappropriate legal intervention.

The Relation Between Legal Liability and the Standards of the Medical Profession

A discussion of the legal effects of standard setting benefits from a clarification of the relation between legal liability and the criteria that the medical profession itself uses to judge the acceptability of a physician's mode of practice. Despite the considerable public and professional attention given to the legal implications of medical malpractice, a surprising degree of misunderstanding exists on the correlation between the independent assessments of the profession and the outcomes they obtain in legal proceedings. A common misperception, not confined to physicians, is that the ultimate goal of the law of medical malpractice is to tell doctors how to practice, or at least to make their professional behavior conform to norms that are legally defined. The goal of the law is actually quite different, however. Ultimately, the law is very deferential to the medical profession's own efforts to define the acceptable level of practice.

The essential points for our purpose can be illustrated by a series of representations. The symbols we use are found in Figure 15-1. The figure with the vertical lines, positioned on the left, depicts the range of legal liability. This is the sphere in which medical professionals are found

to have legal liability to patients in cases involving alleged malpractice. We will identify this area as simply "legal liability" (LL). The other symbol with horizontal lines covers a different field. Here we are concerned only about the professional judgements of the medical profession itself. Our illustration on the right represents actions that would be judged to be unacceptable by the profession quite apart from any legal consequences. This field is denominated "inadequate professional performance" (IPP). Again, the important question for our purposes is the relation between the two assessments represented here, one legal and one medical.[1]

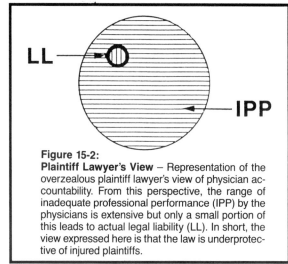

Figure 15-2:
Plaintiff Lawyer's View – Representation of the overzealous plaintiff lawyer's view of physician accountability. From this perspective, the range of inadequate professional performance (IPP) by the physicians is extensive but only a small portion of this leads to actual legal liability (LL). In short, the view expressed here is that the law is underprotective of injured plaintiffs.

Some have a misconception that is illustrated in Figure 15-2. This might be taken, in a bit of understatement, as indicating the view held by overzealous plaintiffs' lawyers. From this perspective, inadequate professional performance abounds, but only a small segment of it ever results in legal liability. In short, physicians are only rarely made to account for their malpractice.

A level of misunderstanding that is equally imbued with hyperbole is shown in Figure 15-3. Here we have the disgruntled physician's view of the world. As seen by this person, a physician experiences tremendous exposure to legal liability, but very little such liability is based on professional performance that is actually inadequate.

Neither of these views need detain us very long, for they represent the emotional extremes of the present malpractice debate. A more serious effort is illustrated in Figure 15-4, which attempts

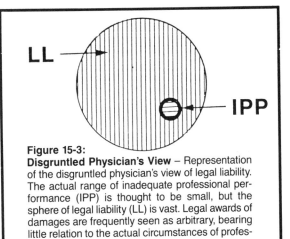

Figure 15-3:
Disgruntled Physician's View – Representation of the disgruntled physician's view of legal liability. The actual range of inadequate professional performance (IPP) is thought to be small, but the sphere of legal liability (LL) is vast. Legal awards of damages are frequently seen as arbitrary, bearing little relation to the actual circumstances of professional malpractice.

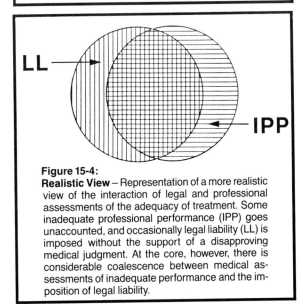

Figure 15-4:
Realistic View – Representation of a more realistic view of the interaction of legal and professional assessments of the adequacy of treatment. Some inadequate professional performance (IPP) goes unaccounted, and occasionally legal liability (LL) is imposed without the support of a disapproving medical judgment. At the core, however, there is considerable coalescence between medical assessments of inadequate performance and the imposition of legal liability.

quate professional performance result in the imposition of liability. Even when cases are taken to litigation, imprecision in our litigation procedures and inadequacy in our fact-finding process often leave the deficient performance unremedied.

But we need not be content with this reality. Indeed, the aspiration of the law is quite different. This is represented by Figure 15-5. The point here is that the goal of the law is to base legal liability on the judgements that are made within the medical profession. The law strives for a rather precise correlation between the assessments of the medical profession as to what is good or bad practice and the instances in which legal liability results.

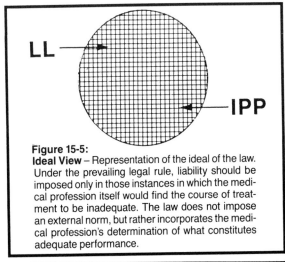

Figure 15-5:
Ideal View – Representation of the ideal of the law. Under the prevailing legal rule, liability should be imposed only in those instances in which the medical profession itself would find the course of treatment to be inadequate. The law does not impose an external norm, but rather incorporates the medical profession's determination of what constitutes adequate performance.

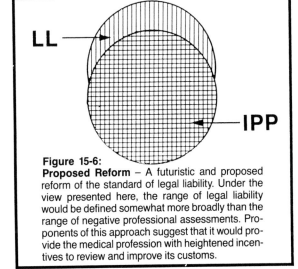

Figure 15-6:
Proposed Reform – A futuristic and proposed reform of the standard of legal liability. Under the view presented here, the range of legal liability would be defined somewhat more broadly than the range of negative professional assessments. Proponents of this approach suggest that it would provide the medical profession with heightened incentives to review and improve its customs.

to depict how the world really works. In this illustration, we are mainly interested in the general relation that is revealed. The details of the configuration will almost certainly be subject to debate. Some will argue that there should be more, or less, overlap. Others might dispute whether the size of the two fields should be shown as equal. But even with these matters unresolved, Figure 15-4 can be taken to suggest that our legal system operates imperfectly. Liability is sometimes imposed when there is little or no support for such an outcome in the internal professional assessment. This is illustrated by the segment on the far left. By the same token, not all instances of inade-

Legal Standards for Defining Liability

This aspiration is reflected in the legal standards that courts announce for defining instances of liability. For example, a common formulation of the physician's duty of care for liability purposes is as follows:

(A) physician is under a duty to use that degree of care and skill which is expected of a reasonably competent practitioner in the same class (or speciality) to which he belongs, acting in the same or similar circumstances.[2]

The important point for our inquiry is that in this statement, all referents for the applicable standard of care are internal to the profession. We are admonished to look to "the degree of care and skill" of "a reasonably competent practitioner." Moreover, the standard is specialty specific, for we are to look to practitioners of "the same class." Notably, what is missing from this test is any suggestion that an external norm is being imposed. Physicians are not told to save patients from all harm. Nor are they directed to take all steps that would reduce harm.[3]

The inward-looking character of the standard for medical malpractice contrasts with that used to define negligence in most other settings. The more common definition of negligence – the one applied to determine liability in industrial accidents and negligence-based products liability cases – does not look solely to custom in identifying the appropriate level of care. Indeed, it is recognized that the prevailing custom may itself give rise to an unacceptable risk of harm.[4]

The rationale for applying a special, more deferential liability standard to physicians is itself the source of some debate.[5] The most plausible explanation is found in the profession's long history of self-regulation. In our Anglo-American legal system, the prerogatives given to the guilds of 16th century London seem to have been particularly influential in shaping later developments.[6] Indeed, the medical profession, perhaps more than any other field of endeavor including the law, has maintained a strong allegiance to the norm of peer governance and internal enforcement.[7] The premise of a guild was that it afforded an adequate mechanism for quality control and that it

was uniquely suited to make knowledgeable judgments in its specialized field of endeavor. As questions of the adequacy of professional performance moved from the tribunal of the guild to the more public venue of the court, the substantive standard did not change drastically.[8]

While the rule in Figure 15-5 is the traditional one, it may be worth noting that there are other potential standards that are debated by those interested in law reform. One alternative is given in Figure 15-6. The premise of this view is that the law should be prepared to extend the range of liability slightly beyond the bounds of existing medical custom. According to the proponents, pure reliance on custom will be too insular at times, and some external mechanism is needed to ensure that the highest priority is given to reducing harm to patients. At least one case gives some credence to this view,[9] but it remains highly controversial.[10]

Yet another approach abandons the insistence on proof of negligence as a deviation from professional custom.[11] Under this standard of so-called strict liability, the critical question is whether the injury that resulted to the patient was preventable. If it was, then proponents of that view would award compensation to the patient.[12] This result would obtain without regard to whether preventive steps be taken. The avowed objective of such an arrangement is to provide a mechanism for spreading the costs of practice-related disabilities among all patients who use medical services. Cost spreading would be achieved as practitioners were forced to raise their fees to all patients to cover the expense of the now more extensive reimbursement system.[13]

But again, for our immediate purpose the traditional rule deferring to prevailing medical custom is the pertinent one. As suggested, this standard does not seek to control or manipulate the medical profession. Rather, it is incorporative: the profession's standard of reasonable care is that which should control legal results.

Pertinence of Custom in Professional Standard Setting

It might reasonably be asked why the real world looks more like Figure 15-4 than Figure 15-5. Why, in short, is the aspiration of the law not achieved?

A full exploration of that issue would be quite elaborate and would most likely excite great controversy. The list of defects, real and debatable, could cover numerous aspects of our litigation system. For our purposes, though, we can identify a few features that are particularly important.

1. Problems in Proving Medical Custom – A central issue in any medical litigation involves the matter of proving the standard of care to be applied. The inquiry is essentially one into the prevailing professional assumptions about what constitutes adequate diagnosis and treatment in the particular case. This issue is subject to an adversarial examination of the sort applied to other disputed points of litigation.

The device typically used to establish the prevailing standard is, of course, the expert witness. Each side is entitled to produce experts to develop its own peculiar – and often self-serving – view of what constitutes good care. The testimony of the competing experts is often conflicting, and the reasons for the conflicts vary. As medical practitioners well know, within the profession itself there will often be differences of opinion as to what amounts to proper caution. Sometimes the uncertainty is a product of incomplete scientific information in an absolute sense. At other times, the differences reflect differences in the training, perspective or skill of the expert. Further, the suspicion that some experts are largely "hired guns" is frequently articulated.

As if these variables did not produce uncertainty enough, the lawyers for the respective parties can have a great effect on the accuracy and completeness of the inquiry. For example, lawyers differ in terms of their access to perceptive, knowledgeable experts. The solo practitioner for whom this is his or her first malpractice case will do less well at producing reliable witnesses than an experienced law firm defending a sophisticated medical center. In addition, lawyers for each side will make strategic judgments that affect the reliability of the evidence on the relevant medical standard. Not all of these judgments will be good. Either lawyer may fail to call a critical witness. Or a strategic error may be made in the lawyers' declining to cross-examine certain witnesses, a choice frequently made for other reasons.[14] Or it may turn out that the jury was greatly influenced by a witness's arrogance, rather than the sub-

stance of what he said. In short, the process of proving medical custom is subject to a wide variety of influences that could undermine the reliability of the results reached.

2. Specific Effects of Standard Setting – It is against this background that the substantive standard setting of this textbook on cardiovascular evaluation of athletes and similar professional efforts can be judged. The most significant legal effect of conscientiously devised standards is likely to be on the process of proving medical custom.[15] There are many respects in which standard setting can be beneficial both to the legal process and to the medical profession that is having its practices reviewed. There are several effects that should be specifically noted.

For example, *carefully devised formal standards will reduce the randomness of legal results*. The point here is implicit in the analysis offered before. Uncertainty as to the relevant medical standard contributes to errors in legal outcomes. In the absence of defined standards, the litigation has an open-ended quality that increases the likelihood that outcomes will be affected by the factors mentioned above, such as the relative experience of the lawyers involved or the strength of strategy decisions that are made. Since litigation is a dynamic process, these influences will never be completely minimized. Nonetheless, the existence of formal professional approved standards will make the proof of prevailing customs much more certain.[16] In short, standards hold the prospect of yielding a reliable and understandable statement of what constitutes prevailing practice.

The medical profession presumably would find it more attractive to define custom through standard setting than through the alternative of definition by litigation. The latter inquiry has a decidedly ad hoc character. The statement of prevailing practice devised in one case will not necessarily have great weight in the next case that is litigated. In addition, a very compelling attraction of formal standard setting is its capacity to increase the control that the profession exercises over the norm against which it will be held to account. In this textbook at least, the process of proposing standards is wholly within the hands of the profession.

A further point can be made:

Standards are inevitable. A significant difference between formal and informal standards is the accuracy with which they can be reproduced in legal proceedings.

In most areas of medical practice, there will be a custom. The custom may emphasize individual discretion and thus be highly idiosyncratic, but it will exist. At its essence, the notion of *custom* is simply description of what knowledgeable practitioners do in diagnosing and treating particular conditions. But as we have suggested, customs become the relevant standards for liability purposes. Since customs are inevitable, standards will also necessarily exist.

An example may be in order. One of the issues addressed in this text concerns the extent to which asymptomatic patients with atherosclerotic coronary artery disease should be discouraged from participating in competitive sports. Let us assume that while there are some cardiologists who would not impose significant restrictions on the activities of such individuals, most practitioners would advise patients with coronary artery disease to refrain from strenuous sports. One can readily imagine the circumstances in which the issue of participation would become important. Assume that a patient with diagnosed coronary artery disease asked his physician if he could regularly play in a basketball league at the local YMCA. Assume that the endeavor was approved, but that the patient later suffered a myocardial infarction and died in the course of play. The patient's estate sues the treating physician, alleging that insufficient professional caution was shown.

If there were a formal standard in existence advising against vigorous competitive activity by patients with coronary artery disease, that measure would provide the focal point for the inquiry into liability. As will be explained below, the formal standard would only be probative, and not determinative, on the question of liability. It would, however, be the starting point from which the liability appraisal proceeded. But in the absence of such a stated norm, each side in the proceeding would attempt to establish the informal or de facto standard that operated in the profession. As we have framed the problem, there is a substantial segment of opinion that would discourage participation even in the absence of a formal statement. And there are some who take a different view. These perspectives would have to

be weighed to determine the norm of the profession. Once that standard is established, it would then be the criterion against which the particular physician's performance was judged.

Thus, the choice facing a professional group is not whether there should be standards. Rather, the important choice, from a legal perspective, is how clearly and accurately those standards will be stated. For some procedures the prevailing practice may be sufficiently clear that little is gained by a formalization of the standard. But for many areas of medical practice, this will not be the case. The setting of formal standards can have the effect of memorializing prevailing customs into a form that can be restated with a level of accuracy that the profession should find desirable.

3. Deviations Between Standards and Custom – Much of what has been said to this point assumes that we have standards that show a strong fidelity to prevailing customs. This premise is, of course, quite optimistic. Formal standards will vary in the degree to which they accurately portray the present state of medical practice. Some may be too general to be useful. Others may be accurate when devised but quickly become dated with subsequent technologic developments. In other cases, the standards will have simply missed the mark. The group devising the standard may have been more – or less – demanding than the profession generally.

The pertinent legal standard will take account of these variations. An important legal concept provides the flexibility needed to deal with deficiencies in the formal standards. As a legal matter, such measures are only "some evidence" of the prevailing standard of the profession.[17] Stated in another way, the ultimate question will always be: what is the prevailing custom? Courts are directed to consider all evidence that contributes to the clarification of that point. A formal standard, if it exists, is certainly relevant evidence. But it is not conclusive. The court will consider all proffers of proof that bear on the matter of custom, including any which limit or qualify the formal criteria.

Several important corollaries flow from these observations.

The actual legal effect of a set of formal standards will depend on the weight of the professional judgment supporting them.

Also,

> A physician's deviation from a formal standard will not automatically result in liability. Liability will result only if the standard in fact conforms to prevailing custom.

The former point can be taken as an assurance that at least from a legal perspective, professionally devised standards will not inhibit further scientific and technologic developments. Each such development will operate as a refinement or qualification of the norm stated in the formal standard. The task for those charged with developing evidence in a legal proceeding will be not only to show the formal standard but also to establish the extent to which it has been qualified in practice.

Goal of Standard Setting

It should also be recognized that standard setting undertaken by a profession often has a different goal from merely codifying or restating existing levels of practice. Indeed, standard setting often is and should be aspirational. That is, the professional pronouncements may seek to advance the state of practice to a level higher than is reflected by the existing norm. Thus, the formally stated standards may seek to quicken the acceptance of new techniques. Or the standards may incorporate respected judgments about which of two or more competing schools of treatment is to be preferred.

Such aspirational standards will not increase the practitioner's exposure to liability if the pertinent legal rules are properly brought to bear. The aspirational character of a rule would itself be a topic for examination through appropriate evidence. The essence of the proof would be that custom had not yet moved to the position of embracing the suggested measure.

To illustrate the point, we might return to the earlier example of the asymptomatic patient with coronary artery disease who is approved for participation in a competitive YMCA basketball league. Recall that we posited that medical opinion was somewhat divided over the question of whether a physician should recommend against participation in these circumstances. However, let us point further that even before the adoption of a formal standard, most practitioners in fact cautioned against strenuous activity in these cir-

cumstances. The point to be made in the present context is that the adoption of a formal standard incorporating the majority position would not automatically invalidate the views of those who had been more permissive in allowing competitive activity by their patients. It is quite conceivable that in some regions of the country the array of expert witnesses supporting an expansive view on participation by patients with coronary artery disease would be sufficiently impressive to support a legal finding that the stated standard was not controlling.

Impact of Formal Standards

Some readers may feel a bit uneasy with one implication of the above analysis. Physicians are not alone in suspecting that the law often drifts in a sea of indeterminancy. The question arises: are the preceding paragraphs to be taken to mean that formal standards have no meaning beyond the separate proof that establishes their relation to existing practice? And if one must show the state of existing practice in any case, what have the standards added? In short, do formal standards really make any difference?

Readers should be assured that from the perspective of the law, formal standards have a significant impact, even though their pertinency is always subject to separate verification. For one thing, formal standards can greatly foreshorten the search for prevailing custom and thus save the energies of courts and litigants. Standards devised by an authoritative group only require modest evidence to establish that they reflect prevailing custom. Of perhaps even greater importance is the fact that formal standards have the effect of significantly narrowing the range of potential inquiry. Where there is no formal standard for the medical procedure in question, the law-trained participants in a legal controversy will be given wide discretion in selecting their offers to proof. Misunderstandings and omissions can have a significant effect on the ultimate outcome. By contrast, with a formal standard, the inquiry into custom does not begin at point zero. Rather, the standard itself establishes an elevated baseline, and the function of other proof is to examine its reflection of actual custom. Deviations between the standard and custom will often be of modest proportion.

A Procedural Concern:
The Wisdom of Updating

The effectiveness of any standard will eventually decrease over time. Increased experience and improved technology will qualify what was formerly the accepted prevailing wisdom. Standards reflecting that wisdom will thus become dated. At some point in this natural aging process, the standards will drop into legal obscurity.

For the reasons given previously for preferring formal over informal standards, it is appropriate for organizations, conferences, and authors of papers and textbooks to consider providing for periodic updating of their recommendations. Such reevaluations are necessary to ensure the currency, and thus the authority, of the standards. Moreover, such periodic review will serve to minimize the extent to which legal strategy and attorney resourcefulness influence liability results.

References and Notes

1. Others have examined this relation from perspectives somewhat different from that presented here. *See* Chapman C, Physicians, Law and Ethics (1984); Havighurst, Decentralizing decision making: private contract versus professional norm. In: Meyer J, ed, Market Reforms in Health Care – Current Issues. New Directions, Strategic Decisions, 22 (1983); McCord, The care required of medical practitioners, 12, Vand L Rev 549 (1959); Pearson, The role of custom in medical malpractice cases, 51, Ind L J 528 (1976).

2. Shilkret v Annapolis Emergency Hosp. Ass'n, 276 Md. 1987, 200, 349 A. 2d 245, 253 (1975). *See also* Waltz J. Inhau F. Medical Jurisprudence, 42 (1971).

3. Such a standard is close to that which would be used in a compensation system premised on strict liability. *See* Ref. 12 and accompanying text.

4. *See* Christie G. Cases and Materials on the Law of Torts 189-93 (1983). The standard used in these other negligence settings is one of reasonableness: did the defendant act reasonably under the circumstance? It is expected that the defendant will not expose the plaintiff to a risk of harm that could be prevented by prudent action.

5. Some suggest that the subject matter of medical negligence cases involves a level of complexity that is not likely to be understood by a lay jury and thus a rule is needed that defers to the judgment of the profession itself. This cannot be the true explanation, however. In nonmedical cases, juries are frequently expected to decide questions of magnitude of complexity well beyond that found in most medically related proceedings. Professor Richard N. Pearson points out, for example, that our legal system assumes that a jury would be competent to determine the reliability of neutron activation analysis. *See* Pearson. The role of custom in medical malpractice cases, 51, Ind L J 528, 535 n.44 (1976), *citing* United States v. Stifel, 433F.2d 431 (6th Cir. 1970), *cert. denied*, 401 U.S. 994 (1971).

6. *See* Chapman C. Physicians, Law and Ethics, 60-63 (1984).

7. Interestingly, even some very modern proposals on cost containment continue the premise of self-governance. *See* Havighurst and Blumstein, Coping with quality/cost tradeoffs in medical care: the role of PSRO's, 70, Nw L Rev 6 (1975).

8. While the internalized nature of the medical liability standard is reasonably clear, not all aspects of the legal test are free from controversy. A debate over whether the test is to use a national norm or the medical customs of the local community has continued for years. The issue seems to have received more attention than it deserves in an age of rapid communication. While the national standard appears to be gaining general acceptance, the evolutionary process has been slow and is not complete. *See* Christie G. Cases and Materials on the Law of Torts 194-202 (1983); Waltz J, Inhau F. Medical Jurisprudence 64-65 (1971); McCord, The care required of medical practitioners, 12, Vand L Rev 549, 569-75 (1959); Note, An evaluation of changes in the medical standard of care, 23, Vand L Rev 729 (1976).

9. *See* Helling v. Carey, 83 Wash.2d 514, 519 P.2d 981 (1974). The Washington legislature subsequently attempted to reverse the substantive rule of *Helling* by statute. *See* Wash Rev Code 4.24.290 (1975).

10. *See* Pearson. The role of custom in medical malpractice cases, 51, Ind L J 528, 552-57 (1976).

11. *See* Gregory. Trespass to negligence to absolute liability, 37, Va L Rev 359 (1951); Havighurst. 'Medical adversity insurance' – has its time come? Duke L J 1233 (1975).

12. At least one commentator writing from a medical perspective manifests some receptivity to the no-fault notion. *See* Chapman C. Physicians, Law and Ethics, 128-29 (1984). For criticisms of this alternative, *see* Calabresi, The problem of malpractice – trying to round out the circle. In: Rottenberg S, ed. The Economics of Medical Malpractice 239 (1978); Epstein, Medical Malpractice: Its Cause and Cure, In: Rottenberg S, ed. The Economics of Medical Malpractice 257 (1978); Havighurst, 'Medical adversity insurance' – has its time come? Duke L J 1233 (1975).

13. Yet another criticism of the traditional liability rule can be found in Havighurst, Decentralizing decision making: private contract versus professional norm. In: Meyer J, ed. Market Reforms in Health Care – Current Issues, New Directions, Strategic Decisions 22 (1983). Professor Havighurst suggests that especially in an era of third party payors, a rule that wholly defers to the profession's definition of the standard of care may result in excessive procedures with limited or uncertain marginal utility. Total medical costs to society will increase significantly and prompt a misallocation of resources.

14. *See also* Calabresi, The problem of malpractice – trying to round out the circle. In: Rottenberg S, ed. The Economics of Medical Malpractice 239 (1978); Havighurst, Decentralizing decision making: private contract versus professional norm. In: Meyer J, ed. Market Reforms in Health Care – Current Issues, New Directions, Strategic Decisions 22 (1983); Havighurst, 'Medical adversity insurance' – has its time come? Duke L J 1233 (1975); Schwartz W, Konesar N. Doctors, Damage, and Deterrence: An Economic View of Malpractice (1978).

15. For a collection of cases on the evidentiary treatment of safety codes and other indicia of custom, *see* Feld, Admissibility in Evidence, on Issue of Negligence, of Codes or Standards of Safety Issued or Sponsored by Governmental Body or by Voluntary Association, 58 ALR3d 148 (1974).

16. There are some settings in which courts are not particularly receptive to a plaintiff's use of a safety code to establish negligence. *See* Ref. 15. It appears, though, that this judicial reticence is fading generally and that within the medical profession specifically, both precedent and policy considerations favor the introduction of professionally devised standards. *See* Darling v. Charleston Community Mem. Hosp., 33 Ill.2d 326, 211 N.E.2d 253, *cert. denied,* 383 U.S. 946 (1965); Cornfeldt v. Tongen, 262 N.W. 2d 684 (Minn. 1977); Stone v. Proctor, 259 N.C. 633, 131 S.E.2d 297 (1963). The various medical specialists have claimed a self-regulatory role for themselves, and practitioners have traditionally looked to their governing groups, for guidance on issues relating to standards of care. Moreover, the diversity of sources of scientific and medical information on treatment techniques requires coordination and assimilation. Professionally devised standards frequently fulfill that role.

17. *See* Darling v. Charleston Community Mem. Hosp., 33 Ill.2d 326, 211 N.E.2d 253, *cert. denied,* 383 U.S. 946 (1965); Cornfeldt v. Tongen, 262 N.W. 2d 684 (Minn. 1977).

APPENDIX 1

MEDICAL EXAMINATION OF SPORT SCUBA DIVERS

SECTION III: COMMON MEDICAL AND SURGICAL CONSIDERATIONS

A. Cardiology

A major concern of diving medicine is to protect those who have medical conditions which could result in increased risk of injury or death. Diminished capacity for aerobic exercise, whether due to poor physical conditioning or disease, could place the diver at increased risk. The spectrum of diminished capacity extends from easy fatigue to exhaustion with sudden loss of consciousness or sudden death as the extreme. Certain cardiovascular conditions can produce sudden incapacitation without warning and if the event occurs while the person is underwater, drowning or pulmonary barotrauma may ensue. A diver with a serious cardiovascular disorder may argue that even sudden death underwater is a risk they are willing to take and that the decision is a personal one. This "decision" does not take into account the hazard they would represent to buddy divers who may also drown in rescue attempts.

In medical decisions on fitness to dive, the physician must consider not only the risk of sudden incapacitation but also the known effects of submersion, temperature, exercise and emotion on cardiovascular function.

The neutrally buoyant scuba diver experiences weightlessness. This is so akin to the zero gravity condition of spaceflight that it is used to allow astronaut candidates to simulate the weightlessness of spaceflight. Potentially adverse effects include diuresis, but weightlessness can be considered favorable in scuba diving. If no emergencies

occur, it is possible for a scuba diver to enjoy underwater activity with very little physiologic cost. We have referred to this as the "deceptively easy" problem of scuba diving because suddenly the diver can be faced with a requirement for vigorous exercise. A diver may need to be able to swim quickly to rescue a buddy diver, provide assistance to the surface and onto a boat or through the surf. Other unplanned environmental problems underwater such as unexpected changes in current, entanglement, threatening marine life or equipment malfunction may impose unexpected significant physiologic and psychologic demands. There must be adequate cardiovascular reserve to allow the diver to respond without either losing consciousness or becoming ineffective because of premature exhaustion.

The scuba diver may expose himself to thermal stress. Scuba diving is often done in tropical or subtropical waters. Long boat trips and donning gear in high temperatures may induce severe thermal stress with large loss of fluid through sweating resulting in dehydration. Significant heat loss can occur in water temperatures of even 72 to 75 degrees F. Skin vasconstriction, muscle shivering to generate heat and increased cardiac output to supply blood to shivering muscles are protective mechanisms to try to preserve core temperature.

A significant demand on the cardiovascular system can come from emotional factors underwater. Danger or perceived danger, even when there is none, can produce panic or near panic reactions with marked elevation in blood pressure and heart rates in excess of 180 per minute. Such events may lead to drowning in otherwise healthy individuals and in a person with heart disease may produce arrhythmias, myocardial infarction or sudden death.

• 1. Coronary Artery Disease (CAD) The growth of scuba diving since it began during the 1950's has produced a large population of divers over the age of 45 years for two reasons. First, those young divers who began diving in the 1950's continue to dive now in their fifth or sixth decade. Second, increasing numbers of people over age 45 are now

Reprinted with permission from "Medical Examination of Sport Scuba Divers"
Edited by Jefferson C. Davis, M.D.
Publisher, Medical Seminars, Inc., San Antonio, Texas

undertaking diving training for the first time. We applaud and want to encourage beginning or continued diving for both groups. If they possess a healthy cardiovascular system and have no other medical contraindications, there is no reason they cannot dive safely. However, some sobering facts require special attention. Despite the encouraging decline in the CAD death rate since 1968, mostly ascribed to preventive medicine and life-style changes, about 650,000 Americans die of CAD and an additional 2 million develop symptoms or signs of CAD each year. Acute myocardial infarction is the most common initial presentation of CAD in the population at large. In some of these patients a detailed history will reveal symptoms of chest discomfort over the preceding days, but these were disregarded by the patient for a variety of reasons. For the remainder of the patients, acute myocardial infarction is their only presenting complaint. The diagnosis of myocardial infarction, whether on the basis of history or abnormal ECG, must be considered a contraindication to diving.

Sudden cardiac death is the presenting symptom of CAD in 15-20% of patients and eventually is the mode of death in nearly 60% of all patients who die due to CAD, the mechanism being a malignant arrhythmia. Silent myocardial infarction, manifested by typical myocardial infarction electrocardiographic findings in the absence of a history of any signs or symptoms is also seen occasionally in the general population.

Despite significant advances in medical and surgical treatment, all authorities agree prevention is most important. We must be certain all divers know the major risk factors and the life-style changes needed to reduce risk of CAD. Cigarette smoking is probably the most potent risk factor. In the Framingham study, men who smoked over one pack of cigarettes per day had a 2.15 times risk of developing CAD compared to non-smokers. Further, discontinuing smoking has been shown to effect a significant reduction in the increased risk. The mechanisms by which smoking produces this increased risk are not fully understood but may be related to decreased high-density lipoprotein (HDL) cholesterol produced by smoking. For this and other reasons specific to diving, smoking is strongly discouraged among divers. The diver should also be advised that the

total cholesterol/HDL ratio can be improved by avoiding saturated fats, participation in a regular exercise program and by not smoking. Elevated blood pressure is a risk factor and must be monitored and maintained below a maximum of 140/90 for any age. Stress and so-called Type A behavior are difficult to quantitate because so often it is part of a life style which incorporates other risk factors. It is considered by some to be a valid risk factor. Diabetes mellitus is an established risk factor for CAD.

A family history of cardiovascular events before age 65 is considered a definite risk factor. While there is nothing the diver can do to affect this factor, it can serve notice that this is a person who must control all other risk factors carefully. The incidence and mortality rates of CAD are greater in men than in women of the same age groups. Obesity and gout are the final risk factors usually considered, hence body weight control and attention to diet are encouraged.

Considering all of this, we come to specific considerations of individual problems. Ideally, one would like to establish a baseline and periodic cardiovascular screening program for all divers which would provide laboratory determination of serum lipids, risk factor analysis, resting and exercise electrocardiography and exercise scintigraphy. This is not practical for sport scuba divers so the diving medicine physician should attempt to identify the high risk population for application of more extensive testing. A suggestion of Bove, et al, in the first edition of this book, was for scuba diving candidates over the age of 40, and poorly conditioned diving candidates under 40, to have an exercise electrocardiogram. To participate in scuba diving, approximately 14 METS should be achieved. In the presence of an abnormal exercise ECG, such a candidate may be tested with exercise ECG with thallium scintigraphy and, if possible, coronary angiography. Exercise scintigraphy, using Thallium-201 to clarify false positive exercise ECG's is of great value. Coronary angiography is the definitive test for CAD and is used if non-invasive testing fails to answer the question of whether significant coronary artery stenoses are present. The guidelines provided above may be considered for recommendation for diving in the asymptomatic individual.

Symptoms of angina pectoris, history or finding of myocardial infarction or arrhythmias due to CAD, represent contraindications to diving in our opinion. Today, we are presented with a growing population of people who are the product of improved understanding of risk factor reduction, coronary artery angioplasty and coronary artery bypass surgery (CAB) for treatment of known CAD. While firm data do not exist to accurately define the risk of coronary events at any given time after intervention for these people at present, we must assume that such a population will remain at increased risk of a subsequent event since atherosclerosis is a progressive disease. While it is estimated there is only a 2% per vessel yearly graft occlusion rate post-CAB, CAD distal to the graft remains and the unpredictable possibility of incapacitating future coronary events must await further follow-up. Again, the risk to the lives of other divers in the water with the afflicted individual must be considered in this decision.

Those exceptional individuals who undergo successful coronary angioplasty and coronary revascularization and those who recover from discrete, non-complicated myocardial infarctions, who have completed rehabilitation programs with life-style and risk-factor modification can be evaluated individually. Their return to diving would be only after the usual non-invasive testing procedures by their cardiologist to rule out myocardial ischemia. They must not require drugs which alter the cardiovascular response to exercise in diving and they must be counseled regarding the risk of drowning and risk to their diving buddies should a cardiac event occur underwater. They should be tested by their cardiologist on an annual basis thereafter and should maintain a high level of physical conditioning to avoid excess cardiovascular stress in diving. It is emphasized that these recommendations are for the exceptional individual for whom sport scuba diving is a central part of their life (e.g., semi-professional underwater photographer, etc.) We would not clear patients in this category to begin scuba training and would not approve diving for those with responsibility for other divers (e.g., scuba instructors, dive guides, divemasters, etc.) and of course, this entire set of guidelines applies only to sport scuba divers.

• **2. Hypertension** – While blood pressure values vary from hour to hour, and there are differences of opinion for upper limits of "normal," the most common opinions set limits at 140/90 for any age. In borderline cases, six blood pressure measurements over a three day period can provide an average value. Hydrostatic pressure of water has no effect on blood pressure which is always relative to ambient pressure. Factors in diving which can cause elevations are cold water, heavy exercise or emotionally disturbing events during the dive. Besides the effect of hypertension on longevity and as a risk factor for CAD, in diving we are especially concerned with the increased risk of sudden incapacitation as would occur in stroke or myocardial ischemia.

Evaluation of the hypertensive diving candidate should seek the etiology and end organ effects involving the eyes, heart or kidney. The next issue is to suspend diving while control of blood pressure is achieved. In those who control blood pressure by weight loss, salt restriction and exercise, diving can be safe. Further, we could clear those who are well-controlled by these measures plus diuretics. The potential need to increase the cardiac output in response to heavy exercise in a diving emergency requires that those taking beta blocking agents or other drugs which produce significant blockade of the nervous system demonstrate adequate performance on an exercise test to 14 METS. Those who have left ventricular hypertrophy, left ventricular dilation or left ventricular dysfunction should not be cleared for diving, even if blood pressure is controlled.

• **3. Electrocardiographic Abnormalities** –

a. Atrioventricular Block: Third degree or complete heart block and Mobitz Type II block should represent disqualifying findings. The problem leading to this recommendation is that the block may prevent response of the heart rate to exercise stress underwater. First degree and Mobitz Type I blocks may be cleared for diving if full cardiac evaluation, including exercise ECG, is normal.

b. Bundle Branch Block: U.S. Air Force studies found right bundle branch block (RBBB) in less than 6 of every 1,000 aviators under the age of 50 and left bundle branch block (LBBB) in less than 2 per 1,000 below that age. The Air Force requires complete evaluation including exercise thallium scintigraphy and coronary angiography in all with acquired LBBB since LBBB is commonly associated with CAD or myocardial disease. RBBB, however, is usually not associated with significant cardiac disease in healthy asymptomatic persons, and if a full cardiac evaluation, including treadmill exercise testing is normal, they may be cleared for sport diving.

c. Sinus Bradycardia: A search for the cause of the slow, 50/min heart rate should be pursued. A common cause at present is use of beta blocking drugs. Well-trained athletes should have bradycardia because of training, and this is a healthy response. The heart rate should increase appropriately with exercise, and if not, cardiac abnormalities should be sought. Abnormal resting or exercise heart rates in a non-conditioned individual should call for further studies. Resting bradycardia can be caused by drugs (beta blocker, digitalis), training and conduction system disease. Inadequate exercise heart rate response can occur from beta blockers, conduction defects, arrhythmias, and myocardial ischemia.

d. Wolf-Parkinson-White (WPW) Syndrome: The unpredictable episodes of atrial tachycardia associated with the short P-R interval, make WPW a disqualifying defect. An episode of tachycardia underwater could lead to unconsciousness and drowning. Although some subjects with ECG evidence of WPW are asymptomatic, only an electrophysiologic study can determine whether a risk of tachycardia is present.

e. Supraventricular Tachycardia (SVT): The concern here as in other cardiac disorders is the threat of sudden loss of consciousness during an episode of tachycardia. Experience has shown that episodes of SVT in otherwise healthy young people are associated with fatigue, alcohol, hunger, caffeine, and seldom recur if the precipitating causes are avoided. If those under age 35 have no syncope with the episode, no recurrence within a 6 month observation period and require no medications, they may be cleared to dive. Those over age 35 should be subjected to studies to rule out cardiac disease.

• **4. Valvular Heart Disease** – Without presenting details of each possible valvular disorder, some basic concerns and discussion of the more common questions will follow.

a. Mild Valvular Regurgitation:

(1) Mitral regurgitation. These patients may be cleared to dive if they are asymptomatic, left ventricular function is normal, there is no left ventricular hypertrophy and minimal left ventricular dilation on ECG and echocardiogram. There must be no evidence that mitral regurgitation is due to ruptured chordae tendinae, papillary muscle dysfunction, or left ventricular dysfunction.

(2) Aortic insufficiency. These patients may be cleared to dive if they are asymptomatic and the aortic insufficiency is hemodynamically insignificant. The ECG and echocardiogram must show no left ventricular hypertrophy, minimal left ventricular dilation, and no left ventricular dysfunction.

b. Any degree of aortic stenosis or mitral stenosis is considered disqualifying for diving since they impede forward flow. The cardiac output is impeded during exercise and pulmonary edema and/or syncope can ensue.

c. Mitral Valve Prolapse (MVP): Usually detected by auscultation of a midsystolic click which may be associated with a late systolic murmur, MVP is found in some 5% of males and 10-12% of females. The mitral valve leaflets are thinned and voluminous and one or both bulge back into the left atrium during ventricular systole. The definitive diagnosis is by echocardiography. Most people with MVP are asymptomatic, but chest pain, palpitations, fatigue, dyspnea or syncope can occur. Uncommon manifestations can be arrhythmias, stroke or endocarditis. Diving is permitted in patients with MVP only if they are totally asymptomatic: i.e., do not have chest pain, palpitations, arrhythmias, syncope, dyspnea and are not taking medications.

A recent report by Nishimura, et al identified the subset of MVP patients with echocardiographically demonstrable redundant mitral valve leaflets as being at significantly increased risk of sudden death, or cerebral embolic event. Such patients should be disqualified for diving.

• **5. Congenital Heart Disease** – Most individuals with severe congenital heart disease will never present for a diving physical examination. There are a few specific problems related to diving which have been seen in recent years.

ANY DEFECT WHICH ALLOWS A COM-

MUNICATION BETWEEN THE RIGHT AND LEFT CIRCULATIONS AT THE LEVEL OF THE HEART OR GREAT VESSELS SHOULD CAUSE DISQUALIFICATION. In decompression from dives which exceed safe limits, venous gas emboli are present in the right side of the circulation. Bubbles are swept back through the right ventricle to the pulmonary circulation and rather large bubble loads can be trapped in the pulmonary vascular bed and dissipated harmlessly. However, in septal defects, even when the net flow is left to right, there are bidirectional flow phases, and if these right sided bubbles are swept to the arterial blood, they have direct access to the arterial circulation and can produce severe central nervous system embolic phenomena.

Patients who have had successful repair of noncyanotic lesions, such as atrial septal defects, patent ductus arteriosus and ventricular septal defect, may be cleared for diving after evaluation by a cardiologist and by a pulmonary medicine specialist in view of the required thoracotomy.

• **6. Peripheral Vascular Disease** – Peripheral vascular disease of either arterial or venous systems of a degree to limit exercise tolerance is a contraindication to diving. Because of cold water, Reynaud's phenomenon is a unique disqualifying disorder.

• **7. Pacemakers** – In general, patients who require permanent pacemakers are disqualified for diving due to their underlying cardiac disease. The only possible exception to this may be the young individual with congenital third degree A-V block who has one of the new dual chamber, A-V sequential pacemakers that allow the sinus rate to increase within certain ranges with exercise. While some pacemakers have been tested in hyperbaric chambers and showed no change in performance or structural integrity under increased barometric pressure, such tests would be required before considering diving with new pacemakers. Also, the patient would need full evaluation by their cardiologist to evaluate their functional status and the pacemaker's ability to perform physiologically.

• **8. Hypertrophic Cardiomyopathy** – An absolute contraindication to diving.

B. Hematology

Unexplained anemia should be disqualifying for diving until studied and corrected. Polycythemia or leukemia and related disorders are disqualifying because of the risk of decompression sickness due to impaired tissue perfusion for gas uptake and elimination. Sickle cell disease and sickle cell trait represent significant concerns in altitude physiology and in commercial diving because of the risk of breathing hypoxic gas mixtures. In sport diving, with compressed air, it is generally agreed there is little risk of a hypoxic episode and scuba diving can be pursued by those with sickle cell trait if they have a normal hemoglobin level and no previous episodes of anemia. Those with sickle cell disease have a hemolytic anemia and are so prone to hemolytic crises during stressful conditions, diving is one of the many stresses they should avoid.

In diving, the only theoretical concern for those with sickle cell trait could be localized areas of tissue hypoxia during a decompression sickness insult with resulting stagnant blood flow. Thus, as with any sport diver, the candidate with sickle cell trait is advised to dive well within the limits of the decompression tables.

C. Pulmonary Medicine

The most dramatic and life-threatening medical emergencies in compressed gas diving are pulmonary overpressure accidents which result from generalized lung overinflation due to breathholding or pathological air trapping in part of the lung during ascents from as shallow as four feet of water. The dire consequences of introduction of high pressure pulmonary gas directly into the pulmonary capillary bed with direct access to the left side of the heart, from there to embolize the coronary or cerebral circulation, produces gas embolism (air embolism in sport scuba divers) with resultant immediate life-threatening incapacitation. The less common pneumothorax and less life-threatening pulmonary interstitial emphysema with mediastinal and subcutaneous emphysema are also seen. All efforts must be to use medical history, physical examination, radiology and pulmonary function tests for prevention of this serious complication. Diving instruction and psychological assessment of diving candidates are the best preventive measures for panic. The remaining challenge is to exclude those from diving who have pulmonary conditions which increase the risk of local air trapping during ascent from depth.

• 1. Bronchial Asthma – The diagnosis of bronchial asthma is usually made by clear cut history of episodic wheezing, dyspnea, cough and pulmonary function studies that demonstrate reversible airflow obstruction. Bronchospasm can be precipitated by a number of triggering factors: infection, inhalation of allergens and irritants (including cold dry air), exercise and strong emotions. Many of these are present in scuba diving: (a) scuba air is dry; (b) in cold water, scuba air can reach quite cold temperatures; (c) bursts of vigorous exercise can be needed in emergencies or in swimming against current; (d) aspiration of salt water can occur. In addition, emotional stress may occur in the event of equipment malfunction or real or imagined emergencies. If bronchospasm occurs while at depth, breathing compressed gas, the stage is set for trapped gas expansion during ascent and the disastrous pulmonary overpressure accident is almost inevitable.

The underlying physiologic mechanisms of bronchial asthma are still not fully understood. People with asthma have altered bronchial reactivity and subclinical bronchospasm may exist even when they are asymptomatic. With the above listed stresses, bronchospasm may intensify.

Asthma is most frequently seen in childhood. It is not uncommon for older children to become asymptomatic. However, the tendency for bronchial hyperactivity persists and a number of these patients will become symptomatic again in early adulthood. Other symptom complexes such as frequent bronchitis, recurrent coughing or bouts of wheezing can be suggestive of undiagnosed or asymptomatic asthma.

Exercise-induced asthma (EIA) is a clinical syndrome of acute, reversible and usually self-limiting airway obstruction which develops after strenuous exercise in patients with asthma or hay fever. The symptoms of wheezing, coughing and dyspnea usually start 5-10 minutes after exercise and peak at about 15 minutes post-exercise. This may last for 1-2 hours. The etiology of EIA involves complex neurophysiologic and biochemical events occurring in the lungs. McFadden, et al showed that drying of the airways with a subsequent loss of heat is the initial stimulus leading to an attack of EIA. Vigorous exercise while breathing cold, dry air intensifies the severity of EIA. Surface swimmers with EIA often have less problems than in other activities, presumably because of humid air breathing, but it must be re-emphasized that scuba air is dry. Because EIA occurs in otherwise healthy, usually athletic young people, we have seen increasing numbers applying for diving training. The frequency of EIA has been estimated as high as 90% of symptomatic asthmatics and there is a population of patients with normal pulmonary function studies and no symptoms of asthma unless they vigorously exercise. Patients with a history of severe allergic rhinitis or seasonal hay fever are also at risk to develop EIA. Patients who had asthma in the past and have been symptom-free for years may develop EIA. The safest way to make the diagnosis is by exercise testing or eucapnic hyperventilation with cold air. Baseline spirometry would typically show an FEV_1 of 75-100% of normal. This may increase briefly during the first 5-10 minutes of exercise, then significantly decrease, lasting for 1-2 hours. While EIA is prevented by such Beta-2 selective bronchodilators as metaproterenol, albuterol, fenoterol or sodium cromolyn, one must be concerned about the side effects of these drugs and that an asymptomatic EIA patient might fail to use them before a dive. Some of the most significant trigger mechanisms for EIA exist on every scuba dive. The consequences of a pulmonary overpressure accident may be life-threatening cerebral gas embolism. For all these reasons, exercise-induced asthma is considered an absolute disqualification for scuba diving.

Any patient with currently active bronchial asthma should be strictly forbidden to dive. Any patient with a history of childhood asthma, symptoms suggestive of asthma within the past year, suspicion of exercise or cold air-induced asthma should be referred to a pulmonary medicine specialist for evaluation to include challenge testing. With the increasing awareness of altered bronchial reactivity, which may become manifest only at depth breathing cold, dry scuba air, the physician should seriously question a history that the candidate "outgrew childhood asthma."

ONE CAUTIOUS REMINDER MUST BE REPEATED: THE GREATEST VOLUME CHANGES IN THE LUNGS OF ANY DIVER WITH AIR TRAPPING OCCUR AT SHALLOW DEPTHS. NEVER CLEAR A PERSON FOR "SHALLOW DIVING ONLY." THE SHALLOWEST FOUR FEET, EVEN IN A SWIMMING POOL IS THE MOST DANGEROUS DEPTH FOR COMPRESSED GAS DIVING FOR A PATIENT WITH A BRONCHOSPASTIC DISORDER.

• **2. Pneumothorax** – A history of spontaneous pneumothorax is considered disqualifying for diving because of the known high risk of recurrence even at ground level without pressure changes encountered in diving. The exact cause or site of air leak is often undetectable, but it is estimated that the most common cause in a healthy 20-40 year old population is rupture of an undetectable apical emphysematous bleb. Considering the dire consequences of a tension pneumothorax during ascent if pneumothorax occurs underwater, the high incidence of recurrence makes even one spontaneous pneumothorax a contraindication to compressed gas diving. In some series, nearly 50% of patients with spontaneous pneumothorax will suffer recurrence. Procedures such as chemical pleurodesis or surgical pleurectomy have been used to try to avoid recurrent pneumothorax. In an Air Force study, Hopkirk, et al followed up 152 aviators who had pleurodesis with 10% silver nitrate. Seven percent suffered recurrences on the same side and 14% had subsequent pneumothorax on the opposite side. Pleurectomy is considered curative for the operated side, but since 14% suffered opposite side pneumothorax after pleurodesis on one side, there is still significant risk. Lobectomy has been used for recurrent pneumothorax but opposite side disease question would still remain.

There are differences of opinion as to whether or not to recommend diving to a candidate who has suffered traumatic hemopneumothorax or has had a thoracotomy for other reasons. The conservative approach is to be concerned about scarring, differential lung stiffness which could cause shearing with pressure imbalance and local air trapping. Our recommendation is that each case be individually evaluated by the thoracic surgeon, pulmonary medicine specialist and diving medicine physician.

• **3. Pulmonary Infection** – Any active pulmonary infection – tuberculosis, mycotic infections, bronchitis, pneumonitis or sequelae such as fibrosis, cavitation, emphysema or calcific bodies in bronchi are disqualifying.

• **4. Chest X-Ray** – We are aware of studies showing low yields of screening chest x-rays in a healthy population. However, we recommend a baseline chest x-ray for all diving candidates.

• **5. Cigarette Smoking** – Cigarette smoking is deleterious in many ways:
   a. Decreased cardiopulmonary efficiency.
   b. Increased risk of mucous plugs and bronchospasm-induced local air trapping.
   c. Nasal irritation which interferes with ear and sinus clearing.
   d. Increased risk of coronary artery disease.
   Divers should be strongly urged to avoid cigarette smoking.

APPENDIX 2

The Official

Position Papers

of the

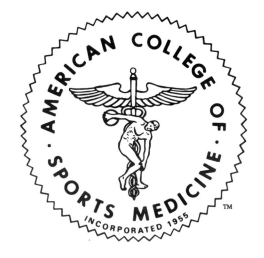

AMERICAN COLLEGE of SPORTS MEDICINE ™

Sixth Edition, First Printing

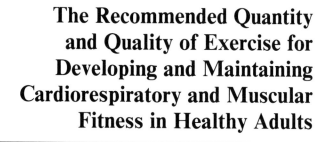

The Recommended Quantity and Quality of Exercise for Developing and Maintaining Cardiorespiratory and Muscular Fitness in Healthy Adults

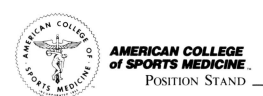

AMERICAN COLLEGE of SPORTS MEDICINE™
POSITION STAND

This Position Stand replaces the 1978 ACSM position paper, "The Recommended Quantity and Quality of Exercise for Developing and Maintaining Fitness in Healthy Adults."

Increasing numbers of persons are becoming involved in endurance training and other forms of physical activity, and, thus, the need for guidelines for exercise prescription is apparent. Based on the existing evidence concerning exercise prescription for healthy adults and the need for guidelines, the American College of Sports Medicine (ACSM) makes the following recommendations for the quantity and quality of training for developing and maintaining cardiorespiratory fitness, body composition, and muscular strength and endurance in the healthy adult:

1. Frequency of training: 3–5 d·wk⁻¹.

2. Intensity of training: 60–90% of maximum heart rate (HR_{max}), or 50–85% of maximum oxygen uptake ($\dot{V}O_{2max}$) or HR_{max} reserve.[1]

3. Duration of training: 20–60 min of continuous aerobic activity. Duration is dependent on the intensity of the activity; thus, lower intensity activity should be conducted over a longer period of time. Because of the importance of "total fitness" and the fact that it is more readily attained in longer duration programs, and because of the potential hazards and compliance problems associated with high intensity activity, lower to moderate intensity activity of longer duration is recommended for the nonathletic adult.

4. Mode of activity: any activity that uses large muscle groups, can be maintained continuously, and is rhythmical and aerobic in nature, e.g., walking-hiking, running-jogging, cycling-bicycling, cross-country skiing, dancing, rope skipping, rowing, stair climbing, swimming, skating, and various endurance game activities.

5. Resistance training: Strength training of a moderate intensity, sufficient to develop and maintain fat-free

---

[1] Maximum heart rate reserve is calculated from the difference between resting and maximum heart rate. To estimate training intensity, a percentage of this value is added to the resting heart rate and is expressed as a percentage of HR_{max} reserve (85).

weight (FFW), should be an integral part of an adult fitness program. One set of 8–12 repetitions of eight to ten exercises that condition the major muscle groups at least 2 d·wk⁻¹ is the recommended minimum.

RATIONALE AND RESEARCH BACKGROUND

Introduction

The questions "How much exercise is enough," and "What type of exercise is best for developing and maintaining fitness?" are frequently asked. It is recognized that the term "physical fitness" is composed of a variety of characteristics included in the broad categories of cardiovascular-respiratory fitness, body composition, muscular strength and endurance, and flexibility. In this context fitness is defined as the ability to perform moderate to vigorous levels of physical activity without undue fatigue and the capability of maintaining such ability throughout life (167). It is also recognized that the adaptive response to training is complex and includes peripheral, central, structural, and functional factors (5,172). Although many such variables and their adaptive response to training have been documented, the lack of sufficient in-depth and comparative data relative to frequency, intensity, and duration of training makes them inadequate to use as comparative models. Thus, in respect to the above questions, fitness is limited mainly to changes in $\dot{V}O_{2max}$, muscular strength and endurance, and body composition, which includes total body mass, fat weight (FW), and FFW. Further, the rationale and research background used for this position stand will be divided into programs for cardiorespiratory fitness and weight control and programs for muscular strength and endurance.

Fitness versus health benefits of exercise. Since the original position statement was published in 1978, an important distinction has been made between physical activity as it relates to health versus fitness. It has been pointed out that the quantity and quality of exercise needed to attain health-related benefits may differ from what is recommended for fitness benefits. It is now clear that lower levels of physical activity than recommended by this position statement may reduce the risk for certain chronic degenerative diseases and yet may not be of sufficient quantity or quality to improve $\dot{V}O_{2max}$ (71,72,98,167). ACSM recognizes the potential health benefits of regular exercise performed more frequently and for a longer duration, but at lower intensities than prescribed in this position statement (13A,71,100,120,160). ACSM will address the issue concerning the proper amount of physical activity necessary to derive health benefits in another statement.

Need for standardization of procedures and reporting results. Despite an abundance of information available concerning the training of the human organism, the lack of standardization of testing protocols and procedures, of methodology in relation to training procedures and experimental design, and of a preciseness in the documentation and reporting of the quantity and quality of training prescribed make interpretation difficult (123,133,139,164,167). Interpretation and comparison of results are also dependent on the initial level of fitness (42,43,58,114,148,151,156), length of time of the training experiment (17,45,125,128,139, 145,150), and specificity of the testing and training (5,43,130,139,145A,172). For example, data from training studies using subjects with varied levels of $\dot{V}O_{2max}$, total body mass, and FW have found changes to occur in relation to their initial values (14,33,109, 112,113,148,151); i.e., the lower the initial $\dot{V}O_{2max}$ the larger the percentage of improvement found, and the higher the FW the greater the reduction. Also, data evaluating trainability with age, comparison of the different magnitudes and quantities of effort, and comparison of the trainability of men and women may have been influenced by the initial fitness levels.

In view of the fact that improvement in the fitness variables discussed in this position statement continues over many months of training (27,86,139,145,150), it is reasonable to believe that short-term studies conducted over a few weeks have certain limitations. Middle-aged sedentary and older participants may take several weeks to adapt to the initial rigors of training, and thus need a longer adaptation period to get the full benefit from a program. For example, Seals et al. (150) exercise trained 60–69-yr-olds for 12 months. Their subjects showed a 12% improvement in $\dot{V}O_{2max}$ after 6 months of moderate intensity walking training. A further 18% increase in $\dot{V}O_{2max}$ occurred during the next 6 months of training when jogging was introduced. How long a training experiment should be conducted is difficult to determine, but 15–20 wk may be a good minimum standard. Although it is difficult to control exercise training experiments for more than 1 yr, there is a need to study this effect. As stated earlier, lower

doses of exercise may improve $\dot{V}O_{2max}$ and control or maintain body composition, but at a slower rate.

Although most of the information concerning training described in this position statement has been conducted on men, the available evidence indicates that women tend to adapt to endurance training in the same manner as men (19,38,46,47,49,62,65,68,90,92,122, 166).

Exercise Prescription for Cardiorespiratory Fitness and Weight Control

Exercise prescription is based upon the frequency, intensity, and duration of training, the mode of activity (aerobic in nature, e.g., listed under No. 4 above), and the initial level of fitness. In evaluating these factors, the following observations have been derived from studies conducted for up to 6–12 months with endurance training programs.

Improvement in $\dot{V}O_{2max}$ is directly related to frequency (3,6,50,75–77,125,126,152,154,164), intensity (3,6,26,29,58,61,75–77,80,85,93,118,152,164), and duration (3,29,60,61,70,75–77,101,109,118,152,162, 164,168) of training. Depending upon the quantity and quality of training, improvement in $\dot{V}O_{2max}$ ranges from 5 to 30% (8,29,30,48,59,61,65,67,69,75–77,82,84,96, 99,101,102,111,115,119,123,127,139,141,143,149, 150,152,153,158,164,168,173). These studies show that a minimum increase in $\dot{V}O_{2max}$ of 15% is generally attained in programs that meet the above stated guidelines. Although changes in $\dot{V}O_{2max}$ greater than 30% have been shown, they are usually associated with large total body mass and FW loss, in cardiac patients, or in persons with a very low initial level of fitness. Also, as a result of leg fatigue or a lack of motivation, persons with low initial fitness may have spuriously low initial $\dot{V}O_{2max}$ values. Klissouras (94A) and Bouchard (16A) have shown that human variation in the trainability of $\dot{V}O_{2max}$ is important and related to current phenotype level. That is, there is a genetically determined pretraining status of the trait and capacity to adapt to physical training. Thus, physiological results should be interpreted with respect to both genetic variation and the quality and quantity of training performed.

Intensity-duration. Intensity and duration of training are interrelated, with total amount of work accomplished being an important factor in improvement in fitness (12,20,27,48,90,92,123,127,128,136,149,151,164). Although more comprehensive inquiry is necessary, present evidence suggests that, when exercise is performed above the minimum intensity threshold, the total amount of work accomplished is an important factor in fitness development (19,27,126,127,149,151) and maintenance (134). That is, improvement will be similar for activities performed at a lower intensity-longer duration compared to higher intensity-shorter duration if the total energy costs of the activities are equal. Higher intensity exercise is associated with greater cardiovascular risk (156A), orthopedic injury (124,139) and lower compliance to training than lower intensity exercise (36,105,124,146). Therefore, programs emphasizing low to moderate intensity training with longer duration are recommended for most adults.

The minimal training intensity threshold for improvement in $\dot{V}O_{2max}$ is approximately 60% of the HR_{max} (50% of $\dot{V}O_{2max}$ or HR_{max} reserve) (80,85). The 50% of HR_{max} reserve represents a heart rate of approximately 130–135 beats·min^{-1} for young persons. As a result of the age-related change in maximum heart rate, the absolute heart rate to achieve this threshold is inversely related to age and can be as low as 105–115 beats·min^{-1} for older persons (35,65,150). Patients who are taking beta-adrenergic blocking drugs may have significantly lower heart rate values (171). Initial level of fitness is another important consideration in prescribing exercise (26,90,104,148,151). The person with a low fitness level can achieve a significant training effect with a sustained training heart rate as low as 40–50% of HR_{max} reserve, while persons with higher fitness levels require a higher training stimulus (35,58,152,164).

Classification of exercise intensity. The classification of exercise intensity and its standardization for exercise prescription based on a 20–60 min training session has been confusing, misinterpreted, and often taken out of context. The most quoted exercise classification system is based on the energy expenditure (kcal·min^{-1}·kg^{-1}) of industrial tasks (40,89). The original data for this classification system were published by Christensen (24) in 1953 and were based on the energy expenditure of working in the steel mill for an 8-h day. The classification of industrial and leisure-time tasks by using absolute values of energy expenditure have been valuable for use in the occupational and nutritional setting. Although this classification system has broad application in medicine and, in particular, making recommendations for weight control and job placement, it has little or no meaning for preventive and rehabilitation exercise training programs. To extrapolate absolute values of energy expenditure for completing an industrial task based on an 8-h work day to 20–60 min regimens of exercise training does not make sense. For example, walking and jogging/running can be accomplished at a wide range of speeds; thus, the relative intensity becomes important under these conditions. Because the endurance training regimens recommended by ACSM for nonathletic adults are geared for 60 min or less of physical activity, the system of classification of exercise training intensity shown in Table 1 is recommended (139). The use of a realistic time period for training and an individual's relative exercise intensity makes this system amenable to young,

TABLE 1. Classification of intensity of exercise based on 20–60 min of endurance training.

| Relative Intensity (%) | | Rating of Perceived Exertion | Classification of Intensity |
HR$_{max}$*	$\dot{V}O_{2max}$* or HR$_{max}$ reserve		
<35%	<30%	<10	Very light
35–59%	30–49%	10–11	Light
60–79%	50–74%	12–13	Moderate (somewhat hard)
80–89%	75–84%	14–16	Heavy
≥90%	≥85%	>16	Very heavy

Table from Pollock, M. L. and J. H. Wilmore. *Exercise in Health and Disease: Evaluation and Prescription for Prevention and Rehabilitation*, 2nd Ed. Philadelphia: W.B. Saunders, 1990. Published with permission.
* HR$_{max}$ = maximum heart rate; $\dot{V}O_{2max}$ = maximum oxygen uptake.

middle-aged, and elderly participants, as well as patients with a limited exercise capacity (3,137,139).

Table 1 also describes the relationship between relative intensity based on percent HR_{max}, percentage of HR_{max} reserve or percentage of $\dot{V}O_{2max}$, and the rating of perceived exertion (RPE) (15,16,137). The use of heart rate as an estimate of intensity of training is the common standard (3,139).

The use of RPE has become a valid tool in the monitoring of intensity in exercise training programs (11,37,137,139). It is generally considered an adjunct to heart rate in monitoring relative exercise intensity, but once the relationship between heart rate and RPE is known, RPE can be used in place of heart rate (23,139). This would not be the case in certain patient populations where a more precise knowledge of heart rate may be critical to the safety of the program.

Frequency. The amount of improvement in $\dot{V}O_{2max}$ tends to plateau when frequency of training is increased above 3 d·wk^{-1} (50,123,139). The value of the added improvement found with training more than 5 d·wk^{-1} is small to not apparent in regard to improvement in $\dot{V}O_{2max}$ (75–77,106,123). Training of less than 2 d·wk^{-1} does not generally show a meaningful change in $\dot{V}O_{2max}$ (29,50,118,123,152,164).

Mode. If frequency, intensity, and duration of training are similar (total kcal expenditure), the training adaptations appear to be independent of the mode of aerobic activity (101A,118,130). Therefore, a variety of endurance activities, e.g., those listed above, may be used to derive the same training effect.

Endurance activities that require running and jumping are considered high impact types of activity and generally cause significantly more debilitating injuries to beginning as well as long-term exercisers than do low impact and non-weight bearing type activities (13,93, 117,124,127,135,140,142). This is particularly evident in the elderly (139). Beginning joggers have increased foot, leg, and knee injuries when training is performed more than 3 d·wk^{-1} and longer than 30 min duration per exercise session (135). High intensity interval training (run-walk) compared to continuous jogging training was also associated with a higher incidence of injury (124,136). Thus, caution should be taken when recommending the type of activity and exercise prescription for the beginning exerciser. Orthopedic injuries as related to overuse increase linearly in runners/joggers when performing these activities (13,140). Thus, there is a need for more inquiry into the effect that different types of activities and the quantity and quality of training has on injuries over short-term and long-term participation.

An activity such as weight training should not be considered as a means of training for developing $\dot{V}O_{2max}$, but it has significant value for increasing muscular strength and endurance and FFW (32,54,107, 110,165). Studies evaluating circuit weight training (weight training conducted almost continuously with moderate weights, using 10–15 repetitions per exercise session with 15–30 s rest between bouts of activity) show an average improvement in $\dot{V}O_{2max}$ of 6% (1,51–54,83,94,108,170). Thus, circuit weight training is not recommended as the only activity used in exercise programs for developing $\dot{V}O_{2max}$.

Age. Age in itself does not appear to be a deterrent to endurance training. Although some earlier studies showed a lower training effect with middle-aged or elderly participants (9,34,79,157,168), more recent studies show the relative change in $\dot{V}O_{2max}$ to be similar to younger age groups (7,8,65,132,150,161,163). Although more investigation is necessary concerning the rate of improvement in $\dot{V}O_{2max}$ with training at various ages, at present it appears that elderly participants need longer periods of time to adapt (34,132,150). Earlier studies showing moderate to no improvement in $\dot{V}O_{2max}$ were conducted over a short time span (9), or exercise was conducted at a moderate to low intensity (34), thus making the interpretation of the results difficult.

Although $\dot{V}O_{2max}$ decreases with age and total body mass and FW increase with age, evidence suggests that this trend can be altered with endurance training (22,27,86–88,139). A 9% reduction in $\dot{V}O_{2max}$ per decade for sedentary adults after age 25 has been shown (31,73), but for active individuals the reduction may be less than 5% per decade (21,31,39,73). Ten or more yr follow-up studies where participants continued training at a similar level showed maintenance of cardiorespiratory fitness (4,87,88,138). A cross-sectional study of older competitive runners showed progressively lower values in $\dot{V}O_{2max}$ from the fourth to seventh decades of life, but also showed less training in the older groups (129). More recent 10-yr follow-up data on these same athletes (50–82 yr of age) showed $\dot{V}O_{2max}$ to be unchanged when training quantity and quality remained unchanged (138). Thus, lifestyle plays a significant role in the maintenance of fitness. More inquiry into the relationship of long-term training (quantity and qual-

ity), for both competitors and noncompetitors, and physiological function with increasing age is necessary before more definitive statements can be made.

Maintenance of training effect. In order to maintain the training effect, exercise must be continued on a regular basis (18,25,28,47,97,111,144,147). A significant reduction in cardiorespiratory fitness occurs after 2 wk of detraining (25,144), with participants returning to near pretraining levels of fitness after 10 wk (47) to 8 months of detraining (97). A loss of 50% of their initial improvement in $\dot{V}O_{2max}$ has been shown after 4–12 wk of detraining (47,91,144). Those individuals who have undergone years of continuous training maintain some benefits for longer periods of detraining than subjects from short-term training studies (25). While stopping training shows dramatic reductions in $\dot{V}O_{2max}$, reduced training shows modest to no reductions for periods of 5–15 wk (18,75–77,144). Hickson et al., in a series of experiments where frequency (75), duration (76), or intensity (77) of training were manipulated, found that, if intensity of training remained unchanged, $\dot{V}O_{2max}$ was maintained for up to 15 wk when frequency and duration of training were reduced by as much as $^2/_3$. When frequency and duration of training remained constant and intensity of training was reduced by $^1/_3$ or $^2/_3$, $\dot{V}O_{2max}$ was significantly reduced. Similar findings were found in regards to reduced strength training exercise. When strength training exercise was reduced from 3 or 2 $d \cdot wk^{-1}$ to at least 1 $d \cdot wk^{-1}$, strength was maintained for 12 wk of reduced training (62). Thus, it appears that missing an exercise session periodically or reducing training for up to 15 wk will not adversely effect $\dot{V}O_{2max}$ or muscular strength and endurance as long as training intensity is maintained.

Even though many new studies have given added insight into the proper amount of exercise, investigation is necessary to evaluate the rate of increase and decrease of fitness when varying training loads and reduction in training in relation to level of fitness, age, and length of time in training. Also, more information is needed to better identify the minimal level of exercise necessary to maintain fitness.

Weight control and body composition. Although there is variability in human response to body composition change with exercise, total body mass and FW are generally reduced with endurance training programs (133,139,171A), while FFW remains constant (123,133,139,169) or increases slightly (116,174). For example, Wilmore (171A) reported the results of 32 studies that met the criteria for developing cardiorespiratory fitness that are outlined in this position stand and found an average loss in total body mass of 1.5 kg and percent fat of 2.2%. Weight loss programs using dietary manipulation that result in a more dramatic decrease in total body mass show reductions in both FW and FFW (2,78,174). When these programs are conducted in conjunction with exercise training, FFW loss is more modest than in programs using diet alone (78,121). Programs that are conducted at least 3 d· wk^{-1} (123,125,126,128,169), of at least 20 min duration (109,123,169), and of sufficient intensity to expend approximately 300 kcal per exercise session (75 kg person)[2] are suggested as a threshold level for total body mass and FW loss (27,64,77,123,133,139). An expenditure of 200 kcal per session has also been shown to be useful in weight reduction if the exercise frequency is at least 4 d·wk^{-1} (155). If the primary purpose of the training program is for weight loss, then regimens of greater frequency and duration of training and low to moderate intensity are recommended (2,139). Programs with less participation generally show little or no change in body composition (44,57,93,123,133,159, 162,169). Significant increases in $\dot{V}O_{2max}$ have been shown with 10–15 min of high intensity training (6,79,109,118,123,152,153); thus, if total body mass and FW reduction are not considerations, then shorter duration, higher intensity programs may be recommended for healthy individuals at low risk for cardiovascular disease and orthopedic injury.

Exercise Prescription for Muscular Strength and Endurance

The addition of resistance/strength training to the position statement results from the need for a well-rounded program that exercises all the major muscle groups of the body. Thus, the inclusion of resistance training in adult fitness programs should be effective in the development and maintenance of FFW. The effect of exercise training is specific to the area of the body being trained (5,43,145A,172). For example, training the legs will have little or no effect on the arms, shoulders, and trunk muscles. A 10-yr follow-up of master runners who continued their training regimen, but did no upper body exercise, showed maintenance of $\dot{V}O_{2max}$ and a 2-kg reduction in FFW (138). Their leg circumference remained unchanged, but arm circumference was significantly lower. These data indicate a loss of muscle mass in the untrained areas. Three of the athletes who practiced weight training exercise for the upper body and trunk muscles maintained their FFW. A comprehensive review by Sale (145A) carefully documents available information on specificity of training.

Specificity of training was further addressed by Graves et al. (63). Using a bilateral knee extension exercise, they trained four groups: group A, first ½ of the range of motion; group B, second ½ of the range of motion; group AB, full range of motion; and a control group that did not train. The results clearly showed that

the training result was specific to the range of motion trained, with group AB getting the best full range effect. Thus, resistance training should be performed through a full range of motion for maximum benefit (63,95).

Muscular strength and endurance are developed by the overload principle, i.e., by increasing more than normal the resistance to movement or frequency and duration of activity (32,41,43,74,145). Muscular strength is best developed by using heavy weights (that require maximum or nearly maximum tension development) with few repetitions, and muscular endurance is best developed by using lighter weights with a greater number of repetitions (10,41,43,145). To some extent, both muscular strength and endurance are developed under each condition, but each system favors a more specific type of development (43,145). Thus, to elicit improvement in both muscular strength and endurance, most experts recommend 8–12 repetitions per bout of exercise.

Any magnitude of overload will result in strength development, but higher intensity effort at or near maximal effort will give a significantly greater effect (43,74,101B,103,145,172). The intensity of resistance training can be manipulated by varying the weight load, repetitions, rest interval between exercises, and number of sets completed (43). Caution is advised for training that emphasizes lengthening (eccentric) contractions, compared to shortening (concentric) or isometric contractions, as the potential for skeletal muscle soreness and injury is accentuated (3A,84A).

Muscular strength and endurance can be developed by means of static (isometric) or dynamic (isotonic or isokinetic) exercises. Although each type of training has its favorable and weak points, for healthy adults, dynamic resistance exercises are recommended. Resistance training for the average participant should be rhythmical, performed at a moderate to slow speed, move through a full range of motion, and not impede normal forced breathing. Heavy resistance exercise can cause a dramatic acute increase in both systolic and diastolic blood pressure (100A,101C).

The expected improvement in strength from resistance training is difficult to assess because increases in strength are affected by the participants' initial level of strength and their potential for improvement (43,66,74,114,172). For example, Mueller and Rohmert (114) found increases in strength ranging from 2 to 9% per week depending on initial strength levels. Although the literature reflects a wide range of improvement in strength with resistance training programs, the average improvement for sedentary young and middle-aged men and women for up to 6 months of training is 25–30%. Fleck and Kraemer (43), in a review of 13 studies representing various forms of isotonic training, showed an average improvement in bench press strength of 23.3% when subjects were tested on the

---

[2] Haskell and Haskell et al. (71,72) have suggested the use of 4 kcal·kg^{-1} of body weight of energy expenditure per day for a minimum standard for use in exercise programs.

equipment with which they were trained and 16.5% when tested on special isotonic or isokinetic ergometers (six studies). Fleck and Kraemer (43) also reported an average increase in leg strength of 26.6% when subjects were tested with the equipment that they trained on (six studies) and 21.2% when tested with special isotonic or isokinetic ergometers (five studies). Results of improvement in strength resulting from isometric training have been of the same magnitude as found with isotonic training (17,43,62,63).

In light of the information reported above, the following guidelines for resistance training are recommended for the average healthy adult. A minimum of 8–10 exercises involving the major muscle groups should be performed a minimum of two times per week. A minimum of one set of 8–12 repetitions to near fatigue should be completed. These minimal standards for resistance training are based on two factors. First, the time it takes to complete a comprehensive, well-rounded exercise program is important. Programs lasting more than 60 min per session are associated with higher dropout rates (124). Second, although greater frequencies of training (17,43,56) and additional sets or combinations of sets and repetitions elicit larger strength gains (10,32,43,74,145,172), the magnitude of difference is usually small. For example, Braith et al. (17) compared training 2 d·wk^{-1} with 3 d·wk^{-1} for 18 wk. The subjects performed one set of 7–10 repetitions to fatigue. The 2 d·wk^{-1} group showed a 21% increase in strength compared to 28% in the 3 d·wk^{-1} group. In other words, 75% of what could be attained in a 3 d·wk^{-1} program was attained in 2 d·wk^{-1}. Also, the 21% improvement in strength found by the 2 d·wk^{-1} regimen is 70–80% of the improvement reported by other programs using additional frequencies of training and combinations of sets and repetitions (43). Graves et al. (62,63), Gettman et al. (55), Hurley et al. (83) and Braith et al. (17) found that programs using one set to fatigue showed a greater than 25% increase in strength. Although resistance training equipment may provide a better graduated and quantitative stimulus for overload than traditional calisthenic exercises, calisthenics and other resistance types of exercise can still be effective in improving and maintaining strength.

SUMMARY

The combination of frequency, intensity, and duration of chronic exercise has been found to be effective for producing a training effect. The interaction of these factors provide the overload stimulus. In general, the lower the stimulus the lower the training effect, and the greater the stimulus the greater the effect. As a result of specificity of training and the need for maintaining muscular strength and endurance, and flexibility of the major muscle groups, a well-rounded training program including resistance training and flexibility exercises is recommended. Although age in itself is not a limiting factor to exercise training, a more gradual approach in applying the prescription at older ages seems prudent. It has also been shown that endurance training of fewer than 2 d·wk^{-1}, at less than 50% of maximum oxygen uptake and for less than 10 min·d^{-1}, is inadequate for developing and maintaining fitness for healthy adults.

In the interpretation of this position statement, it must be recognized that the recommendations should be used in the context of participants' needs, goals, and initial abilities. In this regard, a sliding scale as to the amount of time allotted and intensity of effort should be carefully gauged for both the cardiorespiratory and muscular strength and endurance components of the program. An appropriate warm-up and cool-down, which would include flexibility exercises, is also recommended. The important factor is to design a program for the individual to provide the proper amount of physical activity to attain maximal benefit at the lowest risk. Emphasis should be placed on factors that result in permanent lifestyle change and encourage a lifetime of physical activity.

REFERENCES

1. Allen, T. E., R. J. Byrd, and D. P. Smith. Hemodynamic consequences of circuit weight training. *Res. Q.* 43:299–306, 1976.
2. American College of Sports Medicine. Proper and improper weight loss programs. *Med. Sci. Sports Exerc.* 15:ix–xiii, 1983.
3. American College of Sports Medicine. *Guidelines for Graded Exercise Testing and Exercise Prescription*, 3rd Ed. Philadelphia: Lea and Febiger, 1986.
3A. Armstrong, R. B. Mechanisms of exercise-induced delayed onset muscular soreness: a brief review. *Med. Sci. Sports Exerc.* 16:529–538, 1984.
4. Åstrand, P. O. Exercise physiology of the mature athlete. In: *Sports Medicine for the Mature Athlete*, J. R. Sutton and R. M. Brock (Eds.). Indianapolis, IN: Benchmark Press, Inc., 1986, pp. 3–16.
5. Åstrand, P. O. and K. Rodahl. *Textbook of Work Physiology*, 3rd Ed. New York: McGraw-Hill, 1986, pp. 412–485.
6. Atomi, Y., K. Ito, H. Iwasaski, and M. Miyashita. Effects of intensity and frequency of training on aerobic work capacity of young females. *J. Sports Med.* 18:3–9, 1978.
7. Badenhop, D. T., P. A. Cleary, S. F. Schaal, E. L. Fox, and R. L. Bartels. Physiological adjustments to higher- or lower-intensity exercise in elders. *Med. Sci. Sports Exerc.* 15:496–502, 1983.
8. Barry, A. J., J. W. Daly, E. D. R. Pruett, et al. The effects of physical conditioning on older individuals. I. Work capacity, circulatory-respiratory function, and work electrocardiogram. *J. Gerontol.* 21:182–191, 1966.
9. Benestad, A. M. Trainability of old men. *Acta Med. Scand.* 178:321–327, 1965.
10. Berger, R. A. Effect of varied weight training programs on strength. *Res. Q.* 33:168–181, 1962.

11. BIRK, T. J. and C. A. BIRK. Use of ratings of perceived exertion for exercise prescription. *Sports Med.* 4:1–8, 1987.

12. BLAIR, S. N., J. V. CHANDLER, D. B. ELLISOR, and J. LANGLEY. Improving physical fitness by exercise training programs. *South. Med. J.* 73:1594–1596, 1980.

13. BLAIR, S. N., H. W. KOHL, and N. N. GOODYEAR. Rates and risks for running and exercise injuries: studies in three populations. *Res. Q. Exerc. Sports* 58:221–228, 1987.

13A. BLAIR, S. N., H. W. KOHL, III, R. S. PAFFENBARGER, D. G. CLARK, K. H. COOPER, and L. H. GIBBONS. Physical fitness and all-cause mortality. A prospective study of healthy men and women. *J.A.M.A.* 262:2395–2401, 1989.

14. BOILEAU, R. A., E. R. BUSKIRK, D. H. HORSTMAN, J. MENDEZ, and W. NICHOLAS. Body composition changes in obese and lean men during physical conditioning. *Med. Sci. Sports* 3:183–189, 1971.

15. BORG, G. A. V. Psychophysical bases of perceived exertion. *Med. Sci. Sports Exerc.* 14:377–381, 1982.

16. BORG, G. and D. OTTOSON (Eds.). *The Perception of Exertion in Physical Work.* London, England: The MacMillan Press, Ltd., 1986, pp. 4–7.

16A. BOUCHARD, C. Gene-environment interaction in human adaptability. In: *The Academy Papers*, R. B. Malina and H. M. Eckert (Eds.). Champaign, IL: Human Kinetics Publishers, 1988, pp. 56–66.

17. BRAITH, R. W., J. E. GRAVES, M. L. POLLOCK, S. L. LEGGETT, D. M. CARPENTER, and A. B. COLVIN. Comparison of two versus three days per week of variable resistance training during 10 and 18 week programs. *Int. J. Sports Med.* 10:450–454, 1989.

18. BRYNTESON, P. and W. E. SINNING. The effects of training frequencies on the retention of cardiovascular fitness. *Med. Sci. Sports* 5:29–33, 1973.

19. BURKE, E. J. Physiological effects of similar training programs in males and females. *Res. Q.* 48:510–517, 1977.

20. BURKE, E. J. and B. D. FRANKS. Changes in $\dot{V}O_{2max}$ resulting from bicycle training at different intensities holding total mechanical work constant. *Res. Q.* 46:31–37, 1975.

21. BUSKIRK, E. R. and J. L. HODGSON. Age and aerobic power: the rate of change in men and women. *Fed. Proc.* 46:1824–1829, 1987.

22. CARTER, J. E. L. and W. H. PHILLIPS. Structural changes in exercising middle-aged males during a 2-year period. *J. Appl. Physiol.* 27:787–794, 1969.

23. CHOW, J. R. and J. H. WILMORE. The regulation of exercise intensity by ratings of perceived exertion. *J. Cardiac Rehabil.* 4:382–387, 1984.

24. CHRISTENSEN, E. H. Physiological evaluation of work in the Nykroppa iron works. In: *Ergonomics Society Symposium on Fatigue*, W. F. Floyd and A. T. Welford (Eds.). London, England: Lewis, 1953, pp. 93–108.

25. COYLE, E. F., W. H. MARTIN, D. R. SINACORE, M. J. JOYNER, J. M. HAGBERG, and J. O. HOLLOSZY. Time course of loss of adaptation after stopping prolonged intense endurance training. *J. Appl. Physiol.* 57:1857–1864, 1984.

26. CREWS, T. R. and J. A. ROBERTS. Effects of interaction of frequency and intensity of training. *Res. Q.* 47:48–55, 1976.

27. CURETON, T. K. *The Physiological Effects of Exercise Programs upon Adults.* Springfield, IL: Charles C. Thomas Co., 1969, pp. 3–6, 33–77.

28. CURETON, T. K. and E. E. PHILLIPS. Physical fitness changes in middle-aged men attributable to equal eight-week periods of training, non-training and retraining. *J. Sports Med. Phys. Fitness* 4:1–7, 1964.

29. DAVIES, C. T. M. and A. V. KNIBBS. The training stimulus, the effects of intensity, duration and frequency of effort on maximum aerobic power output. *Int. Z. Angew. Physiol.* 29:299–305, 1971.

30. DAVIS, J. A., M. H. FRANK, B. J. WHIPP, and K. WASSERMAN. Anaerobic threshold alterations caused by endurance training in middle-aged men. *J. Appl. Physiol.* 46:1039–1049, 1979.

31. DEHN, M. M. and R. A. BRUCE. Longitudinal variations in maximal oxygen intake with age and activity. *J. Appl. Physiol.* 33:805–807, 1972.

32. DELORME, T. L. Restoration of muscle power by heavy resistance exercise. *J. Bone Joint Surg.* 27:645–667, 1945.

33. DEMPSEY, J. A. Anthropometrical observations on obese and nonobese young men undergoing a program of vigorous physical exercise. *Res. Q.* 35:275–287, 1964.

34. DEVRIES, H. A. Physiological effects of an exercise training regimen upon men aged 52 to 88. *J. Gerontol.* 24:325–336, 1970.

35. DEVRIES, H. A. Exercise intensity threshold for improvement of cardiovascular-respiratory function in older men. *Geriatrics* 26:94–101, 1971.

36. DISHMAN, R. K., J. SALLIS, and D. ORENSTEIN. The determinants of physical activity and exercise. *Public Health Rep.* 100:158–180, 1985.

37. DISHMAN, R. K., R. W. PATTON, J. SMITH, R. WEINBERG, and A. JACKSON. Using perceived exertion to prescribe and monitor exercise training heart rate. *Int. J. Sports Med.* 8:208–213, 1987.

38. DRINKWATER, B. L. Physiological responses of women to exercise. In: *Exercise and Sports Sciences Reviews*, Vol. 1, J. H. Wilmore (Ed.). New York: Academic Press, 1973, pp. 126–154.

39. DRINKWATER, B. L., S. M. HORVATH, and C. L. WELLS. Aerobic power of females, ages 10 to 68. *J. Gerontol.* 30:385–394, 1975.

40. DURNIN, J. V. G. A. and R. PASSMORE. *Energy, Work and Leisure.* London, England: Heinemann Educational Books, Ltd., 1967, pp. 47–82.

41. EDSTROM, L. and L. GRIMBY. Effect of exercise on the motor unit. *Muscle Nerve* 9:104–126, 1986.

42. EKBLOM, B., P. O. ÅSTRAND, B. SALTIN, J. STENBERG, and B. WALLSTROM. Effect of training on circulatory response to exercise. *J. Appl. Physiol.* 24:518–528, 1968.

43. FLECK, S. J. and W. J. KRAEMER. *Designing Resistance Training Programs.* Champaign, IL: Human Kinetics Books, 1987, pp. 15–46, 161–162.

44. FLINT, M. M., B. L. DRINKWATER, and S. M. HORVATH. Effects of training on women's response to submaximal exercise. *Med. Sci. Sports* 6:89–94, 1974.

45. FOX, E. L., R. L. BARTELS, C. E. BILLINGS, R. O'BRIEN, R. BASON, and D. K. MATHEWS. Frequency and duration of interval training programs and changes in aerobic power. *J. Appl. Physiol.* 38:481–484, 1975.

46. FRANKLIN, B., E. BUSKIRK, J. HODGSON, H. GAHAGAN, J. KOLLIAS, and J. MENDEZ. Effects of physical conditioning on cardiorespiratory function, body composition and serum lipids in relatively normal weight and obese middle-age women. *Int. J. Obes.* 3:97–109, 1979.

47. FRINGER, M. N. and A. G. STULL. Changes in cardiorespiratory parameters during periods of training and detraining in young female adults. *Med. Sci. Sports* 6:20–25, 1974.

48. GAESSER, G. A. and R. G. RICH. Effects of high- and low-intensity exercise training on aerobic capacity and blood lipids. *Med. Sci. Sports Exerc.* 16:269–274, 1984.

49. GETCHELL, L. H. and J. C. MOORE. Physical training: comparative responses of middle-aged adults. *Arch. Phys. Med. Rehabil.* 56:250–254, 1975.

50. GETTMAN, L. R., M. L. POLLOCK, J. L. DURSTINE, A. WARD, J. AYRES, and A. C. LINNERUD. Physiological responses of men to 1,3, and 5 day per week training programs. *Res. Q.* 47:638–646, 1976.

51. GETTMAN, L. R., J. J. AYRES, M. L. POLLOCK, and A. JACKSON. The effect of circuit weight training on strength, cardiorespiratory function, and body composition of adult men. *Med. Sci. Sports* 10:171–176, 1978.

52. GETTMAN, L. R., J. AYRES, M. L. POLLOCK, J. L. DURSTINE, and W. GRANTHAM. Physiological effects of circuit strength training and jogging. *Arch. Phys. Med. Rehabil.* 60:115–120, 1979.

53. GETTMAN, L. R., L. A. CULTER, and T. STRATHMAN. Physiologic changes after 20 weeks of isotonic vs. isokinetic circuit training. *J. Sports Med. Phys. Fitness* 20:265–274, 1980.

54. GETTMAN, L. R. and M. L. POLLOCK. Circuit weight training: a critical review of its physiological benefits. *Phys. Sports Med.* 9:44–60, 1981.

55. GETTMAN, L. R., P. WARD, and R. D. HAGMAN. A comparison of combined running and weight training with circuit weight

training. *Med. Sci. Sports Exerc.* 14:229–234, 1982.

56. GILLAM, G. M. Effects of frequency of weight training on muscle strength enhancement. *J. Sports Med.* 21:432–436, 1981.

57. GIRANDOLA, R. N. Body composition changes in women: effects of high and low exercise intensity. *Arch. Phys. Med. Rehabil.* 57:297–300, 1976.

58. GLEDHILL, N. and R. B. EYNON. The intensity of training. In: *Training Scientific Basis and Application*, A. W. Taylor and M. L. Howell (Eds.). Springfield, IL: Charles C Thomas Co., 1972, pp. 97–102.

59. GOLDING, L. Effects of physical training upon total serum cholesterol levels. *Res. Q.* 32:499–505, 1961.

60. GOODE, R. C., A. VIRGIN, T. T. ROMET, et al. Effects of a short period of physical activity in adolescent boys and girls. *Can. J. Appl. Sports Sci.* 1:241–250, 1976.

61. GOSSARD, D., W. L. HASKELL, B. TAYLOR, et al. Effects of low- and high-intensity home-based exercise training on functional capacity in healthy middle-age men. *Am. J. Cardiol.* 57:446–449, 1986.

62. GRAVES, J. E., M. L. POLLOCK, S. H. LEGGETT, R. W. BRAITH, D. M. CARPENTER, and L. E. BISHOP. Effect of reduced training frequency on muscular strength. *Int. J. Sports Med.* 9:316–319, 1988.

63. GRAVES, J. E., M. L. POLLOCK, A. E. JONES, A. B. COLVIN, and S. H. LEGGETT. Specificity of limited range of motion variable resistance training. *Med. Sci. Sports Exerc.* 21:84–89, 1989.

64. GWINUP, G. Effect of exercise alone on the weight of obese women. *Arch. Int. Med.* 135:676–680, 1975.

65. HAGBERG, J. M., J. E. GRAVES, M. LIMACHER, et al. Cardiovascular responses of 70–79 year old men and women to exercise training. *J. Appl. Physiol.* 66:2589–2594,1989.

66. HAKKINEN, K. Factors influencing trainability of muscular strength during short term and prolonged training. *Natl. Strength Cond. Assoc. J.* 7:32–34, 1985.

67. HANSON, J. S., B. S. TABAKIN, A. M. LEVY, and W. NEDDE. Long-term physical training and cardiovascular dynamics in middle-aged men. *Circulation* 38:783–799, 1968.

68. HANSON, J. S. and W. H. NEDDE. Long-term physical training effect in sedentary females. *J. Appl. Physiol.* 37:112–116, 1974.

69. HARTLEY, L. H., G. GRIMBY, A. KILBOM, et al. Physical training in sedentary middle-aged and older men. *Scand. J. Clin. Lab. Invest.* 24:335–344, 1969.

70. HARTUNG, G. H., M. H. SMOLENSKY, R. B. HARRIST, and R. RUNGE. Effects of varied durations of training on improvement in cardiorespiratory endurance. *J. Hum. Ergol.* 6:61–68, 1977.

71. HASKELL, W. L. Physical activity and health: need to define the required stimulus. *Am. J. Cardiol.* 55:4D–9D, 1985.

72. HASKELL, W. L., H. J. MONTOYE, and D. ORENSTEIN. Physical activity and exercise to achieve health-related physical fitness components. *Public Health Rep.* 100:202–212, 1985.

73. HEATH, G. W., J. M. HAGBERG, A. A. EHSANI, and J. O. HOLLOSZY. A physiological comparison of young and older endurance athletes. *J. Appl. Physiol.* 51:634–640, 1981.

74. HETTINGER, T. *Physiology of Strength.* Springfield, IL: C. C Thomas Publisher, 1961, pp. 18–40.

75. HICKSON, R. C. and M. A. ROSENKOETTER. Reduced training frequencies and maintenance of increased aerobic power. *Med. Sci. Sports Exerc.* 13:13–16, 1981.

76. HICKSON, R. C., C. KANAKIS, J. R. DAVIS, A. M. MOORE, and S. RICH. Reduced training duration effects on aerobic power, endurance, and cardiac growth. *J. Appl. Physiol.* 53:225–229, 1982.

77. HICKSON, R. C., C. FOSTER, M. L. POLLOCK, T. M. GALASSI, and S. RICH. Reduced training intensities and loss of aerobic power, endurance, and cardiac growth. *J. Appl. Physiol.* 58:492–499, 1985.

78. HILL, J. O., P. B. SPARLING, T. W. SHIELDS, and P. A. HELLER. Effects of exercise and food restriction on body composition and metabolic rate in obese women. *Am. J. Clin. Nutr.* 46:622–630, 1987.

79. HOLLMANN, W. *Changes in the Capacity for Maximal and Continuous Effort in Relation to Age. Int. Res. Sports Phys. Ed.*, E. Jokl and E. Simon (Eds.). Springfield, IL: Charles C Thomas Co., 1964, pp. 369–371.

80. HOLLMANN, W. and H. VENRATH. Die Beinflussung von Herzgrösse, maximaler O_2—Aufnahme und Ausdauergranze durch ein Ausdauertraining mittlerer und hoher Intensität. *Der Sportarzt* 9:189–193, 1963.

81. No reference 81 due to renumbering in proof.

82. HUIBREGTSE, W. H., H. H. HARTLEY, L. R. JONES, W. D. DOOLITTLE, and T. L. CRIBLEZ. Improvement of aerobic work capacity following non-strenuous exercise. *Arch. Environ. Health* 27:12–15, 1973.

83. HURLEY, B. F., D. R. SEALS, A. A. EHSANI, et al. Effects of high-intensity strength training on cardiovascular function. *Med. Sci. Sports Exerc.* 16:483–488, 1984.

84. ISMAIL, A. H., D. CORRIGAN, and D. F. MCLEOD. Effect of an eight-month exercise program on selected physiological, biochemical, and audiological variables in adult men. *Br. J. Sports Med.* 7:230–240, 1973.

84A. JONES, D. A., D. J. NEWMAN, J. M. ROUND, and S. E. L. TOLFREE. Experimental human muscle damage: morphological changes in relation to other indices of damage. *J. Physiol. (Lond.)* 375:435–438, 1986.

85. KARVONEN, M., K. KENTALA, and O. MUSTALA. The effects of training heart rate: a longitudinal study. *Ann. Med. Exp. Biol. Fenn* 35:307–315, 1957.

86. KASCH, F. W., W. H. PHILLIPS, J. E. L. CARTER, and J. L. BOYER. Cardiovascular changes in middle-aged men during two years of training. *J. Appl. Physiol.* 314:53–57, 1972.

87. KASCH, F. W. and J. P. WALLACE. Physiological variables during 10 years of endurance exercise. *Med. Sci. Sports* 8:5–8, 1976.

88. KASCH, F. W., J. P. WALLACE, and S. P. VAN CAMP. Effects of 18 years of endurance exercise on physical work capacity of older men. *J. Cardiopulmonary Rehabil.* 5:308–312, 1985.

89. KATCH, F. I. and W. D. MCARDLE. *Nutrition, Weight Control and Exercise*, 3rd Ed. Philadelphia: Lea and Febiger, 1988, pp. 110–112.

90. KEARNEY, J. T., A. G. STULL, J. L. EWING, and J. W. STREIN. Cardiorespiratory responses of sedentary college women as a function of training intensity. *J. Appl. Physiol.* 41:822–825, 1976.

91. KENDRICK, Z. B., M. L. POLLOCK, T. N. HICKMAN, and H. S. MILLER. Effects of training and detraining on cardiovascular efficiency. *Am. Corr. Ther. J.* 25:79–83, 1971.

92. KILBOM, A. Physical training in women. *Scand. J. Clin. Lab. Invest.* 119 (Suppl.):1–34, 1971.

93. KILBOM, A., L. HARTLEY, B. SALTIN, J. BJURE, G. GRIMBY, and I. ÅSTRAND. Physical training in sedentary middle-aged and older men. *Scand. J. Clin. Lab. Invest.* 24:315–322, 1969.

94. KIMURA, Y., H. ITOW, and S. YAMAZAKIE. The effects of circuit weight training on VO_{2max} and body composition of trained and untrained college men. *J. Physiol. Soc. Jpn.* 43:593–596, 1981.

94A. KLISSOURAS, V., F. PIRNAY, and J. PETIT. Adaptation to maximal effort: genetics and age. *J. Appl. Physiol.* 35:288–293, 1973.

95. KNAPIK, J. J., R. H. MAUDSLEY, and N. V. RAMMOS. Angular specificity and test mode specificity of isometric and isokinetic strength training. *J. Orthop. Sports Phys. Ther.* 5:58–65, 1983.

96. KNEHR, C. A., D. B. DILL, and W. NEUFELD. Training and its effect on man at rest and at work. *Am. J. Physiol.* 136:148–156, 1942.

97. KNUTTGEN, H. G., L. O. NORDESJO, B. OLLANDER, and B. SALTIN. Physical conditioning through interval training with young male adults. *Med. Sci. Sports* 5:220–226, 1973.

98. LAPORTE, R. E., L. L. ADAMS, D. D. SAVAGE, G. BRENES, S. DEARWATER, and T. COOK. The spectrum of physical activity, cardiovascular disease and health: an epidemiologic perspective. *Am. J. Epidemiol.* 120:507–517, 1984.

99. LEON, A. S., J. CONRAD, D. B. HUNNINGHAKE, and R. SERFASS. Effects of a vigorous walking program on body composition, and carbohydrate and lipid metabolism of obese young men. *Am. J. Clin. Nutr.* 32:1776–1787, 1979.

100. LEON, A. S., J. CONNETT, D. R. JACOBS, and R. RAURAMAA. Leisure-time physical activity levels and risk of coronary heart disease and death: the multiple risk of coronary heart disease and death: the multiple risk factor intervention trial. *J.A.M.A.* 258:2388–2395, 1987.

100A. LEWIS, S. F., W. F. TAYLOR, R. M. GRAHAM, W. A. PETTINGER,

J. E. SHUTTE, and C. G. BLOMQVIST. Cardiovascular responses to exercise as functions of absolute and relative work load. *J. Appl. Physiol.* 54:1314–1323, 1983.

101. LIANG, M. T., J. F. ALEXANDER, H. L. TAYLOR, R. C. SERFRASS, A. S. LEON, and G. A. STULL. Aerobic training threshold, intensity duration, and frequency of exercise. *Scand. J. Sports Sci.* 4:5–8, 1982.

101A. LIEBER, D. C., R. L. LIEBER, and W. C. ADAMS. Effects of run-training and swim-training at similar absolute intensities on treadmill $\dot{V}O_{2max}$. *Med. Sci. Sports Exerc.* 21:655–661, 1989.

101B. MACDOUGALL, J. D., G. R. WARD, D. G. SALE, and J. R. SUTTON. Biochemical adaptation of human skeletal muscle to heavy resistance training and immobilization. *J. Appl. Physiol.* 43:700–703, 1977.

101C. MACDOUGALL, J. D., D. TUXEN, D. G. SALE, J. R. MOROZ, and J. R. SUTTON. Arterial blood pressure response to heavy resistance training. *J. Appl. Physiol.* 58:785–790, 1985.

102. MANN, G. V., L. H. GARRETT, A. FARHI, et al. Exercise to prevent coronary heart disease. *Am. J. Med.* 46:12–27, 1969.

103. MARCINIK, E. J., J. A. HODGDON, U. MITTLEMAN, and J. J. O'BRIEN. Aerobic/calisthenic and aerobic/circuit weight training programs for Navy men: a comparative study. *Med. Sci. Sports Exerc.* 17:482–487, 1985.

104. MARIGOLD, E. A. The effect of training at predetermined heart rate levels for sedentary college women. *Med. Sci. Sports* 6:14–19, 1974.

105. MARTIN, J. E. and P. M. DUBBERT. Adherence to exercise. In: *Exercise and Sports Sciences Reviews*, Vol. 13, R. L. Terjung (Ed.). New York: MacMillan Publishing Co., 1985, pp. 137–167.

106. MARTIN, W. H., J. MONTGOMERY, P. G. SNELL, et al. Cardiovascular adaptations to intense swim training in sedentary middle-aged men and women. *Circulation* 75:323–330, 1987.

107. MAYHEW, J. L. and P. M. GROSS. Body composition changes in young women with high resistance weight training. *Res. Q.* 45:433–439, 1974.

108. MESSIER, J. P. and M. DILL. Alterations in strength and maximal oxygen uptake consequent to Nautilus circuit weight training. *Res. Q. Exerc. Sport* 56:345–351, 1985.

109. MILESIS, C. A., M. L. POLLOCK, M. D. BAH, J. J. AYRES, A. WARD, and A. C. Linnerud. Effects of different durations of training on cardiorespiratory function, body composition and serum lipids. *Res Q.* 47:716–725, 1976.

110. MISNER, J. E., R. A. BOILEAU, B. H. MASSEY, and J. H. MAYHEW. Alterations in body composition of adult men during selected physical training programs. *J. Am. Geriatr. Soc.* 22:33–38, 1974.

111. MIYASHITA, M., S. HAGA, and T. MITZUTA. Training and detraining effects on aerobic power in middle-aged and older men. *J. Sports Med.* 18:131–137, 1978.

112. MOODY, D. L., J. KOLLIAS, and E. R. BUSKIRK. The effect of a moderate exercise program on body weight and skinfold thickness in overweight college women. *Med. Sci. Sports* 1:75–80, 1969.

113. MOODY, D. L., J. H. WILMORE, R. N. GIRANDOLA, and J. P. ROYCE. The effects of a jogging program on the body composition of normal and obese high school girls. *Med. Sci. Sports* 4:210–213, 1972.

114. MUELLER, E. A. and W. ROHMERT. Die geschwindigkeit der muskelkraft zunahme bein isometrischen training. *Int. Z. Angew. Physiol.* 19:403–419, 1963.

115. NAUGHTON, J. and F. NAGLE. Peak oxygen intake during physical fitness program for middle-aged men. *J.A.M.A.* 191:899–901, 1965.

116. O'HARA, W., C. ALLEN, and R. J. SHEPHARD. Loss of body weight and fat during exercise in a cold chamber. *Eur. J. Appl. Physiol.* 37:205–218, 1977.

117. OJA, P., P. TERASLINNA, T. PARTANEN, and R. KARAVA. Feasibility of an 18 months' physical training program for middle-aged men and its effect on physical fitness. *Am. J. Public Health* 64:459–465, 1975.

118. OLREE, H. D., B. CORBIN, J. PENROD, and C. SMITH. Methods of achieving and maintaining physical fitness for prolonged space flight. Final Progress Rep. to NASA, Grant No. NGR-04-

002-004, 1969.

119. OSCAI, L. B., T. WILLIAMS, and B. HERTIG. Effects of exercise on blood volume. *J. Appl. Physiol.* 24:622–624, 1968.

120. PAFFENBARGER, R. S., R. T. HYDE, A. L. WING, and C. HSIEH. Physical activity and all-cause mortality, and longevity of college alumni. *N. Engl. J. Med.* 314:605–613, 1986.

121. PAVLOU, K. N., W. P. STEFFEE, R. H. LEARMAN, and B. A. BURROWS. Effects of dieting and exercise on lean body mass, oxygen uptake, and strength. *Med. Sci. Sports Exerc.* 17:466–471, 1985.

122. PELS, A. E., M. L. POLLOCK, T. E. DOHMEIER, K. A. LEMBERGER, and B. F. OEHRLEIN. Effects of leg press training on cycling, leg press, and running peak cardiorespiratory measures. *Med. Sci. Sports Exerc.* 19:66–70, 1987.

123. POLLOCK, M. L. The quantification of endurance training programs. In: *Exercise and Sport Sciences Reviews*, J. H. Wilmore (Ed.). New York: Academic Press, 1973, pp. 155–188.

124. POLLOCK, M. L. Prescribing exercise for fitness and adherence. In: *Exercise Adherence: Its Impact on Public Health*, R. K. Dishman (Ed.). Champaign, IL: Human Kinetics Books, 1988, pp. 259–277

125. POLLOCK, M. L., T. K. CURETON, and L. GRENINGER. Effects of frequency of training on working capacity, cardiovascular function, and body composition of adult men. *Med. Sci. Sports* 1:70–74, 1969.

126. POLLOCK, M. L., J. TIFFANY, L. GETTMAN, R. JANEWAY, and H. LOFLAND. Effects of frequency of training on serum lipids, cardiovascular function, and body composition. In: *Exercise and Fitness*, B. D. Franks (Ed.). Chicago: Athletic Institute, 1969, pp. 161–178.

127. POLLOCK, M. L., H. MILLER, R. JANEWAY, A. C. LINNERUD, B. ROBERTSON, and R. VALENTINO. Effects of walking on body composition and cardiovascular function of middle-aged men. *J. Appl. Physiol.* 30:126–130, 1971.

128. POLLOCK, M. L., J. BROIDA, Z. KENDRICK, H. S. MILLER, R. JANEWAY, and A. C. LINNERUD. Effects of training two days per week at different intensities on middle-aged men. *Med. Sci. Sports* 4:192–197, 1972.

129. POLLOCK, M. L., H. S. MILLER, JR., and J. WILMORE. Physiological characteristics of champion American track athletes 40 to 70 years of age. *J. Gerontol.* 29:645–649, 1974.

130. POLLOCK, M. L., J. DIMMICK, H. S. MILLER, Z. KENDRICK, and A. C. LINNERUD. Effects of mode of training on cardiovascular function and body composition of middle-aged men. *Med. Sci. Sports* 7:139–145, 1975.

131. No reference 131 due to renumbering in proof.

132. POLLOCK, M. L., G. A. DAWSON, H. S. MILLER, JR., et al. Physiologic response of men 49 to 65 years of age to endurance training. *J. Am. Geriatr. Soc.* 24:97–104, 1976.

133. POLLOCK, M. L. and A. JACKSON. Body composition: measurement and changes resulting from physical training. Proceedings National College Physical Education Association for Men and Women, January, 1977, pp. 125–137.

134. POLLOCK, M. L., J. AYRES, and A. WARD. Cardiorespiratory fitness: response to differing intensities and durations of training. *Arch. Phys. Med. Rehabil.* 58:467–473, 1977.

135. POLLOCK, M. L., R. GETTMAN, C. A. MILESIS, M. D. BAH, J. L. DURSTINE, and R. B. JOHNSON. Effects of frequency and duration of training on attrition and incidence of injury. *Med. Sci. Sports* 9:31–36, 1977.

136. POLLOCK, M. L., L. R. GETTMAN, P. B. RAVEN, J. AYRES, M. BAH, and A. WARD. Physiological comparison of the effects of aerobic and anaerobic training. In: *Physical Fitness Programs for Law Enforcement Officers: A Manual for Police Administrators*, C. S. Price, M. L. Pollock, L. R. Gettman, and D. A. KENT (Eds.). Washington, D. C.: U. S. Government Printing Office, No. 027-000-00671-0, 1978, pp. 89–96.

137. POLLOCK, M. L., A. S. JACKSON, and C. FOSTER. The use of the perception scale for exercise prescription. In: *The Perception of Exertion in Physical Work*, G. Borg and D. Ottoson (Eds.). London, England: The MacMillan Press, Ltd., 1986, pp. 161–176.

138. POLLOCK, M. L., C. FOSTER, D. KNAPP, J. S. ROD, and D. H. SCHMIDT. Effect of age and training on aerobic capacity and

body composition of master athletes. *J. Appl. Physiol.* 62:725–731, 1987.

139. POLLOCK, M. L. and J. H. WILMORE. *Exercise in Health and Disease: Evaluation and Prescription for Prevention and Rehabilitation*, 2nd Ed. Philadelphia: W. B. Saunders, Co., 1990.

140. POWELL, K. E., H. W. KOHL, C. J. CASPERSEN, and S. N. BLAIR. An epidemiological perspective of the causes of running injuries. *Phys. Sportsmed.* 14:100–114, 1986.

141. RIBISL, P. M. Effects of training upon the maximal oxygen uptake of middle-aged men. *Int. Z. Angew. Physiol.* 26:272–278, 1969.

142. RICHIE, D. H., S. F. KELSO, and P. A. BELLUCCI. Aerobic dance injuries: a retrospective study of instructors and participants. *Phys. Sportsmed.* 13:130–140, 1985.

143. ROBINSON, S. and P. M. HARMON. Lactic acid mechanism and certain properties of blood in relation to training. *Am. J. Physiol.* 132:757–769, 1941.

144. ROSKAMM, H. Optimum patterns of exercise for healthy adults. *Can. Med. Assoc. J.* 96:895–899, 1967.

145. SALE, D. G. Influence of exercise and training on motor unit activation. In: *Exercise and Sport Sciences Reviews*, K. B. Pandolf (Ed.). New York: MacMillan Publishing Co., 1987, pp. 95–152.

145A. SALE, D. G. Neural adaptation to resistance training. *Med. Sci. Sports Exerc.* 20:S135–S145, 1988.

146. SALLIS, J. F., W. L. HASKELL, S. P. FORTMAN, K. M. VRANIZAN, C. B. TAYLOR, and D. S. SOLOMAN. Predictors of adoption and maintenance of physical activity in a community sample. *Prev. Med.* 15:131–141, 1986.

147. SALTIN, B., G. BLOMQVIST, J. MITCHELL, R. L. JOHNSON, K. WILDENTHAL, and C. B. CHAPMAN. Response to exercise after bed rest and after training. *Circulation* 37, 38(Suppl. 7):1–78, 1968.

148. SALTIN, B., L. HARTLEY, A. KILBOM, and I. ÅSTRAND. Physical training in sedentary middle-aged and older men. *Scand. J. Clin. Lab. Invest.* 24:323–334, 1969.

149. SANTIGO, M. C., J. F. ALEXANDER, G. A. STULL, R. C. SERFRASS, A. M. HAYDAY, and A. S. LEON. Physiological responses of sedentary women to a 20-week conditioning program of walking or jogging. *Scand. J. Sports Sci.* 9:33–39, 1987.

150. SEALS, D. R., J. M. HAGBERG, B. F. HURLEY, A. A. EHSANI, and J. O. HOLLOSZY. Endurance training in older men and women. I. Cardiovascular responses to exercise. *J. Appl. Physiol.* 57:1024–1029, 1984.

151. SHARKEY, B. J. Intensity and duration of training and the development of cardiorespiratory endurance. *Med. Sci. Sports* 2:197–202, 1970.

152. SHEPHARD, R. J. Intensity, duration, and frequency of exercise as determinants of the response to a training regime. *Int. Z. Angew. Physiol.* 26:272–278, 1969.

153. SHEPHARD, R. J. Future research on the quantifying of endurance training. *J. Hum. Ergol.* 3:163–181, 1975.

154. SIDNEY, K. H., R. B. EYNON, and D. A. CUNNINGHAM. Effect of frequency of training of exercise upon physical working performance and selected variables representative of cardiorespiratory fitness. In: *Training Scientific Basis and Application*, A. W. Taylor (Ed.). Springfield, IL: Charles C Thomas Co., 1972, pp. 144–188.

155. SIDNEY, K. H., R. J. SHEPHARD, and J. HARRISON. Endurance training and body composition of the elderly. *Am. J. Clin. Nutr.* 30:326–333, 1977.

156. SIEGEL, W., G. BLOMQVIST, and J. H. MITCHELL. Effects of a quantitated physical training program on middle-aged sedentary males. *Circulation* 41:19–29, 1970.

156A. SISCOVICK, D. S., N. S. WEISS, R. H. FLETCHER, and T. LASKY. The incidence of primary cardiac arrest during vigorous exercise. *N. Engl. J. Med.* 311:874–877, 1984.

157. SKINNER, J. The cardiovascular system with aging and exercise. In: *Physical Activity and Aging*, D. Brunner and E. Jokl (Eds.). Baltimore: University Park Press, 1970, pp. 100–108.

158. SKINNER, J., J. HOLLOSZY, and T. CURETON. Effects of a program of endurance exercise on physical work capacity and anthropometric measurements of fifteen middle-aged men. *Am. J. Cardiol.* 14:747–752, 1964.

159. SMITH, D. P. and F. W. STRANSKY. The effect of training and detraining on the body composition and cardiovascular response of young women to exercise. *J. Sports Med.* 16:112–120, 1976.

160. SMITH, E. L., W. REDDAN, and P. E. SMITH. Physical activity and calcium modalities for bone mineral increase in aged women. *Med. Sci. Sports Exerc.* 13:60–64, 1981.

161. SUOMINEN, H., E. HEIKKINEN, and T. TARKATTI. Effect of eight weeks physical training on muscle and connective tissue of the m. vastus lateralis in 69-year-old men and women. *J. Gerontol.* 32:33–37, 1977.

162. TERJUNG, R. L., K. M. BALDWIN, J. COOKSEY, B. SAMSON, and R. A. SUTTER. Cardiovascular adaptation to twelve minutes of mild daily exercise in middle-aged sedentary men. *J. Am. Geriatr. Soc.* 21:164–168, 1973.

163. THOMAS, S. G., D. A. CUNNINGHAM, P. A. RECHNITZER, A. P. DONNER, and J. H. HOWARD. Determinants of the training response in elderly men. *Med. Sci. Sports Exerc.* 17:667–672, 1985.

164. WENGER, H. A. and G. J. BELL. The interactions of intensity, frequency, and duration of exercise training in altering cardiorespiratory fitness. *Sports Med.* 3:346–356, 1986.

165. WILMORE, J. H. Alterations in strength, body composition, and anthropometric measurements consequent to a 10-week weight training program. *Med. Sci. Sports* 6:133–138, 1974.

166. WILMORE, J. Inferiority of female athletes: myth or reality. *J. Sports Med.* 3:1–6, 1974.

167. WILMORE, J. H. Design issues and alternatives in assessing physical fitness among apparently healthy adults in a health examination survey of the general population. In: *Assessing Physical Fitness and Activity in General Population Studies*, T. F. Drury (Ed.). Washington, D.C.: U.S. Public Health Service, National Center for Health Statistics, 1988 (in press).

168. WILMORE, J. H., J. ROYCE, R. N. GIRANDOLA, F. I. KATCH, and V. L. KATCH. Physiological alternatives resulting from a 10-week jogging program. *Med. Sci. Sports* 2:7–14, 1970.

169. WILMORE, J. H., J. ROYCE, R. N. GIRANDOLA, F. I. KATCH, and V. L. KATCH. Body composition changes with a 10-week jogging program. *Med. Sci. Sports* 2:113–117, 1970.

170. WILMORE, J., R. B. PARR, P. A. VODAK, et al. Strength, endurance, BMR, and body composition changes with circuit weight training. *Med. Sci. Sports* 8:58–60, 1976.

171. WILMORE, J. H., G. A. EWY, A. R. MORTAN, et al. The effect of beta-adrenergic blockade on submaximal and maximal exercise performance. *J. Cardiac Rehabil.* 3:30–36, 1983.

171A. WILMORE, J. H. Body composition in sport and exercise: directions for future research. *Med. Sci. Sports Exerc.* 15:21–31, 1983.

172. WILMORE, J. H. and D. L. COSTILL. *Training for Sport and Activity. The Physiological Basis of the Conditioning Process*, 3rd Ed. Dubuque, IA: Wm. C. Brown, 1988, pp. 113–212.

173. WOOD, P. D., W. L. HASKELL, S. N. BLAIR, et al. Increased exercise level and plasma lipoprotein concentrations: a one-year, randomized, controlled study in sedentary, middle-aged men. *Metabolism* 32:31–39, 1983.

174. ZUTI, W. B. and L. A. GOLDING. Comparing diet and exercise as weight reduction tools. *Phys. Sports Med.* 4:49–53, 1976.

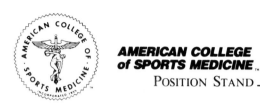

AMERICAN COLLEGE
of SPORTS MEDICINE™
POSITION STAND

Blood Doping
as an Ergogenic Aid

Summary

Blood doping is an ergogenic* procedure wherein normovolemic erythrocythemia is induced via autologous (i.e., reinfusion of athlete's own blood) or homologous (i.e., transfusion of type matched donor's blood) red blood cell (RBC) infusion (11,27,28,34). The resultant hemoconcentration increases arterial oxygen concentration (CaO_2) (9,23). During peak exercise, oxygen delivery [cardiac output ($\dot{Q}$)xCaO_2] to skeletal muscle is enhanced, improving maximal oxygen uptake ($\dot{V}O_{2max}$) and endurance capacity (9,28,29,31). Such terms as blood boosting, blood packing, and induced erythrocythemia are also variously used to describe this ergogenic procedure (11,34).

It is the position of the American College of Sports Medicine that the use of blood doping as an ergogenic aid for athletic competition is unethical and unjustifiable, but that autologous RBC infusion is an acceptable procedure to induce erythrocythemia in clinically controlled conditions for the purpose of legitimate scientific inquiry.

Applications: Experimental and Ergogenic

Blood doping was first used as an experimental procedure to study hematological control mechanisms for systemic transport of oxygen during acute hypoxic exposure (23). Subsequent investigations have experimentally manipulated hemoglobin concentration ([Hb]) via RBC infusion to demonstrate the rate-limiting effect of peak Hb flow rate ($\dot{Q}$x[Hb]) and oxygen delivery on $\dot{V}O_{2max}$ and endurance capacity (4,8,9,13,27–29,31,37). These experimental applications have shown that RBC infusion is a valuable laboratory tool when examining the effect of [Hb] on oxygen transport function during dynamic exercise under both normoxic and hypoxic conditions.

While reports of blood doping for scientific purposes appeared as early as 1947 (23), it was not until the 1976 Olympic Games in Montreal that it was suggested the procedure had been used as an ergogenic aid for endurance events (11,34). Since that time, both athletes and

sports officials have publicly admitted having employed homologous RBC infusion as an ergogenic aid during international competition. These actions prompted a call for an unequivocal statement regarding the *ergogenic, physiological, medical,* and *ethical* implications underlying the use of blood doping as an ergogenic aid. This position statement was prepared by the American College of Sports Medicine in response to these concerns.

Ergogenic Effect

The ergogenic properties of normovolemic erythrocythemia have, in part, been inferred from the increase in oxygen transport capacity that attends prolonged exposure to high altitude. As both $\dot{V}O_{2max}$ and endurance performance are improved under hypoxic conditions following long-term altitude acclimatization, it was hypothesized that artificial production of a normovolemic erythrocythemia via RBC infusion might have a similar ergogenic effect. While documentation of the beneficial effect of blood doping during actual competitive conditions is lacking, a significant amount of experimental evidence supports the ergogenic properties of RBC infusion under both normoxic and hypoxic conditions.

The ergogenic effectiveness of blood doping is dependent on a significant elevation in [Hb] following RBC infusion (11,34). When autologous blood is used, postreinfusion hemoconcentration occurs only if normocythemia has been restored prior to artificial expansion of the RBC mass. In investigations where this methodological criterion was met, the prephlebotomy to postinfusion increase in [Hb] was associated with a significantly higher $\dot{V}O_{2max}$ (i.e., 3.9–12.8%) and/or endurance capacity (i.e., 2.5–35%) (4,23,27–29,31,37). Improvements in maximal aerobic power following blood doping were achieved when subjects received 2,000 ml homologous blood (23) or 900–1,800 ml freeze-preserved autologous blood (4,27–29,37). Infusion of smaller volumes of blood was not sufficient to elevate [Hb] or to significantly improve $\dot{V}O_{2max}$ and/or endurance capacity (7,11,18,27,36).

A number of investigations have not found a statistically significant improvement in maximal aerobic power following blood doping (10,20,25,35). Some reasons for this finding include: improper experimental designs, such as the absence of placebo and control

---

* An ergogenic aid is a physical, mechanical, nutritional, psychological, or pharmacological substance or treatment that either directly improves physiological variables associated with exercise performance or removes subjective restraints which may limit physiological capacity (35).

conditions; the designation of preinfusion (anemic) values rather than prephlebotomy (normocythemic) values as control levels; protocols that could have produced a training effect in the experimental subjects; and most importantly, failure to achieve a significant increase in [Hb] due to an inappropriate storage technique and/or inadequate transfusion volumes and time between phlebotomy and transfusion. Consequently, reviewers of these studies incorrectly concluded that blood doping does not alter $\dot{V}O_{2max}$ or endurance performance (24,33).

Physiological Mechanism

The physiological mechanism underlying the hemoconcentration that attends blood doping involves a shift of protein-free plasma filtrate from the intravascular to interstitial compartment; resolving the immediate postinfusion hypervolemia (16,35). The resulting decrease in plasma volume produces a comparatively rapid restoration of normal blood volume in the presence of a greater [Hb] and CaO_2. Provided hematocrit does not exceed 50%, $\dot{Q}$ during peak exercise is not attenuated by erythrocythemia (9,28–30). As such, the higher CaO_2 following blood doping increases oxygen delivery (i.e., $\dot{Q}xCaO_2$). At peak exercise, augmented oxygen delivery increases the difference between arterial and venous oxygen concentration [$C(a-v)O_2$] (9,28,29,31). The greater tissue respiration increases $\dot{V}O_{2max}$ and endurance capacity. Additionally, both CO_2 transport and acid-base balance are favorably affected by an increase in [Hb]. Such changes in blood-buffering capacity may also contribute to the ergogenic properties of induced erythrocythemia.

Following blood doping, heart rate (4,9,23,27–29), $\dot{Q}$ (28), and lactic acid concentration (4,9,13,29) decrease as $C(a-v)O_2$ increases for a given sub-maximal oxygen uptake. At exercise intensities $\geq$ 40% $\dot{V}O_{2max}$, stroke volume is unaffected by erythrocythemia (28). Although oxygen uptake during sub-maximal exercise is unchanged following blood doping, the relative oxygen (% $\dot{V}O_{2max}$) requirement is reduced as a result of the increased $\dot{V}O_{2max}$.

The blood concentration of 2,3-diphosphoglycerate (4,9,11,28,37) and the oxygen partial pressure at which 50% of Hb is saturated (P_{50}) (28) are not affected by induced erythrocythemia. These findings indicate there is no change in the affinity of the RBC for oxygen when [Hb] is increased.

The time course of the postinfusion hematologic changes is an important consideration for the application of blood doping. Provided normocythemia has been reestablished, both [Hb] and hematocrit are significantly elevated within 24 h following autologous infusion of 900 ml blood (11,12). The erythrocythemia remains relatively constant for 7 d, whereupon hematoligic values return gradually in a linear manner to control levels over a 15-wk period. Thus, increased

oxygen-carrying capacity is observed not just for a brief period following the blood reinfusion, but for many weeks thereafter (4,28). In this context, research involving induced erythrocythemia should be scheduled approximately 120 d (i.e., RBC life span) before an athletic event to insure that normocythemia is restored in experimental subjects prior to their participation in competition.

Procedure for Blood Storage and Reinfusion

Blood is preserved either by refrigeration at 4°C or by a glycerol freezing technique (22). When blood is refrigerated, there is a progressive loss of erythrocytes with a concomitant accumulation of cellular aggregates. As such, regulatory agencies in North America have set 3 wk as the maximum refrigeration storage time for blood. Of concern in an autologous blood doping protocol is that a 3-wk storage period is normally insufficient to restore prephlebotomy [Hb] when more than one unit of blood is removed (11,12). In addition, RBCs are also destroyed in the transfusion process or become so fragile during storage that they hemolyze shortly after they are reinfused. The net result is that only 60% of originally removed cells are viable following reinfusion. The comparatively short storage time and the marked hemolysis associated with storage and transfer make it very difficult to restore normocythemia prior to blood doping when a refrigeration storage procedure is used.

In contrast, when blood is stored as frozen cells, the aging process of the RBC is interrupted, allowing preservation for an indefinite period of time (32). In the context of autologous blood doping, freeze preservation makes it possible to delay reinfusion as long as necessary to insure that normocythemia has been reestablished in the donor. Reestablishing normocythemia following phlebotomy is a primary requisite for postreinfusion erythrocythemia. When used in a blood doping protocol, frozen blood is thawed and reconstituted with physiologic saline to a hematocrit of approximately 50%. The reconstituted blood is usually infused 24 to 48 h prior to laboratory testing or athletic competition.

Medical Implications

While blood doping appears to be an effective ergogenic aid, the safety of its use is suspect. Transfusion of RBCs to the extent of raising the hematocrit over 60% may subject the individual to a hyperviscosity syndrome which includes intravascular clotting, potential heart failure, and death (21). If blood transfusions are performed without adhering to standard medical procedures, severe bacterial infections, air and clot emboli, and major transfusion reactions may occur, in rare instances leading to death (1,15,38).

The medical risks of blood doping can be separated into those associated with homologous transfusions and those associated with autologous transfusions. Homologous transfusions, even under standardized medical procedures, carry several risks. Despite appropriate typing and cross-matching of blood, there is a 3 to 4% incidence of minor transfusion reactions consisting of fever, chills, and malaise (2,19). Delayed reactions can cause destruction of the transfused red cells (26). Both of these reactions can occur without demonstrable incompatibility with the donor cells. Infections transmitted by blood also pose a serious risk with homologous transfusions. Malaria (6), hepatitis (14), acquired immune deficiency syndrome (AIDS) (5), and cytomegalovirus (18) are the most common and dangerous of these infections. Although progress has been made in detecting contaminated blood, there is still a slightly less than 1% chance of acquiring one of these diseases from transfused blood despite the use of the best detection methods (17). All of these infections can be fatal. In contrast, autologous transfusions limited to two units of packed RBC and performed under proper medical supervision carry a substantially lower medical risk (3).

Ethical Considerations

The International Olympic Committee defines doping as "the use of physiological substances in abnormal amounts and with abnormal methods, with the exclusive aim of attaining an artificial and unfair increase of performance in competition" (7). Based on this definition, the International Olympic Committee has banned blood doping as an ergogenic aid. However, techniques to detect an artificially induced erythrocythemia are not available. In addition, if such detection techniques were available, their validity would be confounded by altitude acclimatization, hydration status, and normally occurring individual differences in hematocrit.

Conclusions

A position statement on the use of blood doping must distinguish between scientific and sport applications of the procedure. *Autologous* RBC infusion is considered a scientifically valid and acceptable laboratory procedure to induce erythrocythemia for legitimate scientific inquiry under clinically controlled conditions. However, because RBC infusion (i.e., autologous and homologous) has attendant medical risks and violates doping control regulations, it is the position of the American College of Sports Medicine that the use of blood doping as an ergogenic aid during athletic competition is unethical and unjustifiable.

REFERENCES

1. BRAUDE, A. I. Transfusion reactions from contaminated blood: their recognition and treatment. *N. Engl. J. Med.* 258:1289–1293, 1958.
2. BRITTINGHAM, T. E. and H. CHAPLIN. Febrile transfusion reactions caused by sensitivity to donor leukocytes and platelets. *J.A.M.A.* 165:819–825, 1957.
3. BRAZICA, S. M., A. A. PINEDA, and H. F. TASWELL. Autologous blood transfusion. *Mayo Clin. Proc.* 51:723–737, 1976.
4. BUICK, F. J., N. GLEDHILL, A. B. FROESE, L. SPRIET, and E. C. MEYERS. Effect of induced erythrocythemia on aerobic work capacity. *J. Appl. Physiol.: Respirat. Environ. Exerc. Physiol.* 48:636–642, 1980.
5. CURRAN, J. W., D. N. LAWRENCE, H. JAFFE, et al. Acquired immune-deficiency syndrome (AIDS) associated with transfusion. *N. Engl. J. Med.* 310:69–75, 1984.
6. DOVER, A. S. and W. G. SCHULTZ. Transfusion-induced malaria. *Transfusion* 11:353–357, 1971.
7. DUGAL, R. and M. BERTRAND. Doping. In: *IOC Medical Commission Booklet.* Montreal, Canada: *Comité Orginisateur des Jeux Olympiques* 1976, pp. 1–31.
8. EKBLOM, B., A. N. GOLDBARG, and B. GULLBRING. Response to exercise after blood loss and reinfusion. *J. Appl. Physiol.* 40:379–383, 1972.
9. EKBLOM, B., G. WILSON, and P. O. ÅSTRAND. Central circulation during exercise after venesection and reinfusion of red blood cells. *J. Appl. Physiol.* 40:379–383, 1976.
10. FRYE, A. and R. RUHLING. RBC infusion, exercise, hemoconcentration, and $\dot{V}O_2$ (Abstract). *Med. Sci. Sports* 9:69, 1977.
11. GLEDHILL, N. Blood doping and related issues: a brief review. *Med. Sci. Sports Exerc.* 14:193–189, 1982.
12. GLEDHILL, N., F. J. BUICK, A. B. FROESE, L. SPRIET, and E. C. MEYERS. An optimal method of storing blood for blood boosting. (Abstract) *Med. Sci. Sports* 10:40, 1978.
13. GLEDHILL, N., L. L. SPRIET, A. B. FROESE, D. L. WILKES, and E. C. MEYERS. Acid-base status with induced erythrocythemia and its influence on arterial oxygenation during heavy exercise (Abstract). *Med. Sci. Sports. Exerc.* 12:122, 1980.
14. GRADY, G. F. and T. C. CHALMERS. Risk of post-transfusion viral hepatitis (Abstract). *N. Engl. J. Med.* 271:337, 1964.
15. GREENWALT, T. J. (Ed.). *General Principles of Blood Transfusion.* Chicago, IL: American Medical Association, 1977, pp. 65–74.
16. GREGERSEN, M. and S. CHIEN. Blood volume. In: *Medical Physiology.* V. B. Mountcastle (Ed.). St. Louis, MO: Mosby, 1968, pp. 244–283.
17. HARRISON, T. R. *Harrison's Principles of Internal Medicine.* G. W. Thorn, R. D. Adams, E. Braunwald, K. J. Isselbacher, and R. G. Petersdorf (Eds.). NY: McGraw-Hill, 1977, pp. 1703–1706.
18. HENLE, W., G. HENLE, M. SCRIBA, et al. Antibody responses to the Epstein-Barr virus and cytomegaloviruses after open heart surgery. *N. Engl. J. Med.* 282:1068–1074, 1970.
19. HONIG, C. L. and J. R. BOVE. Transfusion: associated fatalities; review of Biologies reports 1976–1978. *Transfusion* 20:653–661, 1980.
20. KOTS, Y. M., M. M. SHCHERBA, Y. S. KOLNER, V. D. GORODETSKII, and L. D. SIN. Experimental study of the relationship between the blood hemoglobin and physical aerobic working capacity. *Fiziologiya Cheloveka* 4:53–60, 1978.
21. MCGRATH, M. A. and R. PENNY. Paraproteinuria: blood hyperviscosity and clinical manifestations. *J. Clin. Invest.* 58:1155–1162, 1976.
22. MERRYMAN, H. T. and M. HORNBLOWER. A method for freezing and washing red blood cells using a high glycerol concentration. *Transfusion* 12:145–156, 1972.
23. PACE, N., E. L. LOZNER, W. V. CONSOLAZIO, G. C. PITTS, and J. L. PECORA. The increase in hypoxia tolerance of normal men accompanying the polycythemia induced by transfusion of erythrocytes. *Am. J. Physiol.* 148:152–163, 1947.

24. PATE, R. Does the sport need new blood? *Runner's World Magazine* 1976, pp. 25–27, November.

25. PATE, R., J. MCFARLAND, J. V. WYCK, and A. OKOCHA. Effect of blood reinfusion on endurance performance in female distance runners (Abstract). *Med. Sci. Sports* 11:97, 1979.

26. PINEDA, A. A., H. F. TASWELL, and S. M. BRZICA, JR. Delayed hemolytic transfusion reaction: an immunologic hazard of blood transfusion. *Transfusion* 18:1–7, 1978.

27. ROBERTSON, R. J., R. GILCHER, K. F. METZ, et al. Effect of induced erythrocythemia on hypoxia tolerance during physical exercise. *J. Appl. Physiol.: Respirat. Environ. Exerc. Physiol.* 53:490–495, 1982.

28. ROBERTSON, R. J., R. GILCHER, K. F. METZ, et al. Hemoglobin concentration and aerobic work capacity in women following induced erythrocythemia. *J. Appl. Physiol.: Respirat. Environ. Exerc. Physiol.* 57:568–575, 1984.

29. SPRIET, L. L., N. GLEDHILL, A. B. FROESE, and D. L. WILKES. Effect of graded erythrocythemia on cardiovascular and metabolic responses to exercise. *J. Appl. Physiol.* 61:1942–1948, 1986.

30. STONE, H. O., H. K. THOMPSON, and K. SCHMIDT-NIELSEN. Influence of erythrocytes on blood viscosity. *Am. J. Physiol.* 214:913–918, 1968.

31. THOMPSON, J. M., J. A. STONE, A. D. GINSBERG, and P. HAMILTON. O_2 transport during exercise following blood reinfusion. *J. Appl. Physiol.: Respirat. Environ. Exerc. Physiol.* 53:1213–1219, 1982.

32. VALERI, C. R. *Blood Banking and the Use of Frozen Blood Products.* Cleveland, OH: CRC Press, 1976, pp. 9–174.

33. WILLIAMS. M. H. Blood doping in sports. *J. Drug Issues* 3:331–340, 1980.

34. WILLIAMS, M. H. (Ed.). Blood doping. In: *Ergogenic Aids in Sport.* Champaign, IL: Human Kinetics Publishers, 1983, pp. 202–217.

35. WILLIAMS, M. H., A. R. GOODWIN, R. PERKINS, and J. BOCRIE. Effect of blood reinjection upon endurance capacity and heart rate. *Med. Sci. Sports* 5:181–186, 1973.

36. WILLIAMS, M. H., M. LINDHEIM, and R. SCHUSTER. Effect of blood infusion upon endurance capacity and ratings of perceived exertion. *Med. Sci. Sports* 10:113–118, 1978.

37. WILLIAMS, M. H., S. WESSELDINE, T. SOMMA, and R. SCHUSTER. The effect of induced erythrocythemia upon 5-mile treadmill run time. *Med. Sci. Sports Exerc.* 13:169–175, 1981.

38. WILLIAMS, W. J., E. BEUTLER, A. J. ERSLEY, and R. W. RUNDLES. *Hematology.* NY: McGraw-Hill, 1977, pp. 1540–1547.

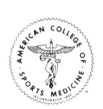

**AMERICAN COLLEGE
of SPORTS MEDICINE.**
POSITION STAND ———————————

The Prevention
of Thermal Injuries
During Distance Running

Purpose of the Position Stand

1. To alert sponsors of distance-running events to potentially serious health hazards during distance running—especially thermal injury.
2. To advise sponsors to consult local weather history and plan events at times when the environmental heat stress would most likely be acceptable.
3. To encourage sponsors to identify the environmental heat stress existing on the day of a race and communicate this to the participants.
4. To educate participants regarding thermal injury susceptibility and prevention.
5. To inform sponsors of preventive actions which may reduce the frequency and severity of this type of injury.

This position stand replaces that of *Prevention of Heat Injury During Distance Running,* published by the American College of Sports Medicine in 1975. It has been expanded to consider thermal problems which may affect the general community of joggers, fun runners, and elite athletes who participate in distance-running events. Although hyperthermia is still the most common serious problem encountered in North American fun runs and races, hypothermia can be a problem for slow runners in long races such as the marathon, in cold and/or wet environmental conditions or following races when blood glucose is low and the body's temperature regulatory mechanism is impaired.

Because the physiological responses to exercise and environmental stress vary among participants, strict compliance with the recommendations, while helpful, will not guarantee complete protection from thermal illness. The general guidelines in this position stand do not constitute definitive medical advice, which should be sought from a physician for specific cases. Nevertheless, adherence to these recommendations should help to minimize the incidence of thermal injury.

Position Stand

It is the position of the American College of Sports Medicine that the following RECOMMENDATIONS be employed by directors of distance runs or community fun runs.

1. Medical Director
A medical director knowledgeable in exercise physiology and sports medicine should coordinate the preventive and therapeutic aspects of the running event and work closely with the race director.

2. Race Organization
a. Races should be organized to avoid the hottest summer months and the hottest part of the day. As there are great regional variations in environmental conditions, the local weather history will be most helpful in scheduling an event to avoid times when an unacceptable level of heat stress is likely to prevail. Organizers should be cautious of unseasonably hot days in the early spring, as entrants will almost certainly not be heat acclimatized.

b. The environmental heat stress prediction for the day should be obtained from the meteorological service. It can be measured as wet bulb globe temperature (WBGT) (see Appendix I), which is a temperature/humidity/radiation index (1). If WBGT is above 28°C (82°F), consideration should be given to rescheduling or delaying the race until safer conditions prevail. If below 28°C, participants may be alerted to the degree of heat stress by using color-coded flags at the start of the race and at key positions along the course (Appendix II; 26).

c. All summer events should be scheduled for the early morning, ideally before 8:00 a.m., or in the evening after 6:00 p.m., to minimize solar radiation.

d. An adequate supply of water should be available before the race and every 2–3 km during the race. Runners should be encouraged to consume 100–200 ml at each station.

e. Race officials should be educated as to the warning signs of an impending collapse. Each official should wear an identifiable arm band or badge and should warn runners to stop if they appear to be in difficulty.

f. Adequate traffic and crowd control must be maintained at all times.

g. There should be a ready source of radio communications from various points on the course to a central organizing point to coordinate responses to emergencies.

3. **Medical Support**
   a. **Medical Organization and Responsibility:**
      The Medical Director should alert local hospitals and ambulance services to the event and should make prior arrangements with medical personnel for the care of casualties, especially those suffering from heat injury. The mere fact that an entrant signs a waiver in no way absolves the organizers of moral and/or legal responsibility. Medical personnel supervising races should have the authority to evaluate, examine, and/or stop a runner who displays the symptoms and signs of impending heat injury, or who appears to be mentally and/or physically out of control for any other reason.
   b. **Medical Facilities:**
      i. Medical support staff and facilities should be available at the race site.
      ii. The facilities should be staffed with personnel capable of instituting immediate and appropriate resuscitation measures. Apart from the routine resuscitation equipment, ice packs and fans for cooling are required.
      iii. Persons trained in first aid, appropriately identified with an arm band, badge, etc., should be stationed along the course to warn runners to stop if they exhibit signs of impending heat injury.
      iv. Ambulances or vans with accompanying medical personnel should be available along the course.
      v. Although the emphasis in this stand has been on the management of hyperthermia, on cold, wet, and windy days athletes may be chilled and require "space blankets," blankets, and warm drinks at the finish to prevent or treat hypothermia (23,45).

4. **Competitor Education**
   The education of fun runners has increased greatly in recent years, but race organizers must not assume that all participants are well informed or prepared. Distributing guidelines at the preregistration, publicizing the event in the press, and holding clinics and/or seminars before runs are valuable.
   The following persons are particularly prone to heat illness: the obese (3,17,43), unfit (13, 29,39,43), dehydrated (6,14,31,37,38,47), those unacclimatized to the heat (20,43), those with a previous history of heat stroke (36,43), and anyone who runs while ill (41). Children perspire less than adults and have a lower heat tolerance (2). Based on the above information, all participants should be advised of the following:
   a. Adequate training and fitness are important for full enjoyment of the run and also to prevent heat-related injuries (13,28,29,39).
   b. Prior training in the heat will promote heat acclimatization and thereby reduce the risk of heat injury. It is wise to do as much training as possible at the time of day at which the race will be held (20).
   c. Fluid consumption before and during the race will reduce the risk of heat injury, particularly in longer runs such as the marathon (6,14,47).
   d. Illness prior to or at the time of the event should preclude competition (41).
   e. Participants should be advised of the early symptoms of heat injury. These include clumsiness, stumbling, excessive sweating (and also cessation of sweating), headache, nausea, dizziness, apathy, and any gradual impairment of consciousness (42).
   f. Participants should be advised to choose a comfortable speed and not to run faster than conditions warrant (18,33).
   g. Participants are advised to run with a partner, each being responsible for the other's well-being (33).

Background for Position Stand

There has been an exponential rise in the number of fun runs and races in recent years and, as would be expected, a similar increase in the number of running-related injuries. Minor injuries such as bruises, blisters and musculoskeletal injuries are most common (41,45). Myocardial infarction or cardiac arrest is, fortunately, very rare and occurs almost exclusively in patients with symptomatic heart disease (44). Hypoglycemia may be seen occasionally in normal runners (11) and has been observed following marathons (21) and shorter fun runs (41).

The most serious injuries in fun runs and races are related to problems of thermoregulation. In the shorter races, 10 km (6.2 miles) or less, hyperthermia with the attendant problems of heat exhaustion and heat syncope dominates, even on relatively cool days (4,5,10,15,16,18,27,41). In longer races, heat problems are common on warm or hot days (31), but on moderate to cold days, hypothermia may be a real risk to some participants (23).

Thermoregulation and hyperthermia. Fun runners may experience hyperthermia or hypothermia, depending on the environmental conditions and clothing worn. The adequately clothed runner is capable of withstanding a wide range of environmental temperatures. Hyperthermia is the potential problem in warm and hot weather, when the body's rate of heat production is greater than its ability to dissipate this heat (1). In cold weather, scanty clothing may provide inadequate protection from the environment and hypothermia may develop, particularly towards the end of a long race when running speed and, therefore, heat production, are reduced.

During intense exercise, heat production in contracting muscles is 15–20 times that of basal metabolism and is sufficient to raise body core temperature in an average-size individual by 1°C every 5 min if no temperature-regulating mechanisms were activated (25). With increased heat production, thermal receptors in the hypothalamus sense the increased body temperature and respond with an increased cutaneous circulation; thus, the excess heat is transferred to the skin surface to be dissipated by physical means, primarily the evaporation of sweat (9). The precise quantitative relationships in heat transfer are beyond the scope of this position stand, but are well reviewed elsewhere (24, 25).

When the rate of heat production exceeds that of heat loss for a sufficient period of time, thermal injury will occur. In long races, sweat loss can be significant and result in a total body water deficit of 6–10% of body weight (47). Such dehydration will subsequently reduce sweating and predispose the runner to hyperthermia, heat stroke, heat exhaustion, and muscle cramps (47). For a given level of dehydration, children have a greater increase in core temperature than do adults (2). Rectal temperatures have been reported above 40.6°C after races and fun runs (7,22,31,35) and as high as 42–43°C in fun run participants who have collapsed (32,34,41,42).

Fluid ingestion before and during prolonged running will minimize dehydration (and reduce the rate of increase in body core temperature) (7,14). However, in fun runs of less than 10 km, hyperthermia may occur in the absence of significant dehydration (41). Runners should avoid consuming large quantities of highly concentrated sugar solution during runs, as this may result in a decrease in gastric emptying (8,12).

Thermoregulation and hypothermia. Heat can be lost readily from the body when the rate of heat production is exceeded by heat loss (46). Even on moderately cool days, if the pace slows and/or if weather conditions become cooler en route, hypothermia may ensue (23). Several deaths have been reported from hypothermia during fun runs in mountain environments (30,40). Hypothermia is common in inexperienced marathon runners who frequently run the second half of the race much more slowly than the first half. Such runners may be able to maintain core temperature initially, but with the slow pace of the second half, especially on cool, wet, or windy days, hypothermia can develop (23).

Early symptoms and signs of hypothermia include shivering, euphoria, and an appearance of intoxication. As core temperature continues to fall, shivering may stop, lethargy and muscular weakness may occur with disorientation, hallucinations, and often a combative nature. If core temperature falls below 30°C, the victim may lose consciousness.

Organizers of distance races and fun runs and their medical support staff should anticipate the medical problems and be capable of responding to significant numbers of hyperthermic and/or hypothermic runners. Thermal injury can be minimized with appropriate education of participants and with adequate facilities, supplies, and support staff.

Appendix I
Measurement of Environmental Heat Stress

Ambient temperature is only one component of environmental heat stress; others are humidity, wind velocity, and radiant heat. Therefore, measurement of ambient temperature, dry bulb alone, is inadequate. The most useful and widely applied approach is web bulb globe temperature (WBGT).

WBGT = (0.7 Twb) + (0.2 Tg) + (0.1 Tdb), where Twb = temperature (web bulb thermometer), Tg = temperature (black globe thermometer), and Tdb = temperature (dry bulb thermometer).

The importance of wet bulb temperature can be readily appreciated, as it accounts for 70% of the index, whereas dry bulb temperature accounts for only 10%. A simple portable heat stress monitor which gives direct WBGT in degrees C or degrees F to monitor conditions during fun runs has proven useful (19).

Alternatively, if a means for readily assessing WBGT is not available from wet bulb, globe, and dry bulb temperatures, one can use the following equation (48):

$$WBGT = (0.567\ Tdb) + (0.393\ Pa) + 3.94$$

where Tdb = temperature (dry bulb thermometer) and Pa = environmental water vapor pressure. These environmental variables should be readily available from local weather or radio stations.

Instruments to measure WBGT are available commercially. Additional information may be obtained from the American College of Sports Medicine.

Appendix II
Use of Color-Coded Flags to Indicate the Risk of Thermal Stress*

1. A RED FLAG: High Risk: When WBGT is 23–28°C (73–82°F).
   This signal would indicate that all runners should be aware that heat injury is possible and any person particularly sensitive to heat or humidity should probably not run.

2. AN AMBER FLAG: Moderate Risk: When WBGT is 18–23°C (65–73°F).
   It should be remembered that the air temperature, probably humidity, and almost certainly the radiant heat at the beginning of the race will increase during the course of the race if conducted in the morning or early afternoon.

3. A GREEN FLAG: Low Risk: When WBGT is below 18°C (65°F).
   This in no way guarantees that heat injury will not occur, but indicates only that the risk is low.

4. A WHITE FLAG: Low Risk for hyperthermia, but possible risk for hypothermia: When WBGT is below 10°C (50°F).

Hypothermia may occur, especially in slow runners in long races, and in wet and windy conditions.

* This scale is determined for runners clad in running shorts, shoes and a T-shirt. In warmer weather, the less clothing the better. For males, wearing no shirt or a mesh top is better than wearing a T-shirt because the surface for evaporation is increased. However, in areas where radiant heat is excessive, a light top may be helpful.

Appendix III
Road Race Checklist

Medical Personnel
1. Have aid personnel available if the race is 10 km (6.2 miles) or longer, and run in warm or cold weather.
2. Recruit back-up personnel from existing emergency medical services (police, fire rescue, emergency medical service).
3. Notify local hospitals of the time and place of the road race.

Aid Stations
1. Provide major aid station at the finish point which is cordoned off from public access.
2. Equip the major aid station with the following supplies:
   —tent
   —cots
   —bath towels
   —water in large containers
   —ice in bag or ice chest or quick-cold packs
   —hose with spray nozzle
   —tables for medical supplies and equipment
   —stethoscopes
   —blood pressure cuffs
   —rectal thermometers or meters (range up to 43°C)
   —dressings
   —blankets
   —aluminum thermal sheets ("space blankets")
   —elastic bandages
   —splints
   —skin disinfectants
   —intravenous fluids (supervision by a physician is required).
3. Position aid stations along the route at 4 km (2.5 mile) intervals for races over 10 km and at the halfway point for shorter races.
4. Stock each aid station with enough fluid (cool water is the optimum) for each runner to have 300–360 ml (10–12 ounces) at each aid station. A margin of 25% additional cups should be available to account for spillage and double usage.

Communications/Surveillance
1. Set up communication between the medical personnel and the major aid station.
2. Arrange for a radio-equipped car or van to follow the race course, and provide radio contact with director.

Instructions to Runners
1. Apprise the race participants of potential medical problems in advance of the race so precautions may be followed.

Table 1. Equipment needed at aid stations and the field hospital (per 1000 runners).

Aid Stations

No.	Item
	ice in small plastic bags or quick-cold packs
5	stretchers (10 at 10 km and beyond)
5	blankets (10 at 10 km and beyond)
6 each	6 inch and 4 inch elastic bandages
½ case	4 × 4 inch gauze pads
½ case	1½ inch tape
½ case	surgical soap
	small instrument kits
	adhesive strips
	moleskin
½ case	petroleum jelly
2 each	inflatable arm and leg splints
	athletic trainer's kit

Field Hospital

No.	Item
10	stretchers
4	sawhorses
10–20	blankets (depending on environmental conditions)
10	intravenous set-ups
2 each	inflatable arm and leg splints
2 cases	1½ inch tape
2 cases each	elastic bandages (2, 4, and 6 inches)
2 cases	sheet wadding underwrap
2 cases	4 × 4 inch gauze pads
	adhesive strips
	moleskin
½ case	surgical soap
2	oxygen tanks with regulators and masks
2	ECG monitors with defibrillators
	ice in small plastic bags
	small instrument kits

Adapted from reference 26.

2. Advise the race director to announce the following information by loudspeaker immediately prior to the race:
   —the flag color; the risks for hyperthermia and/or hypothermia
   —location of aid stations and type of fluid available
   —reinforcement of warm weather or cold weather self-care.
3. Advise the race participants to print their names, addresses, and any medical problems on the back of the registration number.

Appendix IV
Medical Stations
General Guidelines

Staff for Large Races

1. Physician, podiatrist, nurse or EMT, a team of 3 per 1000 runners. Double or triple this number at the finish area.
2. One ambulance per 3000 runners at finish area; one cruising vehicle.
3. One physician to act as triage officer at finish.

Water

Estimate 1 liter (0.26 gallon) per runner per 16 km (10 miles), or roughly, per 60–90 min running time, and depending on number of stations.

For 10 km, the above rule is still recommended.

Cups = (number of entrants × number of stations) + 25% additional per station.

= (2 × number of entrants) extra at finish area.

Double this total if the course is out and back.

In cold weather, an equivalent amount of warm drinks should be available.

REFERENCES

1. ADOLPH, E.I. *Physiology of Man in the Desert.* New York: Interscience, 1947, pp. 5–43.
2. BAR-OR, O. Climate and the exercising child—a review. *Int. J. Sports Med.* 1:53–65, 1980.
3. BAR-OR, O., H.M. LUNDEGREN, and E.R. BUSKIRK. Heat tolerance of exercising lean and obese women. *J. Appl. Physiol.* 26:403–409, 1969.
4. BUSKIRK, E.R., P.F. IAMPIETRO, and D.E. BASS. Work performance after dehydration: effects of physical conditioning and heat acclimatization. *J. Appl. Physiol.* 12:189–194, 1958.
5. CLOWES, G.H.A., JR. and T.F. O'DONNELL, JR. Heat stroke. *N. Engl. J. Med.* 291:564–567, 1974.
6. COSTILL, D.L., R. COTE, E. MILLER, T. MILLER, and S. WYNDER. Water and electrolyte replacement during days of work in the heat. *Aviat. Space Environ. Med.* 46:795–800, 1970.
7. COSTILL, D.L., W.F. KAMMER, and A. FISHER. Fluid ingestion during distance running. *Arch. Environ. Health* 21:520–525, 1970.
8. COSTILL, D.L. and B. SALTIN. Factors limiting gastric emptying during rest and exercise. *J. Appl. Physiol.* 37:679–683, 1974.
9. ELLIS, F.P., A.N. EXTON-SMITH, K.G. FOSTER, and J.S. WEINER. Eccrine sweating and mortality during heat waves in very young and very old persons. *Isr. J. Med. Sci.* 12:815–817, 1976.
10. ENGLAND, A.C., III, D.W. FRASER, A.W. HIGHTOWER, et al. Preventing severe heat injury in runners: suggestions from the 1979 Peachtree Road Race experience. *Ann. Intern. Med.* 97:196–201, 1982.
11. FELIG, P., A. CHERIF, A. MINAGAWA, and J. WAHREN. Hypoglycemia during prolonged exercise in normal men. *N. Engl. J. Med.*
12. FORDTRAN, J.A. and B. SALTIN. Gastric emptying and intestinal absorption during prolonged severe excerise. *J. Appl. Physiol.* 23:331–335, 1967.
13. GISOLFI, C.V. and J. COHEN. Relationships among training, heat acclimation and heat tolerance in men and women: the controversy revisited. *Med. Sci. Sports* 11:56–59, 1979.
14. GISOLFI, C.V. and J.R. COPPING. Thermal effects of prolonged treadmill exercise in the heat. *Med. Sci. Sports* 6:108–113, 1974.
15. HANSON, P.G. and S.W. ZIMMERMAN. Exertional heatstroke in novice runners. *JAMA* 242:154–157, 1979.
16. HART, L.E., B.P. EGIER, A.G. SHIMIZU, P.J. TANDAN, and J.R. SUTTON. Exertional heat stroke: the runner's nemesis. *Can. Med. Assoc. J.* 122:1144–1150, 1980.
17. HAYMES, E.M., R.J. MCCORMICK, and E.R. BUSKIRK. Heat tolerance of exercising lean and obese prepubertal boys. *J. Appl. Physiol.* 39:457–461, 1975.
18. HUGHSON, R.L., H.J. GREEN, M.E. HOUSTON, J.A. THOMSON, D.R. MACLEAN, and J.R. SUTTON. Heat injuries in Canadian mass participation runs. *Can. Med. Assoc. J.* 122:1141–1144, 1980.
19. HUGHSON, R.L., L.A. STANDI, and J.M. MACKIE. Monitoring road racing in the heat. *Phys. Sportsmed.* 11(5):94–105, 1983.
20. KNOCHEI, J.P. Environmental heat illness: an eclectric review. *Arch. Intern. Med.* 133:841–864, 1974.
21. LEVINE, S.A., B. GORDON, and C.L. DERICK. Some changes in the chemical constituents of the blood following a marathon race. *JAMA* 82:1778–1779, 1924.
22. MARON, M.B., J.A. WAGNER, and S.M. HORVATH. Thermoregulatory responses during competitive distance running. *J. Appl. Physiol.* 42:909–914, 1977.
23. MAUGHAN, R.J., I.M. LIGHT, P.H. WHITING, and J.D.B. MILLER. Hypothermia, hyperkalemia, and marathon running. *Lancet* 11:1336, 1982.
24. NADEL, E.R. Control of sweating rate while exercising in the heat. *Med. Sci. Sports* 11:31–35, 1979.
25. NADEL, E.R., C.B. WENGER, M.F. ROBERTS, J.A.J. STOLWIJK, and E. CAFARELLI. Physiological defenses against hyperthermia of exercise. *Ann. NY Acad. Sci.* 301:98–109, 1977.
26. NOBLE, H.B. and D. BACHMAN. Medical aspects of distance race planning. *Phys. Sportsmed.* 7(6):78–84, 1979.
27. O'DONNELL, T.J., JR. Acute heatstroke. Epidemiologic, biochemical, renal and coagulation studies. *JAMA* 234:824–828, 1975.
28. PADOLF, K.B., R.L. BURSE, and R.F. GOLDMAN. Role of physical fitness in heat acclimatization, decay and reinduction. *Ergonomics* 20:399–408, 1977.
29. PIWONKA, R.W., S. ROBINSON, V.L. GAY, and R.S. MANALIS. Preacclimatization of men to heat by training. *J. Appl. Physiol.* 20:379–384, 1965.
30. PUGH, L.G.C.E. Cold stress and muscular exercise with special reference to accidental hypothermia. *Br. Med. J.* 2:333–337, 1967.
31. PUGH, L.G.C.E., J.L. CORBETT, and R.H. JOHNSON. Rectal temperatures, weight losses and sweat rates in marathon running. *J. Appl. Physiol.* 23:347–352, 1967.
32. RICHARDS, D., R. RICHARDS, P.J. SCHOFIELD, V. ROSS, and J.R. SUTTON. Management of heat exhaustion in Sydney's *The Sun* City-to-Surf fun runners. Med. J. Aust. 2:457–461, 1979.
33. RICHARDS, R., D. RICHARDS, P.J. SCHOFIELD, V. ROSS, and J.R. SUTTON. Reducing the hazards in Sydney's *The Sun* City-to-Surf fun runs, 1971 to 1979. *Med. J. Aust.* 2:453–457, 1979.
34. RICHARDS, R., D. RICHARDS, P.J. SCHOFIELD, V. ROSS, and J.R. SUTTON. Organization of *The Sun* City-to-Surf fun run, Sydney, 1979. *Med. J. Aust.* 2:470–474, 1979.
35. ROBINSON, S., S.L. WILEY, L.G. BOUDURANT, and S. MAMLIN, JR. Temperature regulation of men following heatstroke. *Isr. J. Med. Sci.* 12:786–795, 1976.
36. SHAPIRO, Y., A. MAGAZANIK, R. UDASSIN, G. BEN-BARUCH, E. SHVARTZ, and Y. SHOENFELD. Heat tolerance in former heatstroke patients. *Ann. Intern. Med.* 90:913–916, 1979.
37. SHIBOLET, S., R. COLL, T. GILAT, and E. SOHAR. Heatstroke: its clinical picture and mechanism in 36 cases. *Q. J. Med.* 36:525–547, 1967.
38. SHIBOLET, S., M.C. LANCASTER, and Y. DANON. Heat stroke: a review. *Aviat. Space Environ. Med.* 47:280–301, 1976.

306:895–900, 1982.

39. SHVARTZ, E., Y. SHAPIRO, A. MAGAZANIK, et al. Heat acclimation, physical fitness, and responses to exercise in temperate and hot environments. *J. Appl. Physiol.* 43:678–683, 1977.

40. SUTTON, J. Community jogging vs. arduous racing. *N. Engl. J. Med.* 286:951, 1972.

41. SUTTON, J., M.J. COLEMAN, A.P. MILLAR, L. LAZARUS, and P. RUSSO. The medical problems of mass participation in athletic competition. The "City-to-Surf" race. *Med. J. Aust.* 2:127–133, 1972.

42. SUTTON, J.R. Heat illness. In: *Sports Medicine*, R.H. Strauss (Ed.). Philadelphia: W.B. Saunders, 1984, pp. 307–322.

43. SUTTON, J.R. and O. BAR-OR. Thermal illness in fun running. *Am. Heart J.* 100:778–781, 1980.

44. THOMPSON, P.D., M.P. STERN, P. WILLIAMS, K. DUNCAN, W.L. HASKELL, and P.D. WOOD. Death during jogging or running. A study of 18 cases. *JAMA* 242:1265–1267, 1979.

45. WILLIAMS, R.S., D.D. SCHOCKEN, M. MOREY, and F.P. KOISCH. Medical aspects of competitive distance running. *Postgrad. Med.* 70:41–51, 1981.

46. WINSLOW, C.E.A., L.P. HERRINGTON, and A.P. GAGGE. Physiological reactions of the human body to various atmospheric humidities. *Am. J. Physiol.* 120:288–299, 1937.

47. WYNDHAM, C.H. and N.B. STRYDOM. The danger of inadequate water intake during marathon running. *S. Afr. Med. J.* 43:893–896, 1969.

48. YAGLOU, C.P. and D. MINARD. Control of heat casualties at military training centers. *AMA Arch. Ind. Health* 16:302–305, 1957.

**AMERICAN COLLEGE
of SPORTS MEDICINE**™
POSITION STAND

The Use of Anabolic-Androgenic Steroids in Sports

Based on a comprehensive literature survey and a careful analysis of the claims concerning the ergogenic effects and the adverse effects of anabolic-androgenic steroids, it is the position of the American College of Sports Medicine that:

1. Anabolic-androgenic steroids in the presence of an adequate diet can contribute to increases in body weight, often in the lean mass compartment.
2. The gains in muscular strength achieved through high-intensity exercise and proper diet can be increased by the use of anabolic-androgenic steroids in some individuals.
3. Anabolic-androgenic steroids do not increase aerobic power or capacity for muscular exercise.
4. Anabolic-androgenic steroids have been associated with adverse effects on the liver, cardiovascular system, reproductive system, and psychological status in therapeutic trials and in limited research on athletes. Until further research is completed, the potential hazards of the use of the anabolic-androgenic steroids in athletes must include those found in therapeutic trials.
5. The use of anabolic-androgenic steroids by athletes is contrary to the rules and ethical principles of athletic competition as set forth by many of the sports governing bodies. The American College of Sports Medicine supports these ethical principles and deplores the use of anabolic-androgenic steroids by athletes.

This document is a revision of the 1977 position stand of the American College of Sports Medicine concerning anabolic-androgenic steroids (4).

Background

In 1935 the long-suspected positive effect of androgens on protein anabolism was documented (56). Subsequently, this effect was confirmed (53,77), and the development of 19-nortestosterone heralded the synthesis of steroids that have greater anabolic properties than natural testosterone but less of its virilizing effect (39). The use of androgenic steroids by athletes began in the early 1950s (106) and has increased through the years (60,62,83,98,104,106), despite warnings about potential adverse reactions (4,83,106,112) and the banning of these substances by sports governing bodies.

Anabolic-Androgenic Steroids, Body Composition and Athletic Performance

Body composition. Animal studies investigating the effect of anabolic-androgenic steroids on body composition have shown increases in lean body mass, nitrogen retention and muscle growth in castrated males (37,57,58) and normal females (26,37,71). The effects of anabolic-androgenic steroids on the body weights of normal, untrained, male animals (37,40,71,105,114), treadmill-trained (43,97) or isometrically-trained rats (82), or strength-trained monkeys (80) have been minimal to absent; however, the effects of steroids on animals undergoing heavy resistance training have not been adequately studied. Human males who are deficient in natural androgens by castration or other causes have shown significant increases in nitrogen retention and muscular development with anabolic-androgenic steroid therapy (23,58,103). Human males and females involved in experimental (38) and therapeutic trials of anabolic steroids (15,16,93) have shown increases in body weight.

The majority of the strength-training studies in which body weight was reported showed greater increases in weight under steroid treatment than under placebo (17,41,42,50,61,74,94,96,107). Other training studies have reported no significant changes in body weight (21,27,31,34,100,108). The weight gained was determined to be lean body mass in three studies that made this determination with hydrostatic weighing techniques (41,42,107). Four other studies found no significant differences in lean body mass between steroid and placebo treatments (17,21,27,34), but in two of those the mean differences favored the steroid treatment (21,27). The extent to which increased water retention accounts for steroid-induced changes in body composition is controversial (17,42) and has yet to be resolved.

In summary, anabolic-androgenic steroids can contribute to an increase in body weight in the lean mass compartment of the body. The amount of weight gained in the training studies has been small but statistically significant.

Muscular strength. Strength is an important factor in many athletic events. The literature concerning the efficacy of anabolic steroids for promoting strength development is controversial. Many factors contribute to the development of strength, including heredity, intensity of training, diet, and the status of the psyche (112). It is very difficult to control all of these factors in an experimental design. The additional variable of dosage is included when drug research is undertaken. Some athletes claim that doses greater than therapeutic are necessary for strength gains (106) even though positive results have been reported using therapeutic (low-dose) regimens (50,74,94,107). Double-blind studies using anabolic-androgenic steroids are also difficult to conduct because of the physical and/or psychological effects of the drug that, for example, allowed 100% of the participants in one "double-blind" study to correctly identify the steroid phase of the experiment (32). The placebo effect has been shown to be a factor in studies of anabolic-androgenic steroids as in all drug studies (6).

In animal studies, the combination of anabolic-androgenic steroids and overload training has not produced larger gains in force production than training alone (80,97). However, steroid-induced gains in strength have been reported in experienced (42,74, 94,107) and inexperienced weight trainers (50,51,96) with (50,51,74,94) and without dietary control or supplemental protein (42,96). In contrast, no positive effect of steroids on gains in strength over those produced by training alone were reported in other studies involving experienced (21,34,54) and inexperienced weight trainers (17,27,31,41,54,61,100,108) with (21,34,61,100) and without dietary control or supplemental protein (17,27, 31,41,54,108). The studies that reported no changes in strength with anabolic-androgenic steroids have been criticized (112) for the use of inexperienced weight trainers, lack of dietary control, low-intensity training (17,27,31,61), and nonspecific testing of strength (21). The studies that have shown strength gains with the use of anabolic-androgenic steroids have been criticized (83) for inadequate numbers of subjects (74,94,107), improper statistical designs, inadequate execution, and the unsatisfactory reporting of experimental results.

There have been no studies of the effects of the massive doses of steroids used by some athletes over periods of several years. Similarly, there have been no studies of the use of anabolic-androgenic steroids and training in women or children. Theoretically, anabolic and androgenic effects would be greater in women and children because they have naturally lower levels of androgens than men.

Three proposed mechanisms for the actions of the anabolic-androgenic steroids for increases in muscle strength are:

1. Increase in protein synthesis in the muscle as a direct action of the anabolic-androgenic steroid (81,82,92).
2. Blocking of the catabolic effect of glucocorticoids after exercise by increasing the amount of anabolic-androgenic hormone available (1,92,112).
3. Steroid-induced enhancement of aggressive behavior

that promotes a greater quantity and quality of weight training (14).

In spite of the controversial and sometimes contradictory results of the studies in this area, it can be concluded that the use of anabolic-androgenic steroids, especially by experienced weight trainers, can often increase strength gains beyond those seen with training and diet alone. This positive effect on strength is usually small and obviously is not exhibited by all individuals. The explanation for this variability in steroid effects is unclear. When small increments in strength occur, they can be important in athletic competition.

Aerobic capacity. The effect of anabolic-androgenic steroids on aerobic capacity has also been questioned. The potential of these drugs to increase total blood volume and hemoglobin (88) might suggest a positive effect of steroids on aerobic capacity. However, only three studies indicated positive effects (3,51,54), and there has been no substantiation of these results in subsequent studies (27,41,50,52). Thus, the majority of evidence shows no positive effect of anabolic-androgenic steroids on aerobic capacity over aerobic training alone.

Adverse Effects

Anabolic-androgenic steroids have been associated with many undesirable or adverse effects in laboratory studies and therapeutic trials. The effects of major concern are those on the liver, cardiovascular, and reproductive systems, and on the psychological status of individuals who are using the anabolic-androgenic steroids.

Adverse effects on the liver. Impaired excretory function of the liver, resulting in jaundice, has been associated with anabolic-androgenic steroids in a number of therapeutic trials (76,84,90). The possible cause-and-effect nature of this association is strengthened by the observation of jaundice remission after discontinuance of the drug (76,84). In studies of athletes using anabolic-androgenic steroids (65 athletes tested) (89,98,104), no evidence of cholestasis has been found.

Structural changes in the liver following anabolic steroid treatment have been found in animals (95,101) and in humans (73,86). Conclusions concerning the clinical significance of these changes on a short- or long-term basis have not been drawn. Investigations in athletes for these changes have not been performed, but there is no reason to believe that the athlete using anabolic-androgenic steroids is immune from these effects of the drugs.

The most serious liver complications associated with anabolic-androgenic steroids are peliosis hepatis (blood-filled cysts in the liver of unknown etiology) and liver tumors. Cases of peliosis hepatis have been reported in individuals treated with anabolic-androgenic steroids for various conditions (7–10,13,35,65,66,70,88,102).

Rupture of the cysts or liver failure resulting from the condition was fatal in some individuals (9,70,102). In other case reports the condition was an incidental finding at autopsy (8,10,66). The possible cause-and-effect nature of the association between peliosis hepatis and the use of anabolic-androgenic steroids is strengthened by the observation of improvement in the condition after discontinuance of drug therapy in some cases (7,35). There are no reported cases of this condition in athletes using anabolic-androgenic steroids, but investigations specific for this disorder have not been performed in athletes.

Liver tumors have been associated with the use of anabolic-androgenic steroids in individuals receiving these drugs as a part of their treatment regimen (28,29,49,67,69,99,115). These tumors are generally benign (29,67,69,115), but there have been malignant lesions associated with individuals using these drugs (28,99,115). The possible cause-and-effect nature of this association between the use of the drug and tumor development is strengthened by a report of tumor regression after cessation of drug treatment (49). The 17-alpha-alkylated compounds are the specific family of anabolic steroids indicted in the development of liver tumors (46,49). There is one reported case of a 26-year-old male body builder who died of liver cancer after having abused a variety of anabolic steroids for at least four years (75). The testing necessary for discovery of these tumors is not commonly performed, and it is possible that other tumors associated with steroid use by athletes have gone undetected.

Blood tests of liver function have been reported to be unchanged with steroid use in some training studies (31,41,54,94) and abnormal in other training studies (32,51) and in tests performed on athletes known to be using anabolic-androgenic steroids (54,89,104). However, the lesions of peliosis hepatis and liver tumors do not always result in bloot test abnormalities (8,28,29, 49,67,115), and some authors state that liver radioisotope scans, ultrasound, or computed tomography scans are needed for diagnosis (28,29,113).

In summary, liver function tests have been shown to be adversely affected by anabolic-androgenic steroids, especially the 17-alpha-alkylated compounds. The short- and long-term consequences of these changes, though potentially hazardous, have yet to be reported in athletes using these drugs.

Adverse effects on the cardiovascular system. The steroid-induced changes that may affect the development of cardiovascular disease include hyperinsulinism and altered glucose tolerance (111), decreased high-density lipoprotein cholesterol levels (72,98), and elevated blood pressure (68). These effects are variable for different individuals in various clinical situations. Triglycerides are lowered by anabolic-androgenic steroids in certain individuals (24,72) and are increased in others (18,78). Histological examinations of myofibrils and

mitochondria from cardiac tissue obtained from laboratory animals have shown that administration of anabolic steroids leads to pathological alterations in these structures (5,11,12). The cardiovascular effects of the anabolic-androgenic steroids, though potentially hazardous, need further research before any conclusions can be made.

Adverse effects on the male reproductive system. The effects of the anabolic-androgenic steroids on the male reproductive system are oligospermia (small number of sperm) and azoospermia (lack of sperm in the semen), decreased testicular size, abnormal appearance of testicular biopsy material, and reductions in testosterone and gonadotropic hormones. These effects have been shown in training studies (19,41,100), studies of normal volunteers (38), therapeutic trials (44), and studies of athletes who were using anabolic-androgenic steroids (55,79,104). In view of the changes shown in the pituitary-gonadal axis, the dysfunction accounting for these abnormalities is believed to be steroid-induced suppression of gonadotrophin production (19,36,38,79). The changes in these hormones are ordinarily reversible after cessation of drug treatment, but the long-term effects of altering the hypothalamic-pituitary-gonadal axis remain unknown. However, there is a report of residual abnormalities in testicular morphology of healthy men 6 months after discontinuing steroid use (38). It has been reported that the metabolism of androgens to estrogenic compounds may lead to gynecomastia in males (23,58,98,112).

Adverse effects on the female reproductive system. The effects of androgenic steroids on the female reproductive system include reduction in circulating levels of luteinizing hormone, follicle-stimulating hormone, estrogens, and progesterone; inhibition of folliculogenesis and ovulation; and menstrual cycle changes including prolongation of the follicular phase, shortening of the luteal phase, and amenorrhea (20,63,91).

Adverse effects on psychological status. In both sexes, psychological effects of anabolic-androgenic steroids include increases or decreases in libidio, mood swings, and aggressive behavior (38,98), which is related to plasma testosterone levels (25,85). Administration of steroids causes changes in the electroencephalogram similar to those seen with psycho-stimulant drugs (47,48). The possible ramifications of uncontrollably aggressive and possible hostile behavior should be considered prior to the use of anabolic-androgenic steroids.

Other adverse effects. Other side effects associated with the anabolic-androgenic steroids include: ataxia (2); premature epiphysial closure in youths (23,58,64,109,110); virilization in youths and women, including hirsutism (45), clitoromegaly (63,112), and irreversible deepening of the voice (22,33); acne; temporal hair recession; and alopecia (45). These adverse reactions can occur with the use of anabolic-androgenic steroids and are believed to be dependent on the type of steroid, dosage and duration of drug use (58). There is no method for predicting which individuals are more likely to develop these adverse effects, some of which are potentially hazardous.

The Ethical Issue

Equitable competition and fair play are the foundation of athletic competition. If competition is to remain on this foundation, rules are necessary. The International Olympic Committee (IOC) has defined "doping" as "the administration of or the use by a competing athlete of any substance foreign to the body or of any physiological substance taken in abnormal quantity or taken by an abnormal route of entry into the body, with the sole intention of increasing in an artificial and unfair manner his performance in competition." Accordingly, the medically unjustified use of anabolic steroids with the intention of gaining an athletic advantage is clearly unethical. Anabolic-androgenic steroids are listed as banned substances by the IOC in accordance with the rules against doping. The American College of Sports Medicine supports the position that the eradication of anabolic-androgenic steroids use by athletes is in the best interest of sport and endorses the development of effective procedures for drug detection and of policies that exclude from competition those athletes who refuse to abide by the rules.

The "win at all cost" attitude that has pervaded society places the athlete in a precarious situation. Testimonial evidence suggests that some athletes would risk serious harm and even death if they could obtain a drug that would ensure their winning an Olympic gold medal. However, the use of anabolic-androgenic steroids by athletes is contrary to the ethical principles of athletic competition and is deplored.

REFERENCES

1. AAKVAAG, A., O. BENTDOL, K. QUIGSTOD, P. WALSTOD, H. RENNINGEN, and F. FONNUM. Testosterone and testosterone binding globulin (TeBg) in young men during prolonged stress. *Int. J. Androl.* 1:22–31, 1978.
2. AGRAWAL, B. L. Ataxia caused by fluoxymesterone therapy in breast cancer. *Arch. Intern. Med.* 141:953–959, 1981.
3. ALBRECHT, H. and E. ALBRECHT. Ergometric, rheographic, reflexographic and electrographic tests at altitude and effects of drugs on human physical performance. *Fed. Proc.* 28:1262–1267, 1969.
4. American College of Sports Medicine. Position statement on the use and abuse of anabolic-androgenic steroids in sports. *Med. Sci. Sports* 9(4):xi–xiii, 1977.
5. APPELL, H.-J., B. HELLER-UMPFENBACH, M. FERAUDI, and H. WEICKER. Ultrastructural and morphometric investigations on the effects of training and administration of anabolic steroids on the myocardium of guinea pigs. *Int. J. Sports Med.* 4:268–274, 1983.
6. ARIEL, G. and W. SAVILLE. Anabolic steroids: the physiological effects of placebos. *Med. Sci. Sports* 4:124–126, 1972.
7. ARNOLD, G. L. and M. M. KAPLAN. Peliosis hepatis due to oxymetholone—a clinically benign disorder. *Am. J. Gastroenterol.* 71:213–216, 1979.
8. ASANO, A., H. WAKASA, S. KAISE, T. NISHIMAKI, and R. KASUKAWA. Peliosis hepatis. Report on two autopsy cases with a review of literature. *Acta Pathol. Jpn.* 32:861–877, 1982.
9. BAGHERI, S. and J. BOYER. Peliosis hepatis associated with anabolic-androgenic steroid therapy—a severe form of hepatic injury. *Ann. Intern. Med.* 81:610–618, 1974.
10. BANK, J. I., D. LYKKEBO, and I. HAGERSTRAND. Peliosis hepatis in a child. *Acta Ped. Scand.* 67:105–107, 1978.
11. BEHRENDT, H. Effect of anabolic steroid on rat heart muscle cells. I. Intermediate filaments. *Cell Tissue Res.* 180:305–315, 1977.
12. BEHRENDT, H. and H. BOFFIN. Myocardial cell lesions caused by anabolic hormone. *Cell Tissue Res.* 181:423–426, 1977.
13. BENJAMIN, D. C. and B. SHUNK. A fatal case of peliosis of the liver and spleen. *Am. J. Dis. Child.* 132:207–208, 1978.
14. BROOKS, R. V. Anabolic steroids and athletes. *Phys. Sportsmed.* 8(3):161–163, 1980.
15. BUCHWALD, D., S. ARGYRES, R. E. EASTERLING, et al. Effects of Nandrolone Decanoate on the anemia of chronic hemodialysis patients. *Nephron* 18:232–238, 1977.
16. CARTER, C. H. The anabolic steroid, Stanozolol, its evaluation in debilitated children. *Clin. Pediatr.* 4:671–680, 1965.
17. CASNER, S. W., R. G. EARLY, and B. R. CARLSON. Anabolic steroid effects on body composition in normal young men. *J. Sports Med. Phys. Fitness* 11:98–103, 1971.
18. CHOI, E. S. K., T. CHUNG, R. S. MORRISON, C. MYERS, and M. S. GREENBERG. Hypertriglyceridemia in hemodialysis patients during oral dromostanolone therapy for anemia. *Am. J. Clin. Nutr.* 27:901–904, 1974.
19. CLERICO, A., M. FERDEGHINI, C. PALOMBO, et al. Effects of anabolic treatment on the serum levels of gonadotropins, testosterone, prolactin, thyroid hormones and myoglobin of male athletes under physical training. *J. Nuclear Med. Allied Sci.* 25:79–88, 1981.
20. COX, D. W., W. L. HEINRICHS, C. A. PAULSEN, et al. Perturbations of the human menstrual cycle by oxymetholone. *Am. J. Obstet. Gynecol.* 121:121–126, 1975.
21. CRIST, D. M., P. J. STACKPOLE, and G. T. PEAKE. Effects of androgenic-anabolic steroids on neuromuscular power and body composition. *J. Appl. Physiol.* 54:366–370, 1983.
22. DAMSTE, P. H. Voice change in adult women caused by virilizing agents. *J. Speech Hear. Disord.* 32:126–132, 1967.
23. DORFMAN, R. I. and R. A. SHIPLEY. *Androgens: Biochemistry, Physiology and Clinical Significance.* New York: J. Wiley and Sons, 1956.
24. DOYLE, A. E., N. B. PINKUS, and J. GREEN. The use of oxandrolone in hyperlipidaemia. *Med. J. Australia* 1:127–129, 1974.
25. EHRENKRANZ, J., E. BLISS, and M. H. SHEARD. Plasma testosterone correlation with aggressive behavior and social dominance in man. *Psychosom. Med.* 36:469–475, 1974.
26. EXNER, G. U., H. W. STAUDTE, and D. PETTE. Isometric training of rats—effects upon fast and slow muscle and modification by an anabolic hormone (Nandrolone Decanoate) I. Female rats. *Pflügers Arch.* 345:1–14, 1973.
27. FAHEY, T. D. and C. H. BROWN. The effects of an anabolic steroid on the strength, body composition and endurance of college males when accompanied by a weight training program. *Med. Sci. Sports* 5:272–276, 1973.
28. FALK, H., L. THOMAS, H. POPPER, and H. G. ISHAK. Hepatic angiosarcoma associated with anabolic-androgenic steroids. *Lancet* 2:1120–1123, 1979.
29. FARRELL, G. C., D. E. JOSHUA, R. F. UREN, P. J. BAIRD, K. W. PERKINS, and H. KRONENBERG. Androgen-induced hepatoma. *Lancet* 1:430, 1975.
30. FORSYTH, B. T. The effect of testosterone propionate at various protein calorie intakes in malnutrition after trauma. *J. Lab. Clin. Med.* 43:732–740, 1954.
31. FOWLER, W. M., JR., G. W. GARDNER, and G. H. EGSTROM. Effect of an anabolic steroid on physical performance in young men. *J. Appl. Physiol.* 20:1038–1040, 1965.
32. FREED, D. L., A. J. BANKS, D. LONGSON, and D. M. BURLEY. Anabolic steroids in athletics: crossover double-blind trial on weightlifters. *Br. Med. J.* 2:471–473, 1975.
33. GELDER, L. V. Psychosomatic aspects of endocrine disorders of the voice. *J. Commun. Disord.* 7:257–262, 1974.
34. GOLDING, L. A., J. E. FREYDINGER, and S. S. FISHEL. The effect of an androgenic-anabolic steroid and a protein supplement on size, strength, weight and body composition in athletes. *Phys. Sportsmed.* 2(6):39–45, 1974.

35. GROOS, G., O. H. ARNOLD, and G. BRITTINGER. Peliosis hepatis after long-term administration of oxymetholone. *Lancet* 1:874, 1974.

36. HARKNESS, R. A., B. H. KILSHAW, and B. M. HOBSON. Effects of large doses of anabolic steroids. *Br. J. Sports Med.* 9:70–73, 1975.

37. HEITZMAN, R. J. The effectiveness of anabolic agents in increasing rate of growth in farm animals; report on experiments in cattle. In: *Anabolic Agents in Animal Production*, F. C. Lu and J. Rendel (Eds.). Stuttgart: Georg Thieme Publishers, 1976, pp. 89–98.

38. HELLER, C. G., D. J. MOORE, C. A. PAULSEN, W. O. NELSON, and W. M. LAIDLAW. Effects of progesterone and synthetic progestins on the reproductive physiology of normal men. *Fed. Proc.* 18:1057–1065, 1959.

39. HERSHBERGER, J. G., E. G. SHIPLEY, and R. K. MEYER. Myotrophic activity of 19-nortestosterone and other steroids determined by modified levator ani muscle method. *Proc. Soc. Exper. Biol. Med.* 83:175–180, 1953.

40. HERVEY, G. R. and I. HUTCHINSON. The effects of testosterone on body weight and composition in the rat. *J. Endocrinol.* 57:xxiv–xxv, 1973.

41. HERVEY, G. R., I. HUTCHINSON, A. V. KNIBBS, et al. Anabolic effects of methandienone in men undergoing athletic training. *Lancet* 2:699–702, 1976.

42. HERVEY, G. R., A. V. KNIBBS, L. BURKINSHAW, et al. Effects of methandienone on the performance and body composition of men undergoing athletic training. *Clin. Sci.* 60:457–461, 1981.

43. HICKSON, R. C., W. W. HEUSNER, W. D. VAN HUSS, et al. Effects of Diabanol and high-intensity sprint training on body composition of rats. *Med. Sci. Sports* 8:191–195, 1976.

44. HOLMA, P. and H. ALDERCREUTZ. Effect of an anabolic steroid (metandienon) on plasma LH, FSH, and testosterone and on the response to intravenous administration of LRH. *Acta Endocrinol.* 83:856–864, 1976.

45. HOUSSAY, A. B. Effects of anabolic-androgenic steroids on the skin including hair and sebaceous glands. In: *Anabolic-Androgenic Steroids*, C. D. Kochakan (Ed.). New York: Springer-Verlag, 1976, pp. 155–190.

46. ISHAK, K. G. Hepatic lesions caused by anabolic and contraceptive steroids. *Sem. Liver Dis.* 1:116–128, 1981.

47. ITIL, T. M. Neurophysiological effects of hormones in humans: computer EEG profiles of sex and hypothalamic hormones. In: *Hormones, Behavior and Psychotherapy*, E. J. Sachar (Ed.). New York: Raven Press, 1976, pp. 31–40.

48. ITIL, T. M., R. CORA, S. AKPINAR, W. M. HERRMANN, and C. J. PATTERSON. Psychotropic action of sex hormones: computerized EEG in establishing the immediate CNS effects of steroid hormones. *Curr. Ther. Res.* 16:1147–1170, 1974.

49. JOHNSON, F. L., K. G. LERNER, M. SIEGEL, et al. Association of androgenic-anabolic steroid therapy with development of hepatocellular carcinoma. *Lancet* 2:1273, 1972.

50. JOHNSON, L. C., G. FISHER, L. J. SILVESTER, and C. C. HOFHEINS. Anabolic steroid: effects of strength, body weight, oxygen uptake and spermatogenesis upon mature males. *Med. Sci. Sports* 4:43–45, 1972.

51. JOHNSON, L. C. and J. P. O'SHEA. Anabolic steroid: effects on strength development. *Science* 164:957–959, 1969.

52. JOHNSON, L. C., E. S. ROUNDY, P. E. ALLSEN, A. G. FISHER, and L. J. SILVESTER. Effect of anabolic steroid treatment on endurance. *Med. Sci. Sports* 7:287–289, 1975.

53. KENYON, A. T., K. KNOWLTON, and I. SANDIFORD. The anabolic effects of the androgens and somatic growth in man. *Ann. Intern. Med.* 20:632–654, 1944.

54. KEUL, J., H. DEUS, and W. KINDERMAN. Anabole hormone: Schadigung, Leistungsfahigkeit und Stoffwechsel. *Med. Klin.* 71:497–503, 1976.

55. KILSHAW, B. H., R. A. HARKNESS, B. M. HOBSON, and A. W. M. SMITH. The effects of large doses of the anabolic steroid, methandrostenolone, on an athlete. *Clin. Endocrinol.* 4:537–541, 1975.

56. KOCHAKIAN, C. D. and J. R. MURLIN. The effect of male hormones on the protein and energy metabolism of castrate dogs. *J. Nutr.* 10:437–458, 1935.

57. KOCHAKIAN, C. D. and B. R. ENDAHL. Changes in body weight of normal and castrated rats by different doses of testosterone propionate. *Proc. Soc. Exper. Biol. Med.* 100:520–522, 1959.

58. KRUSKEMPER, H. L. *Anabolic Steroids.* New York: Academic Press, 1968, pp. 128–133, 162–164, 182.

59. LANDAU, R. L. The metabolic effects of anabolic steroids in man. In: *Anabolic-Androgenic Steroids*, C. D. Kochakian (Ed.). New York: Springer-Verlag, 1976, pp. 45–72.

60. LJUNGQVIST, A. The use of anabolic steroids in top Swedish athletes. *Br. J. Sports Med.* 9:82, 1975.

61. LOUGHTON, S. J. and R.O. RUHLING. Human strength and endurance responses to anabolic steroid and training. *J. Sports Med.* 17:285–296, 1977.

62. MacDOUGALL, J. D., D. G. SALE, G. C. B. ELDER, and J. R. SUTTON. Muscle ultrastructural characteristics of elite powerlifters and bodybuilders. *Eur. J. Applied Physiol.* 48:117–126, 1982.

63. MAHER, J. M., E. L. SQUIRES, J. L. VOSS, and R. K. SHIDELER. Effect of anabolic steroids on reproductive function of young mares. *J. Am. Vet. Med. Assoc.* 183:519–524, 1983.

64. MASON, A. S. Male precocity: the clinician's view. In: *The Endocrine Function of the Human Testis*, V. H. T. James, M. Serra, and L. Martini (Eds.). New York: Academic Press, 1974, pp. 131–143.

65. McDONALD, E. C.and C. E. SPEICHER. Peliosis hepatis associated with administration of oxymetholone. *JAMA* 240:243–244, 1978.

66. McGIVEN, A. R. Peliosis hepatis: case report and review of pathogenesis. *J. Pathol.* 101:283–285, 1970.

67. MEADOWS, A. T., J. L. NAIMAN, and M. VALDES-DAPENA. Hepatoma associated with androgen therapy for aplastic anemia. *J. Pediatr.* 85:109–110, 1974.

68. MESSERLI, F. H. and E. D. FROHLICH. High blood pressure: a side effect of drugs, poisons, and food. *Arch. Intern. Med.* 139:682–687, 1979.

69. MULVIHILL, J. J., R. L. RIDOLFI, F. R. SCHULTZ, M. S. BROZY, and P. B. T. HAUGHTON. Hepatic adenoma in Fanconi anemia treated with oxymetholone. *J. Pediatr.* 87:122–124, 1975.

70. NADELL, J. and J. KOSEK. Peliosis hepatis. *Arch. Pathol. Lab. Med.* 101:405–410, 1977.

71. NESHEIM, M. C. Some observations on the effectiveness of anabolic agents in increasing the growth rate of poultry. In: *Anabolic Agents in Animal Production*, F. C. Lu and J. Rendel (Eds.). Stuttgart: Georg Thieme Publishers, 1976, pp. 110–114.

72. OLSSON, A. G., L. ORO, and S. ROSSNER. Effects of oxandrolone on plasma lipoproteins and the intravenous fat tolerance in man. *Atherosclerosis* 19:337–346, 1974.

73. ORLANDI, F., A. JEZEQUEL, and A. MELLITI. The action of some anabolic steroids on the structure and the function of human liver cell. *Tijdschr. Gastro-Enterol.* 7:109–113, 1964.

74. O'SHEA, J. P. The effects of an anabolic steroid on dynamic strength levels of weightlifters. *Nutr. Rep. Int.* 4:363–370, 1971.

75. OVERLY, W. L., J. A. DANKOFF, B. K. WANG, and U. D. SINGH. Androgens and hepatocellular carcinoma in an athlete. *Ann. Intern. Med.* 100:158–159, 1984.

76. PALVA, I. P. and C. WASASTJERNA. Treatment of aplastic anaemia with methenolone. *Acta Haematol.* 47:13–20, 1972.

77. PAPANICOLAOU, G. N. and G. A. FALK. General muscular hypertrophy induced by androgenic hormone. *Science* 87:238–239, 1938.

78. REEVES, R. D., M. D. MORRIS, and G. L. BARBOUR. Hyperlipidemia due to oxymetholone therapy. *JAMA* 236:464–472, 1976.

79. REMES, K., P. VUOPIO, M. JARVINEN, M. HARKONEN, and H. ADLERCREUTZ. Effect of short-term treatment with an anabolic steroid (methandienone) and dehydroepiandrosterone sulphate on plasma hormones, red cell volume and 2,3-diphosphoglycerate in athletes. *Scand. J. Clin. Lab. Invest.* 37:577–586, 1977.

80. RICHARDSON, J. H. A comparison of two drugs on strength increase in monkeys. *J. Sports Med. Phys. Fitness* 17:251–254, 1977.

81. ROGOZKIN, V. A. The role of low molecular weight compounds in the regulation of skeletal muscle genome activity during exercise. *Med. Sci. Sports* 8:1–4, 1976.

82. ROGOZKIN, V. A. Anabolic steroid metabolism in skeletal mus-

cle. *J. Steroid Biochem.* 11:923–926, 1979.

83. RYAN, A. J. Anabolic steroids are fool's gold. *Fed. Proc.* 40:2682–2688, 1981.

84. SACKS, P., D. GALE, T. H. BOTHWELL, K. STEVENS. Oxymetholone therapy in aplastic and other refractory anaemias. *S. Afr. Med. J.* 46:1607–1615, 1972.

85. SCARAMELLA, T. J. and W. A. BROWN. Serum testosterone and aggressiveness in hockey players. *Psychosom. Med.* 40:262–265, 1978.

86. SCHAFFNER, F., H. POPPER, and V. PEREZ. Changes in bile canaliculi produced by norethandrolone: electron microscopic study of human and rat liver. *J. Lab. Clin. Med.* 56:623–628, 1960.

87. SHAHIDI, N. T. Androgens and erythropoeisis. *N. Engl. J. Med.* 289:72–80, 1973.

88. SHAPIRO, P., R. M. IKEDO, B. H. RUEBNER, M. H. CONNERS, C. C. HALSTED, and C. F. ABILDGAARD. Multiple hepatic tumors and peliosis hepatitis in Fanconi's anemia treated with androgens. *Am. J. Dis. Child.* 131:1104–1106, 1977.

89. SHEPHARD, R. J., D. KILLINGER, and T. FRIED. Responses to sustained use of anabolic steroid. *Br. J. Sports Med.* 11:170–173, 1977.

90. SKARBERG, K. O., L. ENGSTEDT, S. JAMESON, et al. Oxymetholone treatment in hypoproliferative anaemia. *Acta Haematol.* 49:321–330, 1973.

91. SMITH, K. D., L. J. RODRIGUEZ-RIGAU, R. K. TCHOLAKIAN, and E. STEINBERG. The relation between plasma testosterone levels and the lengths of phases of the menstrual cycle. *Fertil. Steril.* 32:403–407, 1979.

92. SNOCHOWSKI, M., E. DAHLBERG, E. ERIKSSON, and J. A. GUS-TAFSSON. Androgen and glucocorticoid receptors in human skeletal muscle cytosol. *J. Steroid Biochem.* 14:765–771, 1981.

93. SPIERS, A. S. D., S. F. DEVITA, M. J. ALLAR, S. RICHARDS, and N. SEDRANSK. Beneficial effects of an anabolic steroid during cytotoxic chemotherapy for metastatic cancer. *J. Med.* 12:433–445, 1981.

94. STAMFORD, B. A. and R. MOFFATT. Anabolic steroid: effectiveness as an ergogenic aid to experienced weight trainers. J. Sports Med. Phys. Fitness 14:191–197, 1974.

95. STANG-VOSS, C. and H-J. APPEL. Structural alterations of liver parenchyma induced by anabolic steroids. *Int. J. Sports Med.* 2:101–105, 1981.

96. STEINBACH, M. Uber den Einfluss Anaboler wirkstoffe auf Korpergewicht, Muskelkraft und Muskeltraining. *Sportarzt Sportmed.* 11:485–492, 1968.

97. STONE, M. H., M. E. RUSH, and H. LIPNER. Responses to intensive training and methandrostenolone administration: II. Hormonal, organ weights, muscle weights and body composition. *Pflugers Arch.* 375:147–151, 1978.

98. STRAUSS, R. H., H. E. WRIGHT, G. A. M. FINERMAN, and D. H. CATLIN. Side effects of anabolic steroids in weight-trained men. *Phys. Sportsmed.* 11(12):87–96, 1983.

99. STROMEYER, F. W., D. H. SMITH, and K. G. ISHAK. Anabolic steroid therapy and intrahepatic cholangiocarcinoma *Cancer* 43:440–443, 1979.

100. STROMME, S. B., H. D. MEEN, and A. AAKVAAG. Effects of an androgenic-anabolic steroid on strength development and plasma testosterone levels in normal males. *Med. Sci. Sports* 6:203–208, 1974.

101. TAYLOR, W., S. SNOWBALL, C. M. DICKSON, and M. LESNA. Alterations of liver architecture in mice treated with anabolic androgens and diethylnitrosamine. *NATO Adv. Study Inst. Series, Series A* 52:279–288, 1982.

102. TAXY, J. B. Peliosis: a morphologic curiosity becomes an iatrogenic problem. *Hum. Pathol.* 9:331–340, 1978.

103. TEPPERMAN, J. *Metabolic and Endocrine Physiology.* Chicago: Year Book Medical Publishers, 1973, p. 70.

104. THOMSON, D. P., D. R. PEARSON, and D. L. COSTILL. Use of anabolic steroids by national level athletes. *Med. Sci. Sports Exerc.* 13:111, 1981. (Abstract)

105. VANDERWAL, P. General aspects of the effectiveness of anabolic agents in increasing protein production in farm animals, in particular in bull calves. In: *Anabolic Agents in Animal Production,* F. C. Lu and J. Rendel (Eds.). Stuttgart: Georg Thieme Publishers, 1976, pp. 60–78.

106. WADE, N. Anabolic steroids: doctors denounce them, but athletes aren't listening. *Science* 176:1399–1403, 1972.

107. WARD, P. The effect of an anabolic steroid on strength and lean body mass. *Med. Sci. Sports* 5:277–282, 1973.

108. WEISS, V. and H. MULLER. Auf Frage der Beeinflussung des Krafttrainings durch Anabole Hormone. *Schweiz. Z. Sportmed.* 16:79–89, 1968.

109. WHITELAW, M. J., T. N. FOSTER, and W. H. GRAHAM. Methandrostenolone (Diabanol): a controlled study of its anabolic and androgenic effect in children. *Pediatric Pharm. Ther.* 68:291–296, 1966.

110. WILSON, J. D. and J. E. GRIFFIN. The use and misuse of androgens. *Metabolism* 29:1278–1295, 1980.

111. WOODARD, T. L., G. A. BURGHEN, A. E. KITABCHI, and J. A. WILIMAS. Glucose intolerance and insulin resistance in aplastic anemia treated with oxymetholone. *J. Clin. Endocrinol. Metab.* 53:905–908, 1981.

112. WRIGHT, J. E. Anabolic steroids and athletes. *Exerc. Sport Sci. Rev.* 8:149–202, 1980.

113. YAMAGISHI, M., A. HIRAOKA, and H. UCHINO. Silent hepatic lesions detected with computed tomography in aplastic anemia patients administered androgens for a long period. *Acta Haematol. Jpn.* 45:703–710, 1982.

114. YOUNG, M., H. R. CROOKSHANK, and L. PONDER. Effects of an anabolic steroid on selected parameters in male albino rats. *Res. Q.* 48:653–656, 1977.

115. ZEVIN, D., H. TURANI, A. COHEN, and J. LEVI. Androgen-associated hepatoma in a hemodialysis patient. *Nephron* 29:274–276, 1981.

AMERICAN COLLEGE
of SPORTS MEDICINE™

POSITION STAND

Proper and Improper
Weight Loss Programs

Millions of individuals are involved in weight reduction programs. With the number of undesirable weight loss programs available and a general misconception by many about weight loss, the need for guidelines for proper weight loss programs is apparent.

Based on the existing evidence concerning the effects of weight loss on health status, physiologic processes and body composition parameters, the American College of Sports Medicine makes the following statements and recommendations for weight loss programs.

For the purposes of this position stand, body weight will be represented by two components, fat and fat-free (water, electrolytes, minerals, glycogen stores, muscular tissue, bone, etc.):

1. Prolonged fasting and diet programs that severely restrict caloric intake are scientifically undesirable and can be medically dangerous.
2. Fasting and diet programs that severely restrict caloric intake result in the loss of large amounts of water, electrolytes, minerals, glycogen stores, and other fat-free tissue (including proteins within fat-free tissues), with minimal amounts of fat loss.
3. Mild calorie restriction (500–1000 kcal less than the usual daily intake) results in a smaller loss of water, electrolytes, minerals, and other fat-free tissue, and is less likely to cause malnutrition.
4. Dynamic exercise of large muscles helps to maintain fat-free tissue, including muscle mass and bone density, and results in losses of body weight. Weight loss resulting from an increase in energy expenditure is primarily in the form of fat weight.
5. A nutritionally sound diet resulting in mild calorie restriction coupled with an endurance exercise program along with behavioral modification of existing eating habits is recommended for weight reduction. The rate of sustained weight loss should not exceed 1 kg (2 lb) per week.
6. To maintain proper weight control and optimal body fat levels, a lifetime commitment to proper eating habits and regular physical activity is required.

Research Background for the Position Stand

Each year millions of individuals undertake weight loss programs for a variety of reasons. It is well known that obesity is associated with a number of health-related problems (3,4,57). These problems include impairment of cardiac function due to an increase in the work of the heart (2) and to left ventricular dysfunction (1,40); hypertension (6,22,80); diabetes (83,97); renal disease (95); gall bladder disease (55,72); respiratory dysfunction (19); joint diseases and gout (90); endometrial cancer (15); abnormal plasma lipid and lipoprotein concentrations (56,74); problems in the administration of anesthetics during surgery (93); and impairment of physical working capacity (49). As a result, weight reduction is frequently advised by physicians for medical reasons. In addition, there are a vast number of individuals who are on weight reduction programs for aesthetic reasons.

It is estimated that 60–70 million American adults and at least 10 million American teenagers are overfat (49). Because millions of Americans have adopted unsupervised weight loss programs, it is the opinion of the American College of Sports Medicine that guidelines are needed for safe and effective weight loss programs. This position stand deals with desirable and undesirable weight loss programs. Desirable weight loss programs are defined as those that are nutritionally sound and result in maximal losses in fat weight and minimal losses of fat-free tissue. Undesirable weight loss programs are defined as those that are not nutritionally sound, that result in large losses of fat-free tissue, that pose potential serious medical complications, and that cannot be followed for long-term weight maintenance.

Therefore, a desirable weight loss program is one that:

1. Provides a caloric intake not lower than 1200 kcal·d^{-1} for normal adults in order to get a proper blend of foods to meet nutritional requirements. (Note: this requirement may change for children, older individuals, athletes, etc.).
2. Includes foods acceptable to the dieter from the viewpoints of socio-cultural background, usual habits, taste, cost, and ease in acquisition and preparation.
3. Provides a negative caloric balance (not to exceed 500–1000 kcal·d^{-1} lower than recommended), resulting in gradual weight loss without metabolic derangements. Maximal weight loss should be 1 kg·wk^{-1}.
4. Includes the use of behavior modification techniques

to identify and eliminate dieting habits that contribute to improper nutrition.

5. Includes an endurance exercise program of at least 3 d/wk, 20–30 minutes in duration, at a minimum intensity of 60% of maximum heart rate (refer to ACSM Position Stand on the *Recommended Quantity and Quality of Exercise for Developing and Maintaining Fitness in Healthy Adults, Med. Sci. Sports* 10:vii, 1978).

6. Provides that the new eating and physical activity habits can be continued for life in order to maintain the achieved lower body weight.

1. Since the early work of Keys et al. (50) and Bloom (16), which indicated that marked reduction in caloric intake or fasting (starvation or semistarvation) rapidly reduced body weight, numerous fasting, modified fasting, and fad diet and weight loss programs have emerged. While these programs promise and generally cause rapid weight loss, they are associated with significant medical risks.

The medical risks associated with these types of diet and weight loss programs are numerous. Blood glucose concentrations have been shown to be markedly reduced in obese subjects who undergo fasting (18,32,74,84). Further, in obese non-diabetic subjects, fasting may result in impairment of glucose tolerance (10,52). Ketonuria begins within a few hours after fasting or low-carbohydrate diets are begun (53), and hyperuricemia is common among subjects who fast to reduce body weight (18). Fasting also results in high serum uric acid levels with decreased urinary output (59). Fasting and low-calorie diets also result in urinary nitrogen loss and a significant decrease in fat-free tissue (7,11,17,42,101; see section 2). In comparison to ingestion of a normal diet, fasting substantially elevates urinary excretion of potassium (10,32,37,52,53,78). This, coupled with the aforementioned nitrogen loss, suggests that the potassium loss is due to a loss of lean tissue (78). Other electrolytes, including sodium (32,53), calcium (30,84), magnesium (30,84), and phosphate (84), have been shown to be elevated in urine during prolonged fasting. Reductions in blood volume and body fluids are also common with fasting and fad diets (18). This can be associated with weakness and fainting (32). Congestive heart failure and sudden death have been reported in subjects who fasted (48,79,80) or markedly restricted their caloric intake (79). Myocardial atrophy appears to contribute to sudden death (79). Sudden death may also occur during refeeding (25,79). Untreated fasting has also been reported to reduce serum iron binding capacity, resulting in anemia (47,73,89). Liver glycogen levels are depleted with fasting (38,60,63), and liver function (29,31,37,75,76,92) and gastrointestinal tract abnormalities (13,32,53, 65,85,91) are associated with fasting. While fasting and calorically restricted diets have been shown to lower serum cholesterol levels (88,96), a large portion of the cholesterol reduction is a result of lowered HDL-cholesterol levels (88,96). Other risks associated with fasting and low-calorie diets include lactic acidosis (12,26), alopecia (73), hypoalaninemia (34), edema (23,78), anuria (101), hypotension (18,32,78), elevated serum bilirubin (8,9), nausea and vomiting (53), alterations in thyroxine metabolism (71,91), impaired serum triglyceride removal and production (86), and death (25,37,48,61,80).

2. The major objective of any weight reduction program is to lose body fat while maintaining fat-free tissue. The vast majority of research reveals that starvation and low-calorie diets result in large losses of water, electrolytes, and other fat-free tissue. One of the best controlled experiments was conducted from 1944 to 1946 at the Laboratory of Phsyiological Hygiene at the University of Minnesota (50). In this study subjects had their base-line caloric intake cut by 45%, and body weight and body composition changes were followed for 24 wk. During the first 12 wk of semistarvation, body weight declined by 25.4 lb (11.5 kg) with only an 11.6-lb (5.3 kg) decline in body fat. During the second 12-wk period, body weight declined an additional 9.1 lb (4.1kg) with only a 6.1-lb (2.8 kg) decrease in body fat. These data clearly demonstrate that fat-free tissue significantly contributes to weight loss from semistarvation. Similar results have been reported by several other investigators. Buskirk et al. (20) reported that the 13.5-kg weight loss in six subjects on a low-calorie mixed diet averaged 76% fat and 24% fat-free tissue. Similarly, Passmore et al. (64) reported results of 78% of weight loss (15.3 kg) as fat and 22% as fat-free tissue in seven women who consumed a 400-kcal·d^{-1} diet for 45 d. Yang and Van Itallie (101) followed weight loss and body composition changes for the first 5 d of a weight loss program involving subjects consuming an 800-kcal mixed diet, an 800-kcal ketogenic diet, or undergoing starvation. Subjects on the mixed diet lost 1.3 kg of weight (59% fat loss, 3.4% protein loss, 37.6% water loss), subjects on the ketogenic diet lost 2.3 kg of weight (33.2% fat, 3.8% protein, 63.0% water), and subjects on starvation regimens lost 3.8 kg of weight (32.3% fat, 6.5% protein, 61.2% water). Grande (41) and Grande et al. (43) reported similar findings with a 1000-kcal carbohydrate diet. It was further reported that water restriction combined with 1000-kcal·d^{-1} of carbohydrate resulted in greater water loss and less fat loss.

Recently there has been some renewed speculation about the efficacy of the very-low-calorie diet (VLCD). Krotkiewski and associates (51) studied the effects on body weight and body composition after 3 wk on the so-called Cambridge diet. Two groups of obese middle-aged women were studied. One group had a VLCD only, while the second group had a VLCD combined with a 55-min/d, 3-d/wk exercise program. The VLCD-only group lost 6.2 kg in 3 wk, of which only 2.6 kg was fat loss, while the VLCD-plus-exercise group lost

6.8 kg in 3 wk with only a 1.9-kg body fat loss. Thus it can be seen that VLCD results in undesirable losses of body fat, and the addition of the normally protective effect of chronic exercise to VLCD does not reduce the catabolism of fat-free tissue. Further, with VLCD, a large reduction (29%) in HDL-cholesterol is seen (94).

3. Even mild calorie restriction (reduction of 500–1000 kcal·d^{-1} from base-line caloric intake), when used alone as a tool for weight loss, results in the loss of moderate amounts of water and other fat-free tissue. In a study by Goldman et al. (39), 15 female subjects consumed a low-calorie mixed diet for 7–8 wk. Weight loss during this period averaged 6.43 kg (0.85 kg·wk^{-1}), 88.6% of which was fat. The remaining 11.4% represented water and other fat-free tissue. Zuti and Golding (102) examined the effect of 500 kcal·d^{-1} calorie restriction on body composition changes in adult females. Over a 16-wk period the women lost approximately 5.2 kg; however, 1.1 kg of the weight loss (21%) was due to a loss of water and other fat-free tissue. More recently, Weltman et al. (96) examined the effects of 500 kcal·d^{-1} calorie restriction (from base-line levels) on body composition changes in sedentary middle-aged males. Over a 10-wk period subjects lost 5.95 kg, 4.03 kg (68%) of which was fat loss and 1.92 kg (32%) of which was loss of water and other fat-free tissue. Further, with calorie restriction only, these subjects exhibited a decrease in HDL-cholesterol. In the same study, the two other groups who exercised and/or dieted and exercised were able to maintain their HDL-cholesterol levels. Similar results for females have been presented by Thompson et al. (88). It should be noted that the decrease seen in HDL-cholesterol with weight loss may be an acute effect. There are data that indicate that stable weight loss has a beneficial effect on HDL-cholesterol (21,24,46,88).

Further, an additional problem associated with calorie restriction alone for effective weight loss is the fact that it is associated with a reduction in basal metabolic rate (5). Apparently exercise combined with calorie restriction can counter this response (14).

4. There are several studies that indicate that exercise helps maintain fat-free tissue while promoting fat loss. Total body weight and fat weight are generally reduced with endurance training programs (70), while fat-free weight remains constant (36,54,69,70,98) or increases slightly (62,96,102). Programs conducted at least 3 d/wk (66–69,98), of at least 20-min duration (58,69,98) and of sufficient intensity and duration to expend at least 300 kcal per exercise session, have been suggested as a threshold level for total body weight and fat weight reduction (27,44,69,70). Increasing caloric expenditure above 300 kcal per exercise session and increasing the frequency of exercise sessions will enhance fat weight loss while sparing fat-free tissue (54,102). Leon et al. (54) had six obese male subjects walk vigorously for 90 min, 5 d/wk for 16 wk. Work output progressed weekly to an energy expenditure of 1000–1200 kcal/session. At the end of 16 wk, subjects averaged 5.7 kg of weight loss with a 5.9-kg loss of fat weight and a 0.2-kg gain in fat-free tissue. Similarly, Zuti and Golding (102) followed the progress of adult women who expended 500 kcal/exercise session 5d/wk for 16 wk of exercise. At the end of 16 wk the women lost 5.8 kg of fat and gained 0.9 kg of fat-free tissue.

5. Review of the literature cited above strongly indicates that optimal body composition changes occur with a combination of calorie restriction (while on a well-balanced diet) plus exercise. This combination promotes loss of fat weight while sparing fat-free tissue. Data of Zuti and Golding (102) and Weltman et al. (96) support this contention. Calorie restriction of 500 kcal·d^{-1} combined with 3–5 d of exercise requiring 300–500 kcal per exercise session results in favorable changes in body composition (96,102). Therefore, the optimal rate of weight loss should be between 0.45–1 kg (1–2 lb) per wk. This seems especially relevant in light of the data which indicates that rapid weight loss due to low caloric intake can be associated with sudden death (79). In order to institute a desirable pattern of calorie restriction plus exercise, behavior modification techniques should be incorporated to identify and eliminate habits contributing to obesity and/or overfatness (28,33,35,81,87,99,100).

6. The problem with losing weight is that, although many individuals succeed in doing so, they invariably put the weight on again (45). The goal of an effective weight loss regimen is not merely to lose weight. Weight control requires a lifelong commitment, an understanding of our eating habits and a willingness to change them. Frequent exercise is necessary, and accomplishment must be reinforced to sustain motivation. Crash dieting and other promised weight loss cures are ineffective (45).

REFERENCES

1. ALEXANDER, J.K. and J.R. PETTIGROVE. Obesity and congestive heart failure. *Geriatrics* 22:101–108, 1967.
2. ALEXANDER, J.K and K.L. PETERSON. Cardiovascular effects of weight reduction. *Circulation* 45:310–318, 1972.
3. ANGEL, A. Pathophysiologic changes in obesity. *Can. Med. Assoc. J.* 119:1401–1406, 1978.
4. ANGEL, A. and D.A.K. RONCARI. Medical complications of obesity. *Can. med. Assoc. J.* 191:1408–1411, 1978.
5. APPELBAUM, M., J. BOSTSARRON, and D. LACATIS. Effect of caloric restriction and excessive caloric intake on energy expenditure. *Am. J. Clin. Nutr.* 24:1405–1409, 1971.
6. BACHMAN, L., V. FRESCHUSS, D. HALLBERG, and A. MELCHER. Cardiovascular function in extreme obesity. *Acta Med. Scand.* 193:437–446, 1972.
7. BALL, M.F. J.J. CANARY, and L.H. KYLE. Comparative effects of caloric restrictions and total starvation on body composition in obesity. *Ann. Intern. Med.* 67:60–67, 1967.
8. BARRETT, P.V.D. Hyperbilirubinemia of fasting. *JAMA* 217:1349–1353, 1971.
9. BARRETT, P.V.D. The effect of diet and fasting on the serum bilirubin concentration in the rat. *Gastroenterology* 60:572–576, 1971.
10. BECK, P., J.J.T. KOUMANS, C.A. WINTERLING, M.F. STEIN, W.H. DAUGHADAY, and D.M. KIPNIS. Studies on insulin and growth hormone secretion in human obesity. *J. Lab. Clin. Med.* 64:654–667, 1964.

11. BENOIT, F.L., R.L. MARTIN, and R.H. WATTEN. Changes in body composition during weight reduction in obesity. *Ann. Intern. Med.* 63:604–612, 1965.

12. BERGER, H. Fatal lactic acidosis during "crash" reducing diet. *N.Y. State J. Med.* 67:2258–2263, 1967.

13. BILLICH, C., G. BRAY, T.F. GALLAGHER, A.V. HOFFBRAND, and R. LEVITAN. Absorptive capacity of the jejunum of obese and lean subjects; effect of fasting. *Arch. Intern. Med.* 130:377–387, 1972.

14. BJORNTORP, P.L SJOSTROM, and L. SULLIVAN. The role of physical exercise in the management of obesity. In: *The Treatment of Obesity.* J.F. Munro (Ed.). Lancaster, England: MTP Press, 1979.

15. BLITZER, P.H., E. C. BLITZER, and A.A.RIMM. Association between teenage obesity and cancer in 56,111 women. *Prev. Med.* 5:20–31, 1976.

16. BLOOM, W.L. Fasting as an introduction to the treatment of obesity. *Metabolism* 8:214–220, 1959.

17. BOLINGER, R.E., B.P. LUKERT, R.W. BROWN, L. GUEVERA, and R. STEINBERG. Metabolic balances of obese subjects during fasting. *Arch. Intern. Med.* 118:3–8, 1966.

18. BRAY, G.A., M.B. DAVIDSON, and E.J. DRENICK. Obesity: a serious symptom. *Ann. Intern. Med.* 77:779–805, 1972.

19. BURWELL, C.S. E.D. ROBIN, R.D. WHALEY, and A.G. BICKELMANN. Extreme obesity associated with alveolar hypoventilation—a Pickwickian syndrome. *Am. J. Med.* 21:811–818, 1956.

20. BUSKIRK, E.R., R.H. THOMPSON, L. LUTWAK, and G.D. WHEDON. Energy balance of obese patients during weight reduction: influence of diet restriction and exercise. *Ann. NY Acad. Sci.* 110:918–940, 1963.

21. CAGGIULA, A.W., G. CHRISTAKIS, M. FERRAND, et al. The multiple risk factors intervention trial. IV Intervention on blood lipids. *Prev. Med.* 10:443–475, 1981.

22. CHAING, B.M., L.V. PERLMAN, and F.H. EPSTEIN. Overweight and hypertension: a review. *Circulation* 39:403–421, 1969.

23. COLLISON, D.R. Total fasting for up to 249 days. *Lancet* 1:112, 1967.

24. CONTALDO, F., P. STRAZULLO, A. POSTIGLIONE, et al. Plasma high density lipoprotein in severe obesity after stable weight loss. *Atherosclerosis* 37:163–167, 1980.

25. CRUICKSHANK, E.K. Protein malnutrition. In: Proceedings of a conference in Jamaica (1953), J.C. Waterlow (Ed.). Cambridge: University Press, 1955, p. 107.

26. CUBBERLEY, P.T., S.A. POLSTER, and C.L. SHULMAN. Lactic acidosis and death after the treatment of obesity by fasting. *N.Engl. J. Med.* 272:628–633, 1965.

27. CURETON, T.K. *The Physiological Effects of Exercise Programs Upon Adults.* Springfield, IL: C. Thomas Company, 1969.

28. DAHLKOETTER, J., E.J. CALLAHAN, and J. LINTON. Obesity and the unbalanced energy equation: exercise versus eating habit change. *J. Consult. Clin. Psychol.* 47:898–905, 1979.

29. DRENICK, E.J. The relation of BSP retention during prolonged fasts to changes in plasma volume. *Metabolism* 17:522–527, 1968.

30. DRENICK, E.J., I.F. HUNT, and M.E. SWENDSEID. Magnesium depletion during prolonged fasting in obese males. *J. Clin. Endocrinol. Metab.* 29:1341–1348, 1969.

31. DRENICK, E.J., F. SIMMONS, and J.F. MURPHY. Effect on hepatic morphology of treatment of obesity by fasting, reducing diets and small-bowel bypass. *N. Engl. J. Med.* 282:829–834, 1970.

32. DRENICK, E.J., M.E. SWENDSEID, W.H. BLAHD, and S.G. TUTTLE. Prolonged starvation as treatment for severe obesity. *JAMA* 187:100–105, 1964.

33. EPSTEIN, L.H. and R.R. WING. Aerobic exercise and weight. *Addict. Behav.* 5:371–388, 1980.

34. FELIG, P., O.E. OWEN, J. WAHREN, and G.F. CAHILL, JR. Amino acid metabolism during prolonged starvation. *J. Clin. Invest.* 48:584–594, 1969.

35. FERGUSON, J. *Learning to Eat: Behavior Modification for Weight Control.* Palo Alto, CA: Bull Publishing, 1975.

36. FRANKLIN, B., E. BUSKIRK, J. HODGSON, H. GAHAGAN, J. KOLLIAS, and J. MENDEZ. Effects of physical conditioning on cardiorespiratory function, body composition and serum lipids in relatively normal-weight and obese middle-aged women. *Int. J. Obesity* 3:97–109, 1979.

37. GARNETT, E.S., J. FORD, D.L. BARNARD, R.A. GOODBODY, and M.A. WOODEHOUSE. Gross fragmentation of cardiac myofibrils after therapeutic starvation for obesity. *Lancet* 1:914, 1969.

38. GARROW, J.S. *Energy Balance and Obesity in Man.* New York: American Elsevier, 1974.

39. GOLDMAN, R.F., B. BULLEN, and C. SELTZER. Changes in specific gravity and body fat in overweight female adolescents as a result of weight reduction. *Ann. NY Acad. Sci.* 110:913–917, 1963.

40. GORDON, T. and W.B. KANNEL. The effects of overweight on cardiovascular diseases. *Geriatrics* 28:80–88, 1973.

41. GRANDE, F. Nutrition and energy balance in body composition studies In: *Techniques for Meausuring Body Compositions.* J. Brozek and A. Henschel (Eds.). Washington, DC: National Academy of Sciences—National Research Council, 1961. (Reprinted by the Office of Technical Services, U.S. Department of Commerce, Washington, DC as U.S. Government Research Report AD286, 1963, 560.)

42. GRANDE, F. Energy balance and body composition changes. *Ann. Intern. Med.* 68:467–480, 1968.

43. GRANDE, F., H.L. TAYLOR, J.T. ANDERSON, E. BUSKIRK, and A. KEYS. Water exchange in men on a restricted water intake and a low calorie carbohydrate diet accompanied by physical work. *J. Appl. Physiol.* 12:202–210, 1958.

44. GWINUP, G. Effect of exercise alone on the weight of obese women. *Arch. Intern. Med.* 135:676–680, 1975.

45. HAFEN, B.A. *Nutrition, Food and Weight Control.* Boston: Allyn and Bacon. 1981, pp. 271–289.

46. HULLEY, S.B., R. COHEN, and G. WIDDOWSON. Plasma high-density lipoprotein cholesterol level: influence of risk factor intervention. *JAMA* 238:2269–2271, 1977.

47. JAGENBURG, R and A. SVANBORG. Self-induced protein-calorie malnutrition in a healthy adult male. *Acta Med. Scad.* 183:67–71, 1968.

48. KAHAN, A. Death during therapeutic starvation. *Lancet* 1:1378–1379, 1968.

49. KATCH, F.I. and W.B. MCARDLE. *Nutrition, Weight Control and Exercise.* Boston: Houghton Mifflin, 1977.

50. KEYS, A., J. BROZEK, A. HENSHEL, O. MICKELSON, and H.L. TAYLOR. *The Biology of Human Starvation.* Minneapolis: University of Minnesota Press, 1950.

51. KROTKIEWSKI, M., L. TOSS, P. BJORNTORP, and G. HOLM. The effect of a very low-calorie diet with and without chronic exercise on thyroid and sex hormones, plasma proteins, oxygen uptake, insulin and c peptide concentrations in obese women. *Int. J. Obes.* 5:287–293, 1981.

52. LASZLO, J., R.F. KLEIN, and M.D. BOGDONOFF. Prolonged starvation in obese patients, in vitro and in vivo effects. *Clin. Res.* 9:183, 1961. (Abstract).

53. LAWLOR, T. and D.G. WELLS. Metabolic hazards of fasting. *Am. J. Clin. Nutr.* 22:1142–1149, 1969.

54. LEON, A.S., J. CONRAD, D.M. HUNNINGHAKE, and R. SERFASS. Effects of a vigorous walking program on body composition, and carbohydrate and lipid metabolism of obese young men. *Am. J. Clin. Nutr.* 32:1776–1787, 1979.

55. MABEE, F.M., P. MEYER, L. DENBESTEN, and E.E. MASON. The mechanism of increased gallstone formation on obese human subjects. *Surgery* 79:460–468, 1978.

56. MATTER, S., A. WELTMAN, and B.A. STAMFORD. Body fat content and serum lipid levels. *J. Am. Diet. Assoc.* 77:149–152, 1980.

57. MCARDLE, W.D., F.I. KATCH, and V.L. KATCH. *Exercise Physiology: Energy, Nutrition and Human Performance.* Philadelphia: Lea and Febiger, 1981.

58. MILESIS, C.A., M.L. POLLOCK, M.D. BAH, J.J. AYRES, A. WARD, and A.C. LINNERUD. Effects of different durations of training on cardiorespiratory function, body composition and serum lipids. *Res. Q.* 47:716–725, 1976.

59. MURPHY, R. and K. H. SHIPMAN. Hyperuricemia during total fasting. *Arch. Intern. Med.* 112:954–959, 1963.

60. NILSSON, L.H. and E. HULTMAN. Total starvation or a carbohydrate-poor diet followed by carbohydrate refeeding. *Scand. J. Clin. Lab. Invest.* 32:325–330, 1973.

61. NORBURY, F.B. Contraindication of long term fasting. *JAMA* 188:88, 1964.

62. O'HARA, W., C. ALLEN, and R.J. SHEPARD. Loss of body weight and fat during exercise in a cold chamber. *Eur. J. Appl. Physiol.* 37:205–218, 1977.

63. OYAMA, J., J.A. THOMAS, and R.L. BRANT. Effect of starvation

on glucose tolerance and serum insulin-like activity of Osborne-Mendel rats. *Diabetes* 12:332–334, 1963.

64. PASSMORE, R., J.A. STRONG, and F.J. RITCHIE. The chemical composition of the tissue lost by obese patients on a reducing regimen. *Br. J. Nutri.* 12:113–122, 1958.

65. PITTMAN, F.E. Primary malabsorption following extreme attempts to lose weight. *Gut* 7:154–158, 1966.

66. POLLOCK, M.L., T.K. CURETON, and L. GRENINGER. Effects of frequency of training on working capacity, cardiovascular function and body composition of adult men. *Med. Sci. Sports* 1:70–74, 1969.

67. POLLOCK, M.L., J. TIFFANY, L. GETTMAN, R. JANEWAY, and H. LOFLAND. Effects of frequency of training on serum lipids, cardiovascular function and body composition. In: *Exercise and Fitness*, B.D. Franks (Ed.). Chicago: *Athletic Institute*, 1969, pp. 161–178.

68. POLLOCK, M.L., J. BROIDA, Z. KENDRICK, H.S. MILLER, JR., R. JANEWAY, and A.C. LINNERUD. Effects of training two days per week at different intensities on middle aged men. *Med. Sci. Sports* 4:192–197, 1972.

69. POLLOCK, M.L. The quantification of endurance training programs. *Exercise and Sports Sciences Reviews*, J. Wilmore (Ed.). New York: Academic Press, 1973, pp. 155–188.

70. POLLOCK, M.L. and A. JACKSON. Body composition: measurement and changes resulting from physical training. In: *Proceedings National College Physical Education Association for Men and Women*, 1977, pp. 123–137.

71. PORTNAY, G.I., J.T. O'BRIAN, J. BUSH, et al. The effect of starvation on the concentration and binding of thyroxine and triiodothyronine in serum and on the response to TRH. *J. Clin. Endocrinol. Metab.* 39:191–194, 1974.

72. RIMM, A.A., L.H. WERNER, R. BERNSTEIN, and B. VAN YSERLOO. Disease and obesity in 73,532 women. *Obesity Bariatric Med.* 1:77–84, 1972.

73. ROOTH, G. and S. CARLSTROM. Therapeutic fasting. *Acta Med. Scand.* 187:455–463, 1970.

74. ROSSNER, S. and D. HALLBERG. Serum lipoproteins in massive obesity. *Acta Med. Scand.* 204:103–110, 1978.

75. ROZENTAL, P., C. BIARA, H. SPENCER, and H.J. ZIMMERMAN. Liver morphology and function tests in obesity and during starvation. *Am. J. Dig. Dis.* 12:198–208, 1967.

76. RUNCIE, J. Urinary sodium and potassium excretion in fasting obese subjects. *Br. Med. J.* 3:432–435, 1970.

77. RUNCIE, J. and T.J. THOMSON. Total fasting, hyperuricemia and gout. *Postgrad. Med. J.* 45:251–254, 1969.

78. RUNCIE, J. and T.J. THOMSON. Prolonged starvation—a dangerous procedure? *Br. Med. J.* 3:432–435, 1970.

79. SOURS, H.E., V.P. FRATTALI, C.D. BRAND, et al. Sudden death associated with very low calorie weight reduction regimens. *Am. J. Clin. Nutri.* 34:453–461, 1981.

80. SPENCER, I.O.B. Death during therapeutic starvation for obesity. *Lancet* 2:679–680, 1968.

81. STALONAS, P.M., W.G. JOHNSON, and M. CHRIST. Behavior modification for obesity: the evaluation of exercise, contingency, management, and program behavior. *J. Consult. Clin. Psychol.* 46:463–467, 1978.

82. STAMLER, R., J. STAMLER, W.F. RIEDLINGER, G. ALGERA, and R.H. ROBERTS. Weight and blood pressure. Findings in hypertension screening of 1 million Americans. *JAMA* 240:1607–1610, 1978.

83. STEIN, J.S. and J. HIRSCH. Obesity and pancreatic function. In: *Handbook of physiology. Section 1. Endocrinology*. Vol. 1, D. Steener and N. Frankel (Eds.). Washington, DC: American Physiological Society, 1972.

84. STEWART, W.K. and L.W. FLEMING. Features of a successful therapeutic fast of 382 days duration. *Postgrad. Med. J.* 49:203–209, 1973.

85. STEWART, J.S., D.L. POLLOCK, A.V. HOFFBRAND, D.L. MOLLIN, and C.C. BOOTH. A study of proximal and distal intestinal structure and absorptive function in idiopathic steatorrhea. *Q. J. Med.* 36:425–444, 1967.

86. STREJA, D.A., E.B. MARLISS, and G. STEINER. The effects of prolonged fasting on plasma triglyceride kinetics in man. *Metabolism* 26:505–516, 1977.

87. STUART, R.B. and B. DAVIS. *Slim Chance in a Fat World. Behavioral Control of Obesity*. Champaign, IL: Research Press, 1972.

88. THOMPSON, P.D., R.W. JEFFREY, R.R. WING, and P.D. WOOD. Unexpected decrease in plasma high density lipoprotein cholesterol with weight loss. *Am. J. Clin. Nutr.* 32:2016–2021, 1979.

89. THOMSON, T.J., J. RUNCIE, and V. MILLER. Treatment of obesity by total fasting up to 249 days. *Lancet* 2:992–996, 1966.

90. THORN, G.W., M.M. WINTROBE, R.D. ADAMS, E. BRAUNWALD, K.J. ISSELBACHER, and R.G. PETERSDORF. *Harrison's Principles of Internal Medicine*, 8th Edition. New York: McGraw-Hill, 1977.

91. VEGENAKIS, A.G., A. BURGER, G.I. PORTNAY, et al. Diversion of peripheral thyroxine metabolism from activating to inactivating pathways during complete fasting. *J. Clin. Endocrinol. Metab.* 41:191–194, 1975.

92. VERDY, M. B.S.P. retention during total fasting. *Metabolism* 15:769, 1966.

93. WARNER, W.A. and L.P. GARRETT. The obese patient and anesthesia. *JAMA* 205:102–103, 1968.

94. WECHSLER, J.G., V. HUTT, H. WENZEL, H. KLOR, and H. DITSCHUNEIT. Lipids and lipoproteins during a very-low-calorie diet. *Int. J. Obes.* 5:325–331, 1981.

95. WEISINGER, J.R., A. SEEMAN, M.G. HERRERA, J.P. ASSAL, J.S. SOELDNER, and R.E. GLEASON. The nephrotic syndrome: a complication of massive obesity. *Ann. Intern. Med.* 80:332–341, 1974.

96. WELTMAN, A., S. MATTER, and B.A. STAMFORD. Caloric restriction and/or mild exercise: effects on serum lipids and body composition. *Am. J. Clin. Nutr.* 33:1002–1009, 1980.

97. WEST, K. *Epidemiology of Diabetes and its Vascular Lesions*. New York: Elsevier, 1978.

98. WILMORE, J.H., J. ROYCE, R.N. GIRANDOLA, F.I. KATCH, and V. L. KATCH. Body composition changes with a 10 week jogging program. *Med. Sci. Sports* 2:113–117, 1970.

99. WILSON, G.T. Behavior modification and the treatment of obesity. In: *Obesity*. A.J. Stunkard (Ed.). Philadelphia: W.B. Saunders, 1980.

100. WOOLEY, S.C., O.W. WOOLEY, and S.R. DYRENFORTH. Theoretical practical and social issues in behavioral treatments of obesity. *J. Appl. Behav. Anal.* 12:3–25, 1979.

101. YANG, M. and T.B. VAN ITALLIE. Metabolic responses of obese subjects to starvation and low calorie ketogenic and nonketogenic diets. *J. Clin. Invest.* 58:722–730, 1976.

102. ZUTI, W.B. and L.A. GOLDING. Comparing diet and exercise as weight reduction tools. *Phys. Sportsmed.* 4(1):49–53, 1976.

**AMERICAN COLLEGE
of SPORTS MEDICINE**
POSITION STAND

The Use of Alcohol in Sports

Based upon a comprehensive analysis of the available research relative to the effects of alcohol upon human physical performance, it is the position of the American College of Sports Medicine that:

1. The acute ingestion of alcohol can exert a deleterious effect upon a wide variety of psychomotor skills such as reaction time, hand-eye coordination, accuracy, balance, and complex coordination.

2. Acute ingestion of alcohol will not substantially influence metabolic or physiological functions essential to physical performance such as energy metabolism, maximal oxygen consumption ($\dot{V}O_{2max}$), heart rate, stroke volume, cardiac output, muscle blood flow, arteriovenous oxygen difference, or respiratory dynamics. Alcohol consumption may impair body temperature regulation during prolonged exercise in a cold environment.

3. Acute alcohol ingestion will not improve and may decrease strength, power, local muscular endurance, speed, and cardiovascular endurance.

4. Alcohol is the most abused drug in the United States and is a major contributing factor to accidents and their consequences. Also, it has been documented widely that prolonged excessive alcohol consumption can elicit pathological changes in the liver, heart, brain, and muscle, which can lead to disability and death.

5. Serious and continuing efforts should be made to educate athletes, coaches, health and physical educators, physicians, trainers, the sports media, and the general public regarding the effects of acute alcohol ingestion upon human physical performance and on the potential acute and chronic problems of excessive alcohol consumption.

Research Background for the Position Stand

This position stand is concerned primarily with the effects of acute alcohol ingestion upon physical performance and is based upon a comprehensive review of the pertinent international literature. When one interprets these results, several precautions should be kept in mind. First, there are varying reactions to alcohol ingestion, not only among individuals, but also within an individual depending upon the circumstances. Second, it is virtually impossible to conduct double-blind placebo research with alcohol because subjects can always tell when alcohol has been consumed. Nevertheless, the results cited below provide us with some valid

general conclusions relative to the effects of alcohol on physical performance. In most of the research studies, a small dose consisted of 1.5–2.0 ounces (45–60 ml) of alcohol, equivalent to a blood alcohol level (BAL) of 0.04–0.05 in the average-size male. A moderate dose was equivalent to 3–4 ounces (90–120ml), or a BAL of about 0.10. Few studies employed a large dose, with a BAL of 0.15.

1. Athletes may consume alcohol to improve psychological function, but it is psychomotor performance that deteriorates most. A consistent finding is the impairment of information processing. In sports involving rapid reactions to changing stimuli, performance will be affected most adversely. Research has shown that small to moderate amounts of alcohol will impair reaction time (8,25,26,34–36,42) hand-eye coordination (8,9,14,40), accuracy (36,39), balance (3), and complex coordination or gross motor skills (4,8,22,36,41). Thus, while Coopersmith (10) suggests that alcohol may improve self-confidence, the available research reveals a deterioration in psychomotor performance.

2. Many studies have been conducted relative to the effects of acute alcohol ingestion upon metabolic and physiological functions important to physical performance. Alcohol ingestion exerts no beneficial influence relative to energy sources for exercise. Muscle glycogen at rest was significantly lower after alcohol consumption, compared to control (30). However, in exercise at 50% maximal oxygen uptake ($\dot{V}O_{2max}$), total glycogen depletion in the leg muscles was not affected by alcohol (30). Moreover, Juhlin-Dannfelt et al. (29) have shown that although alcohol does not impair lipolysis or free fatty acid (FFA) utilization during exercise, it may decrease splanchnic glucose output, decrease the potential contribution from liver gluconeogenesis, elicit a greater decline in blood glucose levels leading to hypoglycemia, and decrease the leg muscle uptake of glucose during the latter stages of a 3-h run. Other studies (17,19) have supported the theory concerning the hypoglycemic effect of alcohol during both moderate and prolonged exhaustive exercise in a cold environment. These studies also noted a significant loss of body heat and a resultant drop in body temperature and suggested that alcohol may impair temperature regulation. These changes may impair endurance capacity.

In one study (5), alcohol has been shown to increase oxygen uptake significantly during submaximal work and simultaneously to decrease mechanical efficiency, but this finding has not been confirmed by others (6,15,33,44). Alcohol appears to have no effect on maximal or near-maximal $\dot{V}O_2$ (5–7,44).

The effects of alcohol on cardiovascular-respiratory parameters associated with oxygen uptake are variable at submaximal exercise intensities and are negligible at maximal levels. Alcohol has been shown by some investigators to increase submaximal exercise heart rate (5,20,23) and cardiac output (5), but these heart rate findings have not been confirmed by others (6,15,33,36,44). Alcohol had no effect on stroke volume (5), pulmonary ventilation (5,15), or muscle blood flow (16,30) at submaximal levels of exercise, but did decrease peripheral vascular resistance (5). During maximal exercise, alcohol ingestion elicited no significant effect upon heart rate (5–7), stroke volume and cardiac output, arteriovenous oxygen difference, mean arterial pressure, and peripheral vascular resistance, or peak lactate (5), but did significantly reduce tidal volume resulting in a lowered pulmonary ventilation (5).

In summary, alcohol appears to have little or no beneficial effect on the metabolic and physiological responses to exercise. Further, in those studies reporting significant effects, the change appears to be detrimental to performance.

3. The effects of alcohol on tests of fitness components are variable. It has been shown that alcohol ingestion may decrease dynamic muscular strength (24), isometric grip strength (36), dynamometer strength (37), power (20), and ergographic muscular output (28). Other studies (13,20,24,27,43) reported no effect of alcohol upon muscular strength. Local muscular endurance was also unaffected by alcohol ingestion (43). Small doses of alcohol exerted no effect upon bicycle ergometer exercise tasks simulating a 100-m dash or a 1500-m run, but larger doses had a deleterious effect (2). Other research has shown that alcohol has no significant effect upon physical performance capacity (15,16), exercise time at maximal levels (5), or exercise time to exhaustion (7).

Thus, alcohol ingestion will not improve muscular work capacity and may lead to decreased performance levels.

4. Alcohol is the most abused drug in the United States (11). There are an estimated 10 million adult problem drinkers and an additional 3.3 million in the 14–17 age range. Alcohol is significantly involved in all types of accidents—motor vehicle, home, industrial, and recreational. Most significantly, half of all traffic fatalities and one-third of all traffic injuries are alcohol related. Although alcohol abuse is associated with pathological conditions such as generalized skeletal myopathy, cardiomyopathy, pharyngeal and esophageal cancer, and brain damage, its most prominent effect is liver damage (11,31,32).

5. Because alcohol has not been shown to help improve physical performance capacity, but may lead to decreased ability in certain events, it is important for all those associated with the conduct of sports to educate athletes against its use in conjunction with athletic contests. Moreover, the other dangers inherent in alcohol abuse mandate that concomitantly we educate our youth to make intelligent choices regarding alcohol consumption. Anstie's rule, or limit (1), may be used as a reasonable guideline to moderate, safe drinking for adults (12). In essence, no more than 0.5 ounces of pure alcohol per 23 kg body weight should be consumed in any one day. This would be the equivalent of three bottles of 4.5% beer, three 4-ounce glasses of 14% wine, or three ounces of 50% whiskey for a 68-kg person.

REFERENCES

1. ANSTIE, F.E. *On the Uses of Wine in Health and Disease.* London: MacMillan, 1877, pp. 5–6.
2. ASMUSSEN, E. and O. BOJE. The effects of alcohol and some drugs on the capacity for work. *Acta Physiol. Scand.* 15:109–118, 1948.
3. BEGBIE, G. The effects of alcohol and of varying amounts of visual information on a balancing test. *Ergonomics* 9:325–333, 1966.
4. BELGRAVE, B., K. BIRD, G. CHESHER, D. JACKSON, K. LUBBE, G. STARMER, and R. TEO. The effect of cannabidiol, alone and in combination with ethanol, on human performance. *Psychopharmacology* 64:243–246, 1979.
5. BLOMQVIST, G., B. SALTIN, and J. MITCHELL. Acute effects of ethanol ingestion on the response to submaximal and maximal exercise in man. *Circulation* 42:463–470, 1970.
6. BOBO, W. Effects of alcohol upon maximum oxygen uptake, lung ventilation, and heart rate. *Res. Q.* 43:1–6, 1972.
7. BOND, V. Effect of alcohol on cardiorespiratory function. In: *Abstracts: Research Papers of 1979 AAHPER Convention.* Washington, DC: AAHPER, 1979, p. 24.
8. CARPENTER, J. Effects of alcohol on some psychological processes. *Q.J. Stud. Alcohol* 23:274–314, 1962.
9. COLLINS, W., D. SCHROEDER, R. GILSON, and F. GUEDRY. Effects of alcohol ingestion on tracking performance during angular acceleration. *J. Appl. Psychol.* 55:559–563, 1971.
10. COOPERSMITH, S. The effects of alcohol on reaction to affective stimuli. *Q. J. Stud. Alcohol* 25:459–475, 1964.
11. DEPARTMENT OF HEALTH, EDUCATION, AND WELFARE. Third special report to the U.S. Congress on alcohol and health. *NIAAA Information and Feature Service.* DHEW Publication No. (ADM) 78–151, November 30, 1978, pp. 1–4.
12. *Dorland's Illustrated Medical Dictionary.* 24th Edition. Philadelphia: W.B. Saunders, 1974, p. 1370.
13. ENZER, N., E. SIMONSON, and G. BALLARD. The effect of small doses of alcohol on the central nervous system. *Am. J. Clin. Pathol.* 14:333–341, 1944.
14. FORNEY, R., F. HUGHES, and W. GREATBATCH. Measurement of attentive motor performance after alcohol. *Percept. Mot. Skills* 19:151–154, 1964.
15. GARLIND, T., L. GOLDBERG, K. GRAF, E. PERMAN, T. STRANDELL, and G. STROM. Effect of ethanol on circulatory, metabolic, and neurohumoral function during muscular work in man. *Acta Pharmacol. et Toxicol.* 17:106–114, 1960.

16. GRAF, K. and G. STROM. Effect of ethanol ingestion on arm blood flow in healthy young men at rest and during work. *Acta Pharmacol. et Toxicol.* 17:115–120, 1960.

17. GRAHAM, T. Thermal and glycemic responses during mild exercise in +5 to −15°C environments following alcohol ingestion. *Aviat. Space Environ. Med.* 25:517–522, 1981.

18. GRAHAM, T. and J. DALTON. Effect of alcohol on man's response to mild physical activity in a cold environment. *Aviat. Space Environ. med.* 51:793–796, 1980.

19. HAIGHT, J. and W. KEATINGE. Failure of thermoregulation in the cold during hypoglycemia induced by exercise and ethanol. *J. Physiol. (Lond.)* 229:87–97, 1973.

20. HEBBELINCK, M. The effects of a moderate dose of alcohol on a series of functions of physical performance in man. *Arch. Int. Pharmacol.* 120:402–405, 1959.

21. HEBELLINCK, M. The effect of a moderate dose of ethyl alcohol on human respiratory gas exchange during rest and muscular exercise. *Arch. Int. Pharmacod.* 126:214–218, 1960.

22. HEBBELINCK, M. *Spierarbeid en Ethylalkohol.* Brussels: Arsica Uitgaven, N.V., 1961, pp. 81–84.

23. HEBBELINCK, M. The effects of a small dose of ethyl alcohol on certain basic components of human physical performance. The effect on cardiac rate during muscular work. *Arch. Int. Pharmacod.* 140:61–67, 1962.

24. HEBBELINCK, M. The effects of a small dose of ethyl alcohol on certain basic components of human physical performance. *Arch. Int. Pharmacod.* 143:247–257, 1963.

25. HUNTLEY, M. Effects of alcohol, uncertainty and novelty upon response selection. *Psychopharmacologia* 39:259–266, 1974.

26. HUNTLEY, M. Influences of alcohol and S-R uncertainty upon spatial localization time. *Psychopharmacologia* 27:131–140, 1972.

27. IKAI, M. and A. STEINHAUS. Some factors modifying the expression of human strength. *J. Appl. Physiol.* 16:157–161, 1961.

28. JELLINEK, E. Effect of small amounts of alcohol on psychological functions. In Yale University Center for Alcohol Studies. *Alcohol, Science and Society.* New Haven, CT; Yale University, 1954, pp. 83–94.

29. JUHLIN-DANNFELT, A.G. AHLBORG, L. HAGENFELDT, L. JORFELDT, and P. FELIG. Influence of ethanol on splanchnic and skeletal muscle substrate turnover during prolonged exercise in man. *Am. J. Physiol.* 233:E195–E202, 1977.

30. JUHLIN-DANNFELT, A.L. JORFELDT, L. HAGENFELDT, and B. HULTEN. Influence of ethanol on non-esterified fatty acid and carbohydrate metabolism during exercise in man. *Clin. Soc. Mol. Med.* 53:205–214, 1977.

31. LIEBER, C.S. Liver injury and adaptation in alcoholism. *N. Engl. J. Med.* 288:356–362, 1973.

32. LIEBER, C.S. The metabolism of alcohol. *Sci. Am.* 234(March):25–33, 1976.

33. MAZESS, R., E. PICON-REATEGUI, and R. THOMAS. Effects of alcohol and altitude on man during rest and work. *Aerospace Med.* 39:403–406, 1968.

34. MOSKOWITZ, H. and M. BURNS. Effect of alcohol on the psychological refractory period. *Q. J. Stud. Alcohol* 32:782–790, 1971.

35. MOSKOWITZ, H. and S. ROTH. Effect of alcohol on response latency in object naming. *Q. J. Stud. Alcohol* 32:969–975, 1971.

36. NELSON, D. Effects of ethyl alcohol on the performance of selected gross motor tests. *Res. Q.* 30:312–320, 1959.

37. PIHKANEN, T. Neurological and physiological studies on distilled and brewed beverages. *Ann. Med. Exp. Biol. Fenn.* 35:Suppl. 9, 1–152, 1957.

38. RIFF, D., A. JAIN, and H. WILLIAMS. Alcohol and speed-accuracy tradeoff. *Hum. Factors* 21:433–443, 1979.

39. RUNDELL, O. and H. WILLIAMS. Alcohol and sped-accuracy tradeoff. *Hum. Factors* 21:433–443, 1979.

40. SIDELL, F. and J. PLESS. Ethyl alcohol blood levels and performance decrements after oral administration to man. *Psychopharmacologia* 19:246–261, 1971.

41. TANG, P. and R. ROSENSTEIN. Influence of alcohol and Dramamine, alone and in combination, on psychomotor performance. *Aerospace Med.* 39:818–821, 1967.

42. THARP, V., O. RUNDELL, B. LESTER, and H. WILLIAMS. Alcohol and information processing. *psychopharmacologia* 40:33–52, 1974.

43. WILLIAMS, M.H. Effect of selected doses of alcohol on fatigue parameters of the forearm flexor muscles. *Res. Q.* 40:832–840, 1969.

44. WILLIAMS, M.H. Effect of small and moderate doses of alcohol on exercise heart rate and oxygen consumption. *Res. Q.* 43:94–104, 1972.

AMERICAN COLLEGE of SPORTS MEDICINE

POSITION STAND

Weight Loss in Wrestlers

Despite repeated admonitions by medical, educational and athletic groups (2,8,17,22,33), most wrestlers have been inculcated by instruction or accepted tradition to lose weight in order to be certified for a class that is lower than their preseason weight (34). Studies (34,40) of weight losses in high school and college wrestlers indicate that from 3–20% of the preseason body weight is lost before certification or competition occurs. Of this weight loss, most of the decrease occurs in the final days or day before the official weigh-in (34,40) with the youngest and/or lightest members of the team losing the highest percentage of their body weight (34). Under existing rules and practices, it is not uncommon for an individual to repeat this weight losing process many times during the season because successful wrestlers compete in 15–30 matches/year (13).

Contrary to existing beliefs, most wrestlers are not "fat" before the season starts (35). In fact, the fat content of high school and college wrestlers weighing less than 190 lbs. has been shown to range from 1.6–15.1% of their body weight with the majority possessing less than 8% (14,28,31). It is well known and documented that wrestlers lose body weight by a combination of food restriction, fluid deprivation and sweating induced by thermal or exercise procedures (20,22,34,40). Of these methods, dehydration through sweating appears to be the method most frequently chosen.

Careful studies on the nature of the weight being lost show that water, fats, and proteins are lost when food restriction and fluid deprivation procedures are followed (10). Moreover, the proportionality between these constituents will change with continued restriction and deprivation. For example, if food restriction is held constant when the volume of fluid being consumed is decreased, more water will be lost from the tissues of the body than before the fluid restriction occurred. The problem becomes more acute when thermal or exercise dehydration occurs because electrolyte losses will accompany the water losses (16). Even when 1–5 h are allowed for purposes of rehydration after the weigh-in, this time interval is insufficient for fluid and electrolyte homeostasis to be completely reestablished (11,37,39,40).

Since the "making of weight" occurs by combinations of food restriction, fluid deprivation and dehydration, responsible officials should realize that the single or combined effects of these practices are generally associated with 1) a reduction in muscular strength (4,15,30); 2) a decrease in work performance times

(24,26,27,30); 3) lower plasma and blood volumes (6,7,24,27); 4) a reduction in cardiac functioning during submaximal work conditions which are associated with higher heart rates (1,19,23,24,27), smaller stroke volumes (27), and reduced cardiac outputs (27); 5) a lower oxygen consumption, especially with food restriction (15,30); 6) an impairment of thermoregulatory processes (3,9,24); 7) a decrease in renal blood flow (21,25) and in the volume of fluid being filtered by the kidney (21); 8) a depletion of liver glycogen stores (12); and 9) an increase in the amount of electrolytes being lost from the body (6,7,16).

Since it is possible for these changes to impede normal growth and development, there is little physiological or medical justification for the use of the weight reduction methods currently followed by many wrestlers. These sentiments have been expressed in part within Rule 1, Section 3, Article 1 of the *Official Wrestling Rule Book* (18) published by the National Federation of State High School Associations which states, "The Rules Committee recommends that individual state high school associations develop and utilize an effective weight control program which will discourage severe weight reduction and/or wide variations in weight, because this may be harmful to the competitor . . . ." However, until the National Federation of State High School Associations defines the meaning of the terms "severe" and "wide variations," this rule will be ineffective in reducing the abuses associated with the "making of weight."

Therefore, it is the position of the American College of Sports Medicine that the potential health hazards created by the procedures used to "make weight" by wrestlers can be eliminated if state and national organizations will:

1. Assess the body composition of each wrestler several weeks in advance of the competitive season (5,14,28,31,38). Individuals with a fat content less than 5% of their certified body weight should receive medical clearance before being allowed to compete.
2. Emphasize the fact that the daily caloric requirements of wrestlers should be obtained from a balanced diet and determined on the basis of age, body surface area, growth and physical activity levels (29). The minimal caloric needs of wrestlers in high schools and colleges will range from 1200–2400 kcal/d (32); therefore, it is the responsibility of coaches, school officials, physicians and parents to discourage wrestlers from securing less than their

minimal needs without prior medical approval.

3. Discourage the practice of fluid deprivation and dehydration. This can be accomplished by:

   a. Educating the coaches and wrestlers on the physiological consequences and medical complications that can occur as a result of these practices.

   b. Prohibiting the single or combined use of rubber suits, steam rooms, hot boxes, saunas, laxatives, and diuretics to "make weight."

   c. Scheduling weigh-ins just prior to competition.

   d. Scheduling more official weigh-ins between team matches.

4. Permit more participants/team to compete in those weight classes (119–145 lbs.) which have the highest percentages of wrestlers certified for competition (36).

5. Standardize regulations concerning the eligibility rules at championship tournaments so that individuals can only participate in those weight classes in which they had the highest frequencies of matches throughout the season.

6. Encourage local and county organizations to systematically collect data on the hydration state (39,40) of wrestlers and its relationship to growth and development.

REFERENCES

1. ALHMAN, K. and M.J. KARVONEN. Weight reduction by sweating in wrestlers and its effect on physical fitness. *J. Sports Med. Phys. Fit.* 1:58–62, 1961.
2. AMA Committee on the Medical Aspects of Sports, Wrestling and Weight Control. *JAMA* 201:541–543, 1967.
3. BOCK, W.E., E.L. FOX and R. BOWERS. The effect of acute dehydration upon cardiorespiratory endurance. *J. Sports Med. Phys. Fit.* 7:62–72, 1967.
4. BOSCO, J.S., R.L. TERJUNG. J.E. GREENLEAF. Effects of progressive hypohydration of maximal isometric muscular strength. *J. Sports Med. Phys. Fit.* 8:81–86, 1968.
5. CLARKE, K.S. Predicting certified weight of young wrestlers: a field study of the Tcheng-Tipton method. *Med. Sci. Sports* 6:52–57, 1974.
6. COSTILL, D.L. and K. E. SPARKS. Rapid fluid replacement following thermal dehydration. *J. Appl. Physiol.* 34:299–303, 1973.
7. COSTILL, D.L., R. COTE, E. MILLER, T. MILLER and S. WYNDER. Water and electrolyte replacement during repeated days of work in the heat. *Aviat. Space Environ. Med.* 46:795–800, 1975.
8. ERIKSEN, F.G. Interscholastic wrestling and weight control: Current plans and their loopholes. *Proceedings of the Eighth National Conference on The Medical Aspects of Sports.* Chicago: AMA, 1967, pp. 34–39.
9. GRANDE, F., J.E. MONAGLE, E.R. BUSKIR and H.L. TAYLOR. Body temperature responses to exercise in man on restricted food and water intake. *J. Appl. Physiol.* 14:194–198, 1959.
10. GRANDE, F. Nutrition and energy balance in body composition studies. *Techniques for Measuring Body Composition*, edited by J. Brozek and A. Henschel. Washington, D.C., National Acad. Sci. & Nat. Res. Council, pp. 168–188, 1961.
11. HERBERT, W.G. and P.M. RIBISL. Effects of dehydration upon physical work capacity of wrestlers under competitive conditions. *Res. Quart.* 43:416–422, 1972.
12. HULTMAN, E. and L. NILSSON. Liver glycogen as glucose-supplying source during exercise. *Limiting Factors of Physical Performance*, edited by J. Keul. Stuttgart Georg Thieme, pp. 179–189, 1973.

13. Iowa High School Athletic Association. 1975 Program for the 55th State Wrestling Tournament., pp. 7–9.
14. KATCH, F.I. and E.D. MICHAEL, JR. Body composition of high school wrestlers according to age and wrestling weight category. *Med. Sea. Sports* 3:190–194, 1971.
15. KEYS, A.L., J. BROZEK, A. HENSCHEL, O. MICKELSEN and H.L. TAYLOR. *The Biology of Human Starvation.* Minneapolis U of Minn. Press, Vol. 1. pp 718–748, 1950.
16. KOZLOWSKI, S. and B. SALTIN. Effect of sweat loss on body fluids. *J. Appl. Physiol.* 19:1119–1124, 1964.
17. KROLL, W. Guidelines for rules and practices. *Proceedings of the Eighth National Conference on the Medical Aspects of Sports.* Chicago AMA, pp. 40–44, 1967.
18. *The National Federation 1974–75 Wrestling Rule Book.* The National Federation Publications. Elgin, Illinois, p. 6.
19. PALMER, W. Selected physiological responses of normal young men following dehydration and rehydration. *Res. Quart.* 39:1054–1059, 1968.
20. PAUL, W.D. Crash diets in wrestling. *J. Iowa Med. Soc.* 56:835–840, 1966.
21. RADIGAN, L.R. and S. ROBINSON. Effect of environmental heat stress and exercise on renal blood flow and filtration rate. *J. Appl. Physiol.* 2:185–191, 1949.
22. RASCH, P.G. and W. KROLL. *What Research Tells the Coach About Wrestling.* Washington: AAHPER, pp. 41–50, 1964.
23. RIBISL, P.M. and W.G. HERBERT. Effect of rapid weight reduction and subsequent rehydration upon the physical working capacity of wrestlers. *Res. Quart.* 41:536–541, 1970.
24. ROBINSON, S. The effect of dehydration on performance. *Football Injuries.* Washington, DC: Natl. Acad. Sci., pp. 191–197, 1970.
25. ROWELL, L.B. Human cardiovascular adjustments to exercise and thermal stress. *Physiol. Rev.* 54:75–159, 1974.
26. SALTIN, B. Aerobic and anaerobic work capacity after dehydration. *J. Appl. Physiol.* 19:1114–1118, 1964.
27. SALTIN, B. Circulatory response to submaximal and maximal exercise after thermal dehydration. *J. Appl. Physiol.* 19:1125–1132, 1964.
28. SINNING, W.E. Body composition assessment of college wresters. *Med. Sci. Sports* 6:139–145, 1974.
29. Suggested Daily Dietary Requirements. National Research Council Data, published in Oser, B.O. *Hawk's Physiological Chemistry*, 14th Edition, New York: McGraw-Hill, pp. 1370–1371, 1965.
30. TAYLOR, H.L., E.R. BUSKIRK, J. BROZEK, J.T. ANDERSON and F. GRANDE. Performance capacity and effects of caloric restriction with hard physical work on young men. *J. Appl. Physiol.* 10:421–429, 1957.
31. TCHENG, T.K. and C.M. TIPTON. Iowa wrestling study: Anthropometric measurements and the prediction of a "minimal" body weight for high school wrestlers. *Med. Sci. Sports* 5:1–10, 1973.
32. TIPTON, C.M. Unpublished calculations on Iowa High School Wrestlers using a height and weight surface area nomogram. (Consalazio, C.F., R.E. Johnson and L.J. Pecora, *Physiological Measurmeents of Metabolic Functions in Man.* New York: McGraw-Hill, 1963, p. 27, that was constructed from the Dubois-Meech formula published in Arch. Int. Med. 17:863–871, 1916) plus the metabolic standards for age used by the Mayo Foundation Standards that were published by Boothby. Berkson and Dunn in *Am. J. Physiol.* 116:467–484, 1936.
33. TIPTON, C.M. and T.K. TCHENG. Iowa wrestling study: Weight loss in high school students. *JAMA* 2114:1269–1274, 1970.
34. TIPTON, C.M. and T.K. TCHENG. Iowa wrestling study: Weight loss in high school students *JAMA* 2114:1269–1274, 1970.
35. TIPTON, C.M. Current status of the Iowa Wrestling Study. *The Predicament.* 12-30-73, p. 7.
36. TIPTON, C.M., T.K. TCHENG and E.J. ZAMBRASKI. Iowa Wrestling Study: Weight classification systems. *Med. Sci. Sports* 8:101–104, 1976.
37. VACCARO, P., C.W. ZAUNER and J.R. CADE. Changes in body weight, hematocrit and plasma protein concentration due to dehydration and rehydration in wrestlers. *Med. Sci. Sports* 7:76, 1975.

38. WILMORE, J.H. and A. BEHNKE. An anthropometric estimation of body density and lean body weight in young men. *J. Appl. Physiol.* 27:25–31, 1969.

39. ZAMBRASKI, E.J., C.M. TIPTON, T.K. TCHENG, H.R. JORDAN, A.C. VAILAS and A.K. CALLAHAN. Changes in the urinary profiles of wrestlers prior to and after competition. *Med. Sci. Sports.* 7:217–220, 1975.

40. ZAMBRASKI, E.J., D.T. FOSTER, P.M. GROSS and C.M. TIPTON. Iowa wrestling study: Weight loss and urinary profiles of collegiate wrestlers. *Med. Sci. Sports* 8:105–108, 1976.

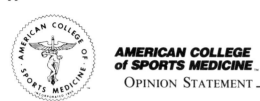

**AMERICAN COLLEGE
of SPORTS MEDICINE™**

OPINION STATEMENT

Physical Fitness in Children and Youth

There is concern about the physical fitness of children and youth in the United States. There is ongoing controversy regarding how much emphasis should be placed on physical fitness in physical education programs, the type and purpose of physical fitness testing, and the structure of awards systems. Physical fitness is primarily determined by physical activity habits and is operationally defined as performance attained on tests of the following: aerobic power, body composition, joint flexibility, and strength and endurance of the skeletal muscles. Physical fitness is important throughout life to develop and maintain functional capability to meet the demands of living and to promote optimal health. The American College of Sports Medicine (ACSM) issues this Opinion Statement in the hope that it will provide direction regarding the structure and scope of physical fitness programs for children and youth.

Opinion Statement

It is the opinion of the ACSM that physical fitness programs for children and youth should be developed with the primary goal of encouraging the adoption of appropriate lifelong exercise behavior in order to develop and maintain sufficient physical fitness for adequate functional capacity and health enhancement.

Recommendations for Action

1. School physical education programs are an important part of the overall education process and should give increased emphasis to the development and maintenance of lifelong exercise habits and provide instruction about how to attain and maintain appropriate physical fitness. The amount of exercise required for optimal functional capacity and health at various ages has not been precisely defined. Until more definitive evidence is available, current recommendations are that children and youth obtain 20–30 minutes of vigorous exercise each day. Physical education classes typically devote instructional time to physical fitness activities, but class time is generally insufficient to develop and maintain optimal physical fitness. Therefore, school programs also must focus on education and behavior change to encourage engagement in appropriate activities outside of class. Recreational and fun aspects of exercise should be emphasized.

2. Home influences are important, and parents should be encouraged to show concern for physical fitness as an important factor that affects their child's health and well-being. Parents should work with local school officials and teachers to promote physical fitness. Parents should strive to be appropriate physical fitness role models.

3. Community opportunities for exercise and physical fitness activities must be expanded. There are many opportunities for children interested in such sports as baseball, basketball, football, swimming, soccer, and gymnastics. Other activities, especially those that are individual in nature and likely to be performed throughout life, need to be more widely available and packaged and promoted in an attractive manner.

4. The health care professions need to become more actively involved in promoting physical fitness for children and youth. More continuing education programs on childhood and youth physical activity and physical fitness should be offered to health professionals. Medical and public health authorities should view the physical fitness of children and youth as being within their sphere of responsibility in addition to traditional undertakings such as immunization and scoliosis screening. Physicians can have a major impact in promoting and supporting physical fitness programs for children and youth.

5. Physical fitness testing is a highly visible and important part of physical fitness programs. School, community, state, and national organizations must adopt a logical, consistent, and scientifically sound approach to physical fitness testing. The focus of physical fitness testing should be health-related rather than athletic-related. Characteristics such as speed, muscular power, and agility are important for athletic success and are primarily genetically determined. These traits should not be assessed in physical fitness testing, although physical education teachers and coaches may wish to measure them for other purposes. Aerobic power, body composition, joint flexibility, and strength and endurance of the skeletal muscles are partly influenced by heredity but can be changed significantly by appropriate exercise patterns.

6. Educational programs designed to increase knowledge and appreciation of the role and value of exercise on physical fitness and health are virtually nonexistent in schools, although such programs are common at colleges and universities. Professional efforts need to be taken to develop, pretest, and publish educational ma-

terials suitable for use in schools. Training programs need to be developed and initiated to provide school teachers with the knowledge and skills to help their students achieve cognitive, affective, and behavioral skills objectives associated with exercise, health and fitness. Teachers also need assistance in ways to integrate other aspects of health promotion (good nutrition and not smoking, for example) into instruction about exercise and physical fitness. The educational components of testing, teaching physical fitness activities, and recognition through awards should be complementary and need to be coordinated for a comprehensive program.

7. The ACSM recommends that physical fitness test scores be interpreted in relation to acceptable standards, rather than by normative comparison. It is illogical to declare that American children and youth are physically unfit as a group and then use group norms to interpret a student's fitness test scores. A standards approach establishes a desirable physical fitness score for each fitness component. Current research is inadequate to establish with scientific precision acceptable standards for all fitness components, but preliminary standards should be developed based on the best available evidence and professional opinion. Additional research to refine, modify, and validate standards is a crucial need.

8. Awards systems that require excellent or exemplary performance on physical fitness tests are inadequate. Awards attainable only by students with superior athletic ability may discourage the majority of children and youth because they cannot qualify. A graduated awards system that rewards exercise behavior and achievement in relation to achievable physical fitness standards should be developed and implemented.

**AMERICAN COLLEGE
of SPORTS MEDICINE**™

Street Address: 401 West Michigan Street • Indianapolis, IN 46202-3233 USA
Mailing Address: P.O. Box 1440 • Indianapolis, IN 46206-1440 USA

APPENDIX 3

Special Report

RECREATIONAL AND OCCUPATIONAL RECOMMENDATIONS FOR YOUNG PATIENTS WITH HEART DISEASE

A Statement for Physicians by the Committee on Congenital Cardiac Defects of the Council on Cardiovascular Disease in the Young, American Heart Association

Howard P. Gutgesell, MD, Chairman
Ira H. Gessner, MD
Victoria L. Vetter, MD
Steven M. Yabek, MD
J.B. Norton Jr., MD
Members

The physician who counsels young patients with heart disease often makes recommendations for both recreational and occupational activities. This statement updates and expands the recommendations published by the American Heart Association in 1971.*

---

*American Heart Association: *Recreational and Occupational Recommendations for Use by Physicians Counseling Young Patients with Heart Disease.* A Statement of the Ad Hoc Committee on Habilitation of the Young Cardiac of the Counsel on Cardiovascular Disease in the Young of the American Heart Association, New York, AHA, 1971.

Correspondence regarding this statement should be directed to the Office of Scientific Affairs, American Heart Association, 7320 Greenville Avenue, Dallas, TX 75231.

Single reprints of this report are free; ask for No. 72-2012.

Classification of Recreational Activity

Category I

No Restrictions
Activities may include endurance training, interscholastic athletic competition, contact sports.

Category II

Moderate Exercise
Activities include regular physical education classes, tennis, baseball.

Category III

Light Exercise
Activities include nonstrenuous team games, recreational swimming, jogging, cycling, golf.

Category IV

Moderate Limitation
Activities include attending school, but no participation in physical education classes.

Category V

Extreme Limitation
Activities include homebound or wheelchair activities only.

Classification of Occupational Activity

The *Dictionary of Occupational Titles*† offers the most comprehensive data on the physical demands of specific occupations. Four thousand jobs have been evaluated, using the five grades defined below. The categories are analogous to those for recreational activities.

Category I

Very Heavy Work
Peak load of 7.6 cal/min and above. Involves lifting objects in excess of 100 lb, with frequent lifting and/or carrying of objects weighing 50 lbs or more.

---

† *Dictionary of Occupational Titles*, ed 3, suppl 2. Washington, DC, US Department of Labor, 1968, p A-1.

Category II

Heavy Work

Peak load of 7.6 cal/min and above. Involves lifting 100 lb maximum, with frequent lifting and/or carrying of objects weighing up to 50 lb.

Category III

Medium Work

Peak load of 5.0 to 7.5 cal/min. Involves lifting 50 lb maximum, with frequent lifting and/or carrying of objects weighing up to 25 lb.

Category IV

Light Work

Peak load of 2.6 to 4.9 cal/min. Involves lifting 20 lb maximum, with frequent lifting and/or carrying of objects weighing up to 10 lb. Even though the weight may be negligible, a job is also in this category if it requires considerable walking or standing, or if it involves sitting most of the time with some pushing and pulling of arm and/or leg controls.

Category V

Sedentary Work

Peak load of 2.5 cal/min and below. Involves lifting 10 lb maximum and occasionally lifting and/or carrying such articles as dockets, ledgers, and small tools. Although a sedentary job is defined as one that involves sitting, a certain amount of walking and standing is often necessary. Jobs are sedentary if walking and standing are required only occasionally and other sedentary criteria are met.

Defects and Restrictions

Diagnosis	Recreational	Occupational
Aortic Insufficiency		
Mild (normal heart size)	I	II
Moderate	III	III
Severe	IV	IV
Aortic Stenosis (with or without surgery)		
Mild	I	II
Moderate	III	III
Severe	IV	IV
Atrial Septal Defect (with or without surgery)		
No pulmonary vascular obstructive disease (PVOD)	I	I
Mild to moderate PVOD	III	III
Moderate to severe PVOD	IV	IV
Cardiomyopathy		
Congestive (dilated)	IV	V
Hypertrophic	III	IV
*Coarctation of the Aorta**		
Operated, normal blood pressure	I	I
Hypertensive (with or without surgery)	III	III
Hypertension (with or without treatment)		
Mild	I	II
Moderate to severe	III	III
Mitral Insufficiency		
Mild, without cardiac enlargement	I	II
Moderate (mild to moderate cardiac enlargement)	II	III
Severe (marked cardiac enlargement and/or atrial fibrillation)	IV	V
Mitral Stenosis		
Mild (normal heart size, no symptoms)	II	III
Moderate (mild to moderate cardiac enlargement)	IV	IV
Severe (marked cardiac enlargement, and/or atrial fibrillation)	IV	V
Mitral Valve Prolapse		
Mild, no symptoms* (*see also* mitral insufficiency, arrhythmia)	I	I

Diagnosis	Recreational	Occupational
Myocarditis		
Active	V	V
Chronic (over 3 months' duration)	IV	V
Patent Ductus Arteriosus (with or without surgery)		
No PVOD	I	I
Mild to moderate PVOD	III	III
Moderate to severe PVOD	IV	IV
Pulmonary Stenosis (with or without surgery)		
Mild	I	I
Moderate	III	III
Severe	IV	IV
Pulmonary Hypertension (idiopathic)		
Pulmonary artery pressure <0.50 systemic	III	IV
Pulmonary artery pressure ≥0.50 systemic	IV	V
Tetralogy of Fallot		
Postoperative, RV pressure <50 mm Hg*	I	II
Postoperative, RV pressure ≥50 mm Hg or marked cardiomegaly	III	III
Ventricular Septal Defect (operated or unoperated)		
No PVOD	I	I
Mild to moderate PVOD	III	III
Moderate to severe PVOD	IV	IV

Diagnosis	Recreational	Occupational
*Other Major Defects** (unoperated or palliated only [e.g., tricuspid atresia, pulmonary atresia, Ebstein's anomaly])*	III	IV
*Other Major Defects** postoperative intracardiac repair [e.g., transposition of the great arteries, tricuspid atresia])*	II	III
Cardiac Arrhythmias		
Complete heart block	II	II
Pacemaker (artificial)	II	II
Premature atrial contractions	I	I
Premature ventricular contractions		
Normal heart	I	I
Congenital or acquired heart disease, with or without operation	III	III
Supraventricular tachycardia	I	II
Ventricular tachycardia		
Normal heart	II	II
Congenital or acquired heart disease, with or without operation	IV	IV
Wolff-Parkinson-White Syndrome	I	I

*Exercise testing recommended prior to athletic competition.
**Marked individual variation exists for these categories. Recommendations should be adjusted for individual requirements.

Additional Considerations

Exercise Testing. Treadmill or bicycle exercise testing with electrocardiographic and blood pressure monitoring may be used to assess exercise capacity and the likelihood of serious cardiac arrhythmias precipitated by exercise. Such testing should be strongly considered in the recommendations for cardiac patients wishing to participate in Category I or II activities.

Cardiac Rehabilitation. Widely used for adults following myocardial infarction, cardiac rehabilitation programs for young cardiac patients have been developed in several areas. Supervised exercise programs increase exercise capacity and help patients (and parents) overcome their fear of exercise.

Nature of Work or Exercise. The nature of the work, i.e., isometric (static) or isotonic (dynamic), significantly affects the circulatory response. Isometric exercise (weight lifting, wrestling, and gymnastics) and isometric work (lifting, holding, or carrying heavy objects) is associated with a much larger increase in systemic blood pressure than isotonic exercise at a similar level of oxygen uptake. Although no specific data are available showing effects secondary to such pressure elevation, it seems prudent to discourage these activities in patients with lesions affecting the left ventricle, e.g., aortic stenosis or coarctation of the aorta.

Risk of Dizziness or Syncope. In certain recreational or occupational activities, the risks of even brief periods of dizziness or syncope create hazards much greater than might be implied by the degree of work itself. Examples include unsupervised swimming, aircraft piloting, and high-rise construction. Consideration of such hazards is necessary in making recommendations for patients with conditions in which dizziness or syncope are recognized symptoms (e.g., patients with ventricular arrhythmias or left ventricular outflow obstruction).

Appendix

Below and on the following page are forms that can be used to record the physician's recommendations for patients' recreational and occupational activities.

Recommendations for Recreational Activity

Name _____

Diagnosis _____

Date _____

[ ] Category I   No Restrictions
                     Activities may include endurance training, interscholastic athletic competition, contact sports.

[ ] Category II   Moderate Exercise
                     Activities include regular physical education classes, tennis, baseball.

[ ] Category III   Light Exercise
                     Activities include nonstrenuous team games, recreational swimming, jogging, cycling, golf.

[ ] Category IV   Moderate Limitation
                     Activities include attending school, but no participation in physical education classes.

[ ] Category V   Extreme Limitation
                     Activities include homebound or wheelchair activities only.

Additional Comments _____

_____

_____

_____

Physician _____

Address _____

_____

_____

_____

Phone _____

Recommendations for Occupational Activity

Name _____

Diagnosis _____

Date _____

[ ] Category I   Very Heavy Work
                   Peak load of 7.6 cal/min and above. Involves lifting objects in excess of 100 lb, with frequent lifting and/or carrying of objects weighing 50 lb or more.

[ ] Category II   Heavy Work
                   Peak load of 7.6 cal/min and above. Involves lifting 100 lb maximum, with frequent lifting and/or carrying of objects weighing up to 50 lb.

[ ] Category III Medium Work
                   Peak load of 5.0 to 7.5 cal/min. Involves lifting 50 lb maximum, with frequent lifting and/or carrying of objects weighing up to 25 lb.

[ ] Category IV   Light Work
                   Peak load of 2.6 to 4.9 cal/min. Involves lifting 20 lb maximum, with frequent lifting and/or carrying of objects weighing up to 10 lb. Even though the weight may be negligible, a job is also in this category if it requires considerable walking or standing, or if it involves sitting most of the time with some pushing and pulling of arm and/or leg controls.

[ ] Category V   Sedentary Work
                   Peak load of 2.5 cal/min and below. Involves lifting 10 lb maximum and occasionally lifting and/or carrying such articles as dockets, ledgers, and small tools. Although a sedentary job is defined as one that involves sitting, a certain amount of walking and standing is often necessary. Jobs are sedentary if walking and standing are required only occasionally and other sedentary criteria are met.

Additional Comments _____

_____

_____

Physician _____

Address _____

_____

_____

_____

Phone _____